The Paroxysmal Disorders

The Paroxysmal Disorders

Edited by

Bettina Schmitz
Vivantes Humboldt-Klinikum and Charité University Hospital, Berlin, Germany

Barbara Tettenborn
Kantonsspital St. Gallen, Switzerland, and Johannes Gutenberg University, Mainz, Germany

Donald L. Schomer
Beth Israel Deaconess Medical Center, Harvard University, Boston, Massachusetts, USA

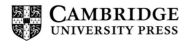

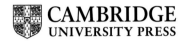

Shaftesbury Road, Cambridge CB2 8EA, United Kingdom

One Liberty Plaza, 20th Floor, New York, NY 10006, USA

477 Williamstown Road, Port Melbourne, VIC 3207, Australia

314–321, 3rd Floor, Plot 3, Splendor Forum, Jasola District Centre, New Delhi – 110025, India

103 Penang Road, #05–06/07, Visioncrest Commercial, Singapore 238467

Cambridge University Press is part of Cambridge University Press & Assessment, a department of the University of Cambridge.

We share the University's mission to contribute to society through the pursuit of education, learning and research at the highest international levels of excellence.

www.cambridge.org
Information on this title: www.cambridge.org/9780521895293

© Cambridge University Press & Assessment 2010

First published 2010

A catalogue record for this publication is available from the British Library

Library of Congress Cataloging-in-Publication data
Paroxysmale Störungen in der Neurologie. English.
The paroxysmal disorders / edited by Bettina Schmitz,
Barbara Tettenborn, Don Schomer.
    p. ; cm.
Includes bibliographical references and index.
ISBN 978-0-521-89529-3 (hardback)
1. Convulsions.   2. Headache.   3. Epilepsy.   4. Vertigo.
I. Schmitz, Bettina, 1960–   II. Tettenborn, Barbara.
III. Schomer, Donald L.   IV. Title.
[DNLM: 1. Neurologic Manifestations. WL 340 P257 2010a]
RC394.C77.P3713   2010
616.8´45 – dc22   2009039047

ISBN   978-0-521-89529-3   Hardback

....

Contents

The color plates are between pages 88 and 89.

Contributors

Hans-Christoph Diener, MD, PhD, FAHA
Department of Neurology, University of Essen, Essen, Germany

Marianne Dieterich, MD, PhD
Department of Neurology, Johannes Gutenberg-University Mainz, Germany

Thomas Grunwald, MD, PhD
Swiss Epilepsy Center, Zurich, Switzerland

Peter Henningsen, MD, PhD
Department of Psychosomatic Medicine and Psychotherapy, Technical University of Munich, Munich, Germany

Monika Jeub, MD
Department of Neurology, University of Bonn Medical Center, Bonn, Germany

Thomas Klockgether, MD, PhD
Department of Neurology, University of Bonn Medical Center, Bonn, Germany

Christina Kölmel, MD
Department of Psychiatry, Schlosspark-Klinik, Berlin, Germany

Hans Wolfgang Kölmel, MD, PhD
Department of Neurology, Helios Clinic, Erfurt, Germany

Günter Krämer, MD
Swiss Epilepsy Center, Zurich, Switzerland

Gerhard Kurlemann, MD, PhD
Department of Neuropediatrics, University Children's Hospital, University of Münster, Münster, Germany

Thomas Lempert, MD, PhD
Department of Neurology, Schlosspark-Klinik, Berlin, Germany

Hans-Michael Meinck, MD, PhD
Department of Neurology, University of Heidelberg, Heidelberg, Germany

Ian Mothersill, MSc
Swiss Epilepsy Center, Zurich, Switzerland

Soheyl Noachtar, MD, PhD
Epilepsy Center, Department of Neurology, University of Munich, Munich, Germany

Jan Rémi, MD
Epilepsy Center, Department of Neurology, University of Munich, Munich, Germany

Ludwig D. Schelosky, MD
Consultant, Medizinische Klinik, Kantonsspital Münsterlingen, Münsterlingen, Switzerland

Bettina Schmitz, MD, PhD
Department of Neurology, Humboldt-University Berlin, Charité Campus, Berlin, Germany

Marc Andre Slomke, MD
Department of Radiology, Alfred-Krupp Krankenhaus, Essen, Germany

Michael Strupp, MD, PhD
Department of Neurology, Ludwig-Maximilians University, Munich, Germany

Barbara Tettenborn, MD, PhD
Department of Neurology, Kantonsspital St. Gallen, St. Gallen, Switzerland; Johannes Gutenberg-University Mainz, Germany

Peter P. Urban, MD, PhD
Department of Neurology, Asklepios Klinik Barmbek, Hamburg, Germany

Florian Weissinger, MD
Postdoctoral Fellow, Epilepsy Research Laboratory, The Children's Hospital of Philadelphia, Philadelphia, PA, USA

Konrad J. Werhahn, MD, PhD
Section on Epilepsy, Department of Neurology, Johannes Gutenberg-University Mainz, Germany

Peter Wolf, MD, PhD
Epilepsy Hospital, Dianalund, Denmark

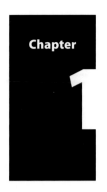

Paroxysmal attacks: diagnostic gold standards and history-taking

Peter Wolf

Gold standard case history

Can the case history ever be considered a gold standard? Generally, a gold standard is a firmly established reference that serves as a reliable comparison for other measures or procedures. We think of gold standards as hard, quantitative and cross-checked data. By comparison, the case history is soft, subjective and carries numerous risks of misunderstandings, prejudices and even the possibility of leading questioning. However, there is no doubt that the results of even the most exact and advanced investigations are of clinical significance only when they make sense in the context of the clinical background as provided by the history. In other words, the history is used in the same way as a gold standard, that is, as a counter-check for the plausibility of the findings.

Specific aspects of the case histories for paroxysmal disorders

The case history is of particularly high importance in paroxysmal disorders because many seizures may comprise a variety of subjective symptoms or may even consist exclusively of these symptoms. Because of their transient character, these symptoms are often difficult to document or can only be discovered through a detailed clinical history of the event. This, too, is not always straightforward because patients relate their experiences in their own language, which may be naïve, imprecise, or metaphorical and may need further interpretation to be correctly understood (Surmann 2005). This level of interpreter involvement can vary from structuring, to clarification by cross-questioning, to veritable "translation." In such a situation, it is very important that the doctor avoids asking questions that lead to answers which conform to his

or her preconceived hypotheses and prejudices, rather than realistically reflecting patients' experiences. On the other hand, to get any result it is often necessary to structure the interview, which will rely on the background of the doctor's knowledge of typical seizure symptoms. It is important to find the correct balance of critically reflecting the physician's own experience with epilepsy but always be prepared to reconsider a working hypothesis if the patient's report does not reflect it. Ideally, the doctor taking the history should be absolutely neutral and block out his or her subjectivity so as not to influence the patient's free flow of remembering the events in question. This sounds difficult to achieve, but it is the method used in the project that established the linguistic criteria in the differential diagnosis of epilepsy from psychogenic non-epileptic seizures (PNES) and is currently used in clinical trials to define the differences experientially between various types of epilepsy. In these studies, the patient is invited by two or three standardized initial questions to speak freely about his or her experiences. The reports are recorded and transcribed, and undergo a detailed analysis using formal linguistic criteria. The method was first developed in Germany (Wolf et al. 2000) and the results have since been duplicated in England (Schwabe et al. 2007). The method used in the research is time-consuming but may end with the development of software programs to provide rapid, even online, diagnostic conclusions.

With this method, it is possible to generate objective and quantitative data based on the patient's subjective reports. It examines exclusively one of several aspects of these reports: their linguistic form, not their contents. However, this aspect is one that has hitherto been neglected. It seems highly questionable whether a similar degree of objectivity can be attained with respect to contents.

The Paroxysmal Disorders, ed. Bettina Schmitz, Barbara Tettenborn and Donald L. Schomer. Published by Cambridge University Press. © Cambridge University Press 2010.

Taking a seizure history is primarily for diagnostic purposes, largely to differentiate epilepsy from other seizure-like disorders but also to distinguish between different types of epileptic seizures and to understand the anatomy and etiology of these events. Hypotheses are formed, followed-up or refuted, and they determine the subsequent course of the interview. The questions asked in a differential diagnosis of epileptic seizures versus migraine accompagnée are entirely different from those to distinguish focal from generalized epileptic seizures. Even if the latter differentiation is only preliminary, it needs to become much more detailed; it can require rather sophisticated history-taking in and of itself. This may be the case when the patient reports some subjective experiences at or near the onset of the seizure. Are these auras indicating a focal seizure onset, absences immediately preceding a generalized tonic-clonic seizure, or non-specific sensations preceding a seizure? In addition to such difficulties inherent in the matter in question, the linguistic abilities of the patients may additionally require adjustments of the interview technique.

Taking a seizure history can and should lead far into the diagnostic process. For example, at the end of taking a history of focal epileptic seizures the doctor should develop a relatively precise hypothesis about where in the brain the seizures originate and how they spread. For this, it is essential to know the exact sequence of seizure symptoms. But this is not necessarily the way they are spontaneously described by the patients, whose reports may instead reflect hierarchies of symptoms according to their subjective importance. They are not aware that symptoms which appear minor to them may provide pivotal anatomical information. Taking a seizure history is therefore typically a structuring process, the dynamics of which are the result of an interaction between doctor and patient, and the course of which is fundamentally unpredictable.

Such an in-depth dialogue also opens up perspectives beyond diagnostics. Most patients are not used to being interrogated by somebody who has a detailed understanding of their subjective experiences and is interested in them. They often feel they are taken seriously in a way they are not accustomed to, so they are often very appreciative. This attitude goes a long way to establish the necessary interpersonal confidence for a subsequent therapeutic relationship.

Beyond providing diagnostic clues and anatomical understanding, another frequent consequence of these interviews is indications for the best further therapeutic strategy. Examples are the development of self-control strategies to avoid specific or non-specific seizure triggers (which the patient needs to be asked about) or to prevent traumas or clusters of seizures.

Verbal communication is only successful when the partners in dialogue find a common language. This is highly important in the diagnostic interview. A doctor who takes a case history or seizure history should be aware that the dialogue is asymmetrical, with the doctor holding the more dominant role. Therefore it is the doctor's responsibility that the communication works, and they need to be aware that misunderstandings may occur in either direction.

To be understood by the patient

To get useful answers from the patient, the doctor needs to ask questions which the patient can understand. Very few patients have studied medicine and know its professional language. To express a complex medical matter to lay people in plain language is not always easy but it is not only a matter of politeness – it is a basic requirement for communication.

In this asymmetrical dialogue situation, the patient cannot be expected to question something he or she has not understood. He or she may be too shy or embarrassed to do that. It is the doctor who needs to make sure that he or she has been understood by the patient (in a polite way, of course). "Did I express myself understandably?" is a much better way to ask the question as opposed to, "Do you follow me?"

To understand the patient

It is by no means trivial to point out that the patient's reports also need to be understood correctly. There may be dialects, accents and colloquialisms which do not have the same meaning everywhere. However, much more important are vague terms and undeclared similes and metaphors. Here are some examples.

- A patient who reports during a seizure to "stand beside himself/herself" may be using a relatively common metaphor for reduced presence of mind, and the interlocutor may understand it like this and pass on. But it may actually need to be understood literally and signify the experience of a double. This is a rare but characteristic possible symptom of parietal lobe seizures and is often described in this way. In a seizure history, it needs to be followed up by the question, "On which side of yourself do you stand?" If it is a double experience, the patient will usually be able to promptly tell the side (typically, contralateral to the focus). If he or she was using a metaphor, the question will not make sense to them and it may be necessary to explain that you were not joking.

- The subjective experiences in epileptic auras are often so unnatural and different from common experiences that they are extremely difficult to describe. Quite a few patients are in the habit of using surrogate terms to get around this difficulty. These are often not descriptive, even if they may seem so to the patient. Dizziness and giddiness are such terms. They should never be taken at face value. The patient should always be asked to be as descriptive as possible. If it turns out that the symptoms are indescribable and cannot be compared to any natural experiences, this is helpful because it is a quality well-known from epileptic seizures and otherwise extremely rare.

- One of the best-known traditional terms in epilepsy – aura – is probably a misunderstanding which arose in such a situation. According to Temkin (1971), "this word, taken from the Greek, originally meant a 'breeze.' It was introduced into medical terminology not by a physician but by a patient. When still a young man, Galen, together with other physicians, visited a 13-year-old boy. The patient told them that the condition originated in the lower leg, and that 'from there it climbed upwards in a straight line through the thigh and further through the flank and side to the neck and as far as the head: but as soon as it had touched the latter he was no longer able to follow.' When the physicians asked him what exactly rose up to the head, he could not tell, but another youth, who was a better observer, said 'that it was like a cold breeze.'" The story in this version does not really make sense because it was a subjective experience, and there was nothing for the other youth to "observe." The scene can easily be imagined. Being interrogated by several physicians and having described the march of a sensory Jacksonian seizure, the boy was embarrassed because he was unable to set words an indescribable quality of the sensation and gratefully grasped the first way out that was presented to him. I have never met a patient who compared his or her aura experience to a cold breeze.

Patients with ictal hallucinations and illusions typically do not report them spontaneously because they are afraid of being considered either mentally disturbed or of becoming so. This is not only true for epileptic hallucinations but also for hypnagogic hallucinations, which the patient needs to be asked about if the differential diagnosis is in the field of narcolepsy or cataplexy. It is important in the interview to create an atmosphere of confidence where the patient can talk about such matters freely. Nonetheless, it is usually necessary to ask directly about them, and this should not be forgotten whenever there is a possibility that these conditions are present – for example, if there are other indications of an epileptic focus in the parieto-occipital area.

A checklist for seizure histories

Taking a seizure history does not necessarily need to follow a rigid scheme; however, it is useful to have an internal standard checklist of topics and questions, both when the history is taken from the patient themselves and/or from witnesses.

The patient

Patients often do not spontaneously report all seizure symptoms but only the most prominent ones. Also, the first symptom mentioned is not always the first in a sequence of symptoms but the one which impresses or bothers the patient the most. A dialogue is frequently necessary to get the full picture of all subjective seizure symptoms and their sequence.

Questions for the patients:

- What is the very first indication of a commencing seizure? Patients sometimes misunderstand the question and report a suspected seizure trigger.
- Can this first symptom be preceded by something else? Many patients understand auras not as part of the seizure but as a warning that precedes it.
- What is the sequence of symptoms? Triggers of seizures (e.g., reflex epileptic seizures); syncope triggered by cough, micturition, pain; emotional triggers of cataplectic fits; movements in kinesigenic paroxysmal choreoathetosis.
- Is this dependent on certain postures? (e.g., orthostatic syncope)
- Can the patient arrest his or her seizures? Sometimes? Always? How?
- What is the duration of the seizure? Relation to time-of-day or sleep-wake cycle (e.g., generalized

3

tonic-clonic seizures or myoclonic seizures after awaking); frontal lobe epileptic seizures in sleep; REM and non-REM sleep parasomnias; sleep paralysis; PNES never in sleep but perhaps at night.

- Are there patterns of recurrence (e.g., clusters at intervals in temporal lobe epilepsy)?

The witnesses

Some witnesses are in the habit of stubbornly not reporting what they have observed but how they reacted to it. Patience is needed to get a seizure description. However, the witness may have some knowledge which may save a lot of unnecessary investigations.

Questions for the witnesses:

- What drew the observer's attention first to the seizure?
- What was the first observed seizure sign?
- What was the sequence of signs and symptoms?
- What movements were observed, including extent, speed and direction?
- Were there jerks? Stiffness? Where was it? Was it unilateral or bilateral? How long did it last?
- Did it spread?
- Were there automatisms? These are often not spontaneously described even if they are quite prominent.
- Was there a fall? If so, in what direction? Did the patient's tone change, and did he or she become flaccid or rigid?
- Were their eyes open or closed? Was there deviation of the eyes?
- What was their facial expression? Did they stare?
- Was there a change of color?
- Did they salivate?
- Did they bite their tongue? If so was it lateral or apical? Does that happen always, often or occasionally?
- Was the patient incontinent or enuretic?
- What was the level of responsiveness?
- Was there speech during and/or after the seizure, or was there speech arrest – speech similar to a foreign language – or speech that was

grammatically correct but nonsensical or paraphasic?

- What was the duration of the seizure? Was that an estimate or was it accurately timed? Most observers often tend to overestimate duration, especially with severe seizures or with the first observed seizure. Most often, they include the postictal phase.
- Were the onset and offset sudden or phased?
- Were there postictal symptoms such as a speech disturbance, a paresis or weakness, disorientation or aggressive-defensive behavior?
- If they have observed many seizures in the same person, are the events stereotyped or variable?

It is often a good idea to take the seizure history from patients and witnesses together in one setting and point out that many seizures have both subjective symptoms which are only known to the patient and objective signs which can be visible to the observer, even as the patient may be unaware of them. This helps all parties to understand the weighting of their observations. For many patients, this is novel because their experience is often that their own knowledge is not appreciated. For every sign and symptom, it needs to be clarified if it is only subjective or only objective, or has both aspects.

References

Schwabe M, Howell S, Reuber M. Differential diagnosis of seizure disorders: a conversation analytic approach. *Social Science and Medicine* 2007; **65**:712–724.

Surmann V. Anfallsbilder. *Metaphorische Konzepte im Sprechen anfallskranker Menschen*. Königshausen & Neumann, Würzburg 2005.

Temkin O. *The Falling Sickness. A History of Epilepsy from the Greeks to the Beginnings of Modern Neurology*. 2nd edn. rev., Johns Hopkins University Press, Baltimore & London 1971.

Wolf P, Schöndienst M, Gülich E. Experiential auras. In: Lüders HO, Noachtar S, (eds.). *Epileptic Seizures: Pathophysiology and Clinical Semiology*. Churchill Livingstone, New York 2000, p. 336–348.

Paroxysmal disorders in childhood

Gerhard Kurlemann

Introduction

Non-epileptic infantile paroxysmal dyskinesia is a common disorder that is not easily distinguished from epileptic seizures at first glance. Whenever parents can provide a good description of symptoms or it is possible to observe the incident firsthand or with video, one can usually diagnose the disorder correctly and distinguish it from epilepsy, which is often the initial diagnosis.

Between 0.8% and 1.0% of the population suffer from epilepsy. Epileptic seizures in infancy are widespread, occurring with an incidence between 80 and 100 per 100,000. Prevalence studies of active epilepsy in infancy show rates between 3 and 6 per 1000 children.

An epileptic seizure is diagnosed according to clinical findings, including a thorough history and neurological examination with corresponding diagnostic studies, for example, electroencephalography (EEG). An exact observation/description and the corresponding EEG result are indispensable for the diagnosis of an epileptic seizure, as for all movement disorders. If the EEG matches the clinical findings – for example, violent tonic dyskinetic arm movement in a six-month-old infant together with a documented hypsarrhythmia during sleep and wake EEG – then West's syndrome with salaam convulsions can be diagnosed reliably.

Absence epilepsy is a frequent cause for children presenting with the observation of paroxysmal "daydreaming." It can often be diagnosed in a primary care setting without the corroborative evidence of an EEG by requesting the patient to perform controlled hyperventilation. Most often the frequent symptoms of absence epilepsy become obvious during hyperventilation, which is interrupted by the discontinuous breathing pattern so elicited. Most frequently, the patient will develop open and upturned eyes, have some mild smacking of the lips and fiddling hand movement. Final corroboration can be provided by the presence of the typical EEG pattern of 3-Hz spike-and-wave discharges. Shoulder girdle localized myoclonus is associated with the Janz syndrome variant. These can be either symmetrical or asymmetrical in nature (Fig. 2.1). This myoclonus in particular can precede grand mal seizures by years. The myoclonic form of this type of epilepsy is accompanied by generalized poly-spike-and-wave discharges on the EEG. Whenever clinical symptoms are not consistent with EEG findings, the wide spectrum of non-epileptic, age-linked movement disorders should be borne in mind, especially where infants are concerned (Table 2.1).

Up to 20% of patients in large representative groups presumed to have epilepsy in fact do not have epilepsy but rather one of the numerous forms of paroxysmal dyskinesia (Scheepers et al. 1998; Uldall et al. 2006). A diagnosis of epilepsy should not rely solely on the EEG. The combination of clinical picture and EEG findings allows a more definitive diagnostic differentiation when viewed as a whole. The EEG is a valuable tool when diagnosing epilepsy; however, an interictal EEG alone can neither prove nor rule out epilepsy reliably. A single, awake EEG showing no typical epileptic pattern is seen in up to 50% of epileptic patients. As a corollary, 3%–5% of routine EEGs performed on children show patterns typical for epilepsy, even though they have not suffered an epileptic fit. If in doubt, it is advisable to wait and see how things develop and broaden the angle of diagnostic possibilities. A false-positive diagnosis of epilepsy with all its consequences is more detrimental to both child and family than waiting for the next possible epileptic fit.

The Paroxysmal Disorders, ed. Bettina Schmitz, Barbara Tettenborn and Donald L. Schomer. Published by Cambridge University Press. © Cambridge University Press 2010.

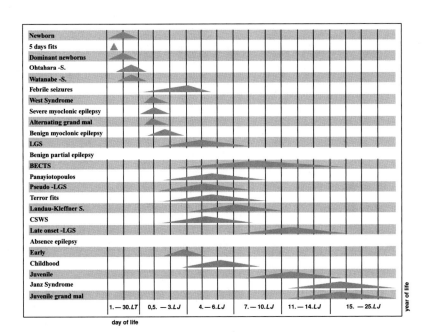

Fig. 2.1. Spectrum and age of manifestation for infant epilepsy syndromes.

Table 2.1 Differential diagnosis of paroxysmal dyskinesia

Altered state of consciousness
Syncope
Affective respiratory spasms – breath-holding spells – cyanotic vs. pale
Narcolepsy / cataplexy
Cardiac dysrhythmia – supraventricular
Atypical migraine / "confusion" migraine

Reflex pattern in sleep
Nightmare
Jactatio capitis / corporis nocturna
Benign infantile sleep myoclonus

Unaltered state of consciousness
Tics
Shuddering attacks
Benign paroxysmal dizziness
Self-stimulation / auto-stimulation
Benign paroxysmal torticollis
Nodding spasm
Sandifer syndrome
Benign paroxysmal upward gaze
Kinesigenic choreoathetosis
Hyperekplexia
Transient infantile dystonia
Kinsbourne syndrome
Alternating infantile hemiplegia
Hyperventilation attacks
Panic attacks
Psychogenic non-epileptic fits
Pulse synchronous bulbus movement in spheno-orbital dysplasia
Munchausen syndrome by proxy

The clinical symptoms of the most frequently occurring movement disorders that should be considered in differential diagnosis are described herein.

Jactatio capitis/corporis nocturna

Jactatio capitis/corporis nocturna is characterized by rhythmic stereotype head-rolling or body-rocking movements while falling asleep during sleep stage I, or during short arousals during sleep stage II. The most frequent movement is head-rolling or banging. Head-banging can occasionally even cause callus formation on the forehead if the bed head and sides are not padded. Jactatio duration varies from between 30 seconds and 30 minutes, and in more than 60% of cases it starts around the age of nine months and generally persists until the age of five years (DiMario 2006).

Key symptoms: Rhythmic head/body movements during light sleep

Syncope

Syncope is frequently experienced by infants and adolescents, although the exact incidence is not known. It has been estimated that about 30% to 50% of children will have experienced a syncopal episode by the time they reach adolescence. A syncope is a brief, temporary loss of consciousness due to a transient reduction of cerebral perfusion. Diminished cerebral perfusion

Table 2.2 Syncope symptoms vs. epileptic seizure

	Syncope	Epileptic seizure
Onset	Sudden	Prodromes: sweating, lightheadedness, dizziness, palpitations
Position	Variable	Standing, more seldom sitting
Muscle activity	Variable	Predominantly hypotensive
Skin color	Pale	Variable – cyanotic
Tonic phase	Brief	Pronounced
Myoclonus	Brief, multifocal	Violent, symmetrical, rhythmic
Reorientation	Rapid	Variable – longer
Tongue bite	3%	Lateral, 30%
Injury	Frequent	Seldom
Bed-wetting	25%	25%

of less than 30 ml/100 g brain tissue per minute causes a syncopal episode, which in turn involves loss of posture followed by spontaneous recovery.

A distinction is made between cardiovascular and vasovagal syncope. The most frequent form in infancy is the vasovagal syncope. It is extremely rare for an epileptic fit to be triggered by a syncope episode. Depending on the clinical symptoms, in particular when violent multifocal myoclonus and bed-wetting occur, an epileptic fit is the most likely diagnosis.

A comprehensive history should always be obtained. Prodromes – such as lightheadedness or ringing in the ears in situations involving, for example, long periods of standing upright in poorly ventilated rooms – are immediately suggestive of syncope. Syncope that occurs during physical exercise could

be associated with a long QT syndrome and, as such, should be ruled out (Paolicchi 2002).

Table 2.2 distinguishes syncope symptoms from those of an epileptic fit; Table 2.3 lists the possible symptoms of syncope in order of frequency.

Key symptoms: See Table 2.2

Breath-holding spell attacks

Breath-holding spell attacks typically occur in infants. It is estimated that up to 4% of children under five years of age are so affected. A distinction is made between the frequently cyanotic form (80%) and pale breath-holding form (20%). Cyanotic attacks are brought on by different triggers, for example, the child cannot have its own way. There is a long run-up to loss of consciousness due to dead-volume ventilation. Brief shoulder myoclonus is common during the final phase of a cerebral hypoxia, when the rising CO_2 concentration is already beginning to activate the respiration reflex, marking the start of the recovery phase. However, this type of myoclonus must not be mistaken for an epileptic seizure. In contrast, the pale syncope occurs abruptly and is frequently pain-induced. The long-term prognosis is favorable, the symptoms are generally self-limiting and therapy is not necessary (Lombroso & Lerman 1967; Evans 1997; Kuhle et al. 2000).

Children who have breath-holding spell attacks should be examined to systematically rule out iron-deficiency anemia. If such an anemia is diagnosed, iron substitution is recommended (Mocan et al. 1999; Hüdaoglu et al. 2006). The mental prognosis for breath-holding spell attacks is good. A detailed history often shows familial incidence. Table 2.3

Table 2.3 Breath-holding spell attacks vs. epileptic fits

	Cyanotic breath-holding spell attacks	Pale breath-holding spell attacks	Tonic-clonic seizures
Family history	Frequent +	Frequent +	Variable
Age	Baby – infant	Baby – infant	Any age
Trigger	Anger, vexation, pain	Sudden unexpected stimulus	Sleep deprivation
Symptoms	Loud crying, dead-space ventilation, apnea, loss of consciousness, opisthotonus, short muscle spasms	All shorter	Tonic-clonic spasms, loss of consciousness
ECG	Primary tachycardia	Primary bradycardia / asystole	Ictal neuronal discharges
EEG	Normal	Normal	Typical epilepsy pattern

compares the symptoms of breath-holding spell attacks with those of epileptic fits.

Key symptoms: Emotionally triggered, dead-space ventilation, longer "run-up" time, cyanosis, loss of consciousness.

Cataplexy/narcolepsy

Narcolepsy is a disorder rarely seen in infants; however, single cases have been reported in patients under four years of age. In 30% of all cases, the disorder begins under 15 years of age with emotionally triggered cataplectic states. The full-blown syndrome includes symptoms such as increased drowsiness during the daytime, cataplexy, hypnagogic hallucinations and sleep paralysis. Sleep paralysis is characterized by persisting muscular atonia from REM sleep, which can be interrupted by body contact (Black et al. 2004). Diagnosis can be made using the multiple sleep latency test and by detection of the HLA antigen DR2 and Dqw1, found in 90% of affected patients, combined with reduced hypocretin (Overeem et al. 2002).

Key symptoms: Emotionally triggered loss of tone, sleep paralysis.

Benign sleep myoclonus

Benign sleep myoclonus in babies can only be diagnosed clinically. The main symptoms are focal, multifocal or generalized bilateral synchronous myoclonus. Myoclonus commonly affects the upper extremities and occurs in non-REM sleep, beginning often when the baby is only a few days old. It can occur in frequent clusters. An EEG reveals no pathological discharges. Myoclonus can be interrupted immediately by waking the infant. The children have no neurological impairment. The myoclonus generally ceases when the child reaches an age of about six months, and symptoms seldom persist longer (Coulter & Allen 1982).

Key symptoms: Myoclonus during non-REM sleep, interruptible by waking the infant.

Benign early infantile myoclonus

Benign early infantile myoclonus occurs in healthy children during the first year of life (age 3 to 15 months). Characteristic symptoms are neck-bending movements accompanied by shaking of the head and contraction of the axial muscles.

Symptoms occur only when the child is awake, several times a day, and frequently in clusters, which makes it easy to mistake for infantile spasms caused by West's syndrome. It may be accompanied by facial grimacing. EMG examinations have shown tonic discharges lasting longer than 200 ms. These tonic discharges are not typical for myoclonus, and the term "myoclonus" is incorrect in this case. Affected children never show focal signs of a movement disorder and remain fully conscious. There is no accompanying eye deviation, and an EEG is always normal. A 24-hour EEG is only necessary to safely rule out epilepsy in exceptionally rare cases. The syndrome is self-limiting; occasionally, it only lasts for a few weeks, but always ceases by the age of two years (Preblick-Salib & Jagoda 1997).

Key symptoms: Self-limiting myoclonus of head and axial muscles in an awake state.

Pavor nocturnus

Paroxysmal panic attacks at night occur in 3.5% of children aged between 4 and 12 years. These attacks are frequently of a dramatic nature and are accompanied by frightened crying containing quite articulate speech. The children "wake up" 1 to 2 hours after falling asleep, sit up scared in bed, wander about the room and often refuse to be comforted by their parents. Their eyes are wide open and the pupils dilated. Amnesia exists for this time span. Pavor nocturnus is linked to the transition phase from non-REM to REM sleep (phase 3 and 4) and thus does not influence dreaming. The typical behavior shown by these children allows a clinical diagnosis to be made.

The syndrome is self-limiting. Stress has repeatedly been discussed as a possible trigger; however, this has not been verified. Frontal lobe epileptic seizures at night, which are often stereotypic, associated with hypermotoric features can resemble pavor nocturnus. If symptoms also occur during the day, then they can be interpreted correctly. Attacks generally cease spontaneously and seldom persist into adulthood.

Key symptoms: Occurring in first two hours after onset of sleep, agitation and confusion, refusal of parental comfort and retrograde amnesia.

Tic disorders

The clinical spectrum of infantile tic disorders is varied and ranges from simple "nervous" tics to complex disorders that frequently show clinical manifestations that are not easily recognized (Kotagal et al. 2002).

Often bizarre movement patterns exist, with the frequency increasing with attention and decreasing when ignored. They are often of an inconsistent pattern. The most frequent movement pattern for girls is rhythmic knee buckling. There also exists the ability to suppress the tic at will for short periods of time.

Additional diagnostic measures such as EEG and further electrophysiological examinations produce no tangible pathological results. Many tic disorders are self-limiting. Depending on the psychological strain, which is often more of a problem for the parents than for the child, psychotherapy may be helpful, and in particularly persistent cases medication may be indicated (Alsaadi & Marquez 2005).

Key symptoms: Bizarre uncoordinated movement patterns, more pronounced in certain situations, can be suppressed at will.

Shuddering attacks

These episodes present as a sudden change in posture, as if cold water was being poured over the body, with brief muscle contraction and shaking movements (Vanasse et al. 1976). The head is bowed or inclined to the side, the arms and legs are close to the body and the arms may be bent. The condition begins in babies and infants with varying frequency of occurrence. Attacks are self-limiting, and an EEG is always negative (Holmes & Russman 1986).

Key symptoms: Paroxysmal tension, entire body shudders.

Benign paroxysmal dizziness

This condition is a sudden emergence of dizziness, occurring between the ages of 1 and 3, in short spells of generally up to one minute duration without aura. Affected children are pale, anxious, cling to their parent or lie down so that they do not fall over, frequently accompanied by nystagmus. Children are fully conscious. Functional disorders of the labyrinth have been reported. The disorder is self-limiting by the time children reach school age. There is no need for therapy.

As with paroxysmal torticollis, a connection between benign paroxysmal dizziness and migraine is also suspected. In the history, it should always be asked if migraines run in the family. Due to the inability of a young child to give an exact description

of their condition, the symptoms can easily be mistaken for a complex partial seizure. However, normal postictal behavior and the fact that there is no loss of consciousness should enable the correct classification of symptoms.

Key symptoms: Brief dizziness with vegetative symptoms, patient fully conscious.

Benign paroxysmal torticollis

Benign paroxysmal torticollis becomes manifest during the first year of life and is probably closely related to benign paroxysmal dizziness. Torticollis attacks can last between several minutes or hours and days accompanied by relapsing vomiting. Rolling eye movements may occur when the labyrinth is affected. The syndrome is self-limiting. Cerebral diagnostic imaging is required to rule out any pathological intracerebral processes when the first attack occurs.

The syndrome may run in families. A relationship to migraine is possible as many children suffer from migraines in later life, and it is therefore advisable to routinely ask whether there is a history of migraines in the family. In the differential diagnosis of an initial attack, this syndrome may be confused with the Sandifer syndrome or paroxysmal vertigo, as the symptoms are similar (Deonna & Martin 1981).

Key symptoms: Paroxysmal wryneck of varying duration, vomiting, seldom eye movement disorders.

Sandifer syndrome

Sandifer syndrome is associated with spasmodic torsional dystonia, chiefly involving the neck and back, accompanied by body-rocking movements and mood changes. There is often a time link to meals, with symptoms developing 30 minutes following ingestion. Further symptoms include regurgitation or retching. Diagnostic examinations should concentrate on gastroesophageal reflux, hiatus hernia or esophageal dysmotility, as incidence of these symptoms is common. Symptoms cease following operative correction of reflux or hernia. In many cases, vomiting persists into infancy (Somijit et al. 2004; Lehwald et al. 2007).

Sandifer syndrome is frequently mistaken for tonic epileptic fits, particularly in retarded children with epilepsy or dystonic seizures. An isolated tonic increase has only been determined as an epileptic phenomenon in 30% of cases (Kabakus & Kurt 2006; Kostakis et al. 2008).

Key symptoms: Paroxysmal tonic increase involving body-rocking, time link to ingestion, no loss of consciousness.

Benign tonic upward gazing

This rare paroxysmal upward gazing in infancy is characterized by tonic upward eye movement of varying duration or intermittent occurrence (Ouvrier & Billson 1998). If a downward glance is attempted during attack, a down-beat nystagmus occurs; horizontal eye movement is normal. Occasionally, this eye movement disorder is accompanied by ataxia. There may rarely be a family history of the disorder, and the syndrome is self-limiting. L-DOPA therapy has been reported to have positive effects (Echenne & Rivior 1992).

Key symptoms: Paroxysmal upward gazing, self-limiting.

Self-stimulation

Self-stimulation or masturbation in infancy is characterized by paroxysmal stereotypical movement patterns involving pressing the thighs together rhythmically and rocking the body to-and-fro simulating copulation, and is found more frequently in girls than in boys. In addition, vegetative symptoms such as sweating, reddened face or irregular breathing can occur; children are fully conscious – girls more frequently than boys. The children never stimulate their genitals manually (Nechay et al. 2004).

Self-stimulation frequently occurs in situations where the children receive no attention. The children do not like being interrupted during self-stimulation and often react irritably. They seem to enjoy the situation. The EEG is always normal and the syndrome is self-limiting. Parental reassurance is most important. Of course, self-stimulation also occurs in children with epilepsy, where the symptoms are frequently mistaken for an epileptic seizure (Yang et al. 2005).

Key symptoms: Rhythmic pressing together of thighs, lack of manual genital stimulation, autonomous accompanying phenomena.

Nodding spasm – spasmus nutans

As with many paroxysmal movement disorders, nodding spasms are a self-limiting disorder affecting infants that involves the triad of head-nodding, tor-ticollis and asymmetric ocular nystagmus; monocular or dissociated nystagmus can also occur. Head-nodding is a compensatory vestibulo-ocular reflex required to avoid visual distortion. The symptoms persist in older children only in exceptional cases. As various retinal and intracerebral complications such as retinitis or diencephalic processes have been reported, an ophthalmological examination and an MRI of the CNS should be performed to rule out associated disorders.

Key symptoms: Head-nodding, torticollis and nystagmus

Paroxysmal kinesigenic choreoathetosis

Characteristic symptoms for this condition are short, bizarre, dystonic choreiform movements of single or whole muscle groups, occasionally with ballism initiated by abrupt body movements. Emotional situations or hyperventilation are seldom the trigger. Patients remain fully conscious during an attack, occasionally experiencing a brief aura, but there is no postictal impairment. The attacks are of short duration and can occur up to 100 times a day. Children between 5 and 15 years of age can be affected. An EEG shows no epileptic pattern.

Symptoms can be suppressed by low-level doses of antiepileptic medication such as phenytoin, carbamazepine/oxcarbazepine or valproic acid. The syndrome ceases spontaneously between the third and fourth decade of life. The disorder is hereditary and is autosomal dominant; if parents have no symptoms, they should be questioned about symptoms during childhood (Vidaillhet 2000).

Table 2.4 shows the differential diagnosis of paroxysmal dystonic – choreoathetoid movement disorders.

Key symptoms: Dystonia, always triggered by movement, patients remain fully conscious.

Psychogenic non-epileptic seizures

Up to 20% of epileptic children suffer from psychogenic, non-epileptic seizures. Young age does not prevent psychogenic seizures, so this diagnosis must also be borne in mind where children under six years of age are concerned (Scheepers et al. 1998; Uldall et al. 2006). Whenever the described symptoms give reason to doubt whether it is a true form of epilepsy and the EEG findings produce no pathological findings,

Table 2.4 Differential diagnosis of paroxysmal dystonic choreoathetoid movement disorders

Feature	Paroxysmal dystonic choreoathetosis (non-kinesigenic)	Paroxysmal kinesigenic choreoathetosis	Paroxysmal exercise-induced choreoathetosis
Age at onset	Baby – mid-adulthood	Baby – early adulthood	Infant – mid-adulthood
Ratio child : adult	1.5 : 1	4 : 1	1 : 4
Trigger	Excitement, fatigue, heat, alcohol, cold, caffeine	Sudden movements	Sustained physical exercise, sudden movement, cold
Attack	Arms, legs, face	Arms, legs, face	Particularly legs
– Duration	2 min–4 hrs	seconds –<5 min	5–30 min
– Frequency	20/day–2/year	110/day–1/month	1/day–1/month
EEG	Normal	Normal	Normal
Therapy	Benzodiazepine, valproate	DPH, CBZ, VAL	CLZ
Genetics	Autosomal dominant, Chr. 2q	Autosomal dominant	Autosomal dominant

non-epileptic psychogenic seizures should be considered as a possible cause in young children. If in doubt, double-image videotaping of an epileptic fit should be made wherever possible to facilitate analysis. Only conclusive EEG findings may be used for diagnostic purposes where physiological variations are known (Bleasel & Kotagal 2005; Beach & Reading 2005).

Depending on seizure duration, the assumption of a non-epileptic psychogenic seizure can be corroborated by no increase in the hormone prolactin. A two- to three-fold increase in prolactin 20 minutes after seizure onset indicates an epileptic fit. Prolactin levels should be measured postictal 24 hours later, if not already available. Measuring creatine kinase (CK) and neurone-specific enolase as a marker of neuronal activity is not as effective as postictal prolactin. Non-epileptic psychogenic seizures require a completely different therapeutic approach, which must be followed just as rigorously as an epilepsy treatment regimen (Egger et al. 2003).

Table 2.5 shows the most important differences between epileptic and non-epileptic psychogenic seizures.

Key symptoms: Dramatic in character, patient fully conscious, longer than epileptic fit, eyes frequently closed.

Pulse synchronous bulbus movement in spheno-orbital dysplasia

If no chemosis or other alterations to the eye can be found, pulse synchronous bulbus movement – frequently one-sided – can be attributed to a spheno-

Table 2.5 Psychogenic non-epileptic seizure (PNES) vs. epileptic seizure

Feature	PNES	Epileptic
Depending on situation	Frequent	Seldom – never
Slow onset	Not infrequent	Seldom – never
Undulating neurology	Frequent	Seldom
Asynchronous movement of extremities	Frequent	Seldom – never
Head-shaking	Frequent	Seldom
Tongue bite	Seldom – tip	Frequent – lateral
Eyes	Closed	Open
Resistance to eye opening	Frequent	Seldom
Quick recovery	Frequent	Seldom
Duration of seizure	≫2 min	<2 min
Nocturnal occurrence	Seldom	Frequent
Cyanosis	Seldom – never	Frequent
Opisthotonos	Seldom in children	Never
Reactivity during apparent unconsciousness	Frequent	Seldom – never

orbital dysplasia. Spheno-orbital dysplasia is a rare but important symptom of neurofibromatosis type 1 (NF1), the most frequent neurocutaneous illness in infancy and adulthood occurring with a frequency of 1 : 2300. The eyelid is often slanted outward on the affected side. Impaired function is rare and only occurs at maximum protrusio bulbi. A clinical examination reveals café-au-lait spots, axillary or inguinal freckling, Lisch nodes in the iris, and further NF1 symptoms. In the case of autosomal dominant inheritance, the parents should also be examined. Therapy is not necessary, as the intensity of pulse synchronous bulbus movement diminishes with increasing age due to increasing fibrosis and hardening of the orbital periphery.

Key symptoms: Pulse synchronous bulbus movement without trauma.

Hyperekplexia

Symptoms of hyperekplexia include an abnormal startle reaction to external, frequently acoustic, stimuli with accompanying loss of muscle tone and posture, causing the patient to fall to the ground without losing consciousness (Tijssen et al. 2002). It is most frequently falsely diagnosed as atonic or myoclonic astatic epileptic seizure. Stimulus response is not self-habituating. Neonates show hyperekplexia in the characteristic triad of (i) increased muscle tone (stiff baby syndrome), which improves spontaneously by the age of one year; (ii) non-habituating startle reaction – a simple clinical test consists of triggering the glabella reflex; and (iii) myoclonic attacks during sleep, which can be life-threatening but which also cease spontaneously after the age of one year. Inheritance is autosomal dominant. Other characteristic features can be identified with the help of the startle reaction, for example, a minimum response to the glabella reflex can manifest itself as a tensing of the neck muscles. Pathological glycine receptors (chromosome 5q) can be effectively treated with GABA-ergic substances (Zhou et al. 2002, Rees et al. 2002).

Key symptoms: Exaggerated non-habituating startle response to external stimuli; paroxysmal muscle tone with loss of posture, patient remains fully conscious.

Munchausen syndrome by proxy

Mothers recount various incongruent symptoms their child supposedly has with this syndrome, simulating a serious illness for which there is no clinical correlation. Symptoms of paroxysmal movement disorders frequently play an important role. Munchausen syndrome by proxy should always be kept in mind if all clinical findings do not match up at all (Schreier 2004). The parents, usually the mother, frequently work in the medical profession and insist on invasive diagnostics. The child usually has already been presented in several clinics or seen a number of doctors. For further discussion of Munchausen syndrome by proxy, see Galvin, Newton and Vandeven (2005).

Key symptoms: Child healthy, mother ill.

References

Alsaaadi TM, Marquez AV. Psychogenic nonepileptic seizures. *Am Fam Physician* 2005, **72**:849–856.

Beach R, Reading R. The importance of acknowledging clinical uncertainty in the diagnosis of epilepsy and non-epileptic events. *Arch Dis Child* 2005, **90**:1219–1222.

Black JE, Brooks SN, Nishino S. Narcolepsy and syndromes of primary excessive daytime somnolence. *Semin Neurol* 2004, **24**:271–282.

Bleasel A, Kotagal P. Paroxysmal nonepileptic disorders in children and adolescents. *Semin Neurol 2005*, **15**:203–217.

Coulter DL, Allen RJ. Benign neonatal sleep myoclonus. *Arch Neurol* 1982, **39**:191–192.

Deonna T, Martin D. Benign paroxysmal torticollis in infancy. *Arch Dis Child* 1981, **56**:956–959.

DiMario FJ. Paroxysmal nonepileptic events of childhood. *Semin Pediatr Neurol* 2006, **13**:208–221.

Echenne B, Rivier F. Benign paroxysmal tonic upward gaze. *Pediatr Neurol* 1992, **8**:154–155.

Egger J, Grossmann G, Auchterlonie A. Benign sleep myoclonus in infancy mistaken for epilepsy. *BMJ* 2003, **326**:975–976.

Evans OB. Breath – holding spells. *Pediatr Ann* 1997, **26**:312–316.

Galvin HK, Newton AW, Vandeven AM. Update on Munchausen syndrome by proxy. *Curr Opin Pediatr* 2005, **17**:252–257.

Holmes GL, Russman BS. Shuddering attacks. *Am J Dis Child* 1986, **140**:72–73.

Hüdaoglu O, Dirik E, Yis U, Kurul S. Parental attitude of mothers, iron deficiency anemia, and breath – holding spells. *Pediatr Neurol* 2006, **35**:18–20.

Kabakus N, Kurt A. Sandifer syndrome: a continuing problem of misdiagnosis. *Pediatr Int* 2006, **48**: 622–625.

Kostakis A, Manjunatha NP, Kumar A, Moreland ES. Abnormal head posture in a patient with normal ocular motilità: Sandifer syndrome. *J Pediatr Ophthalmol Strabismus* 2008, **45**:57–58.

Kotagal P, Costa M, Wyllie E, Wolgamuth B. Paroxysmal nonepileptic events in children and adolescents. *Pediatrics* 2002, **110**:46.

Kuhle S, Tiefenthaler M, Seidl R, Hauser E. Prolonged generalized epileptic seizures triggered by breath-holding spells. *Pediatr Neurol* 2000, **23**:271–273.

Lehwald N, Krausch M, Franke C, Assmann B, Adam R; Knoefel WT. Sandifer syndrome – a multidisciplinary diagnostic and therapeutic challenge. *Eur J Pediatr Surg* 2007, **17**:203–206.

Lombroso C, Lerman P. Breath-holding spells (cyanotic and pallid infantile syncope). *Pediatrics* 1967, **39**:563–581.

Mocan H, Yildiran A, Orhan F, Erduran E. Breath holding spells in children and response to treatment with iron. *Arch Dis Child* 1999, **81**:261–262.

Nechay A, Ross LM, Stephenson JB, O'Regan M. Gratification disorder ("infantile masturbation"). A review. *Arch Dis Child* 2004, **89**:225–226.

Ouvrier RA, Billson F. Benign paroxysmal tonic upgaze of childhood. *J Child Neurol* 1988, **3**:177–180.

Overeem S, Scammell TE, Jan Lammers G. Hypocretin/orexin and sleep: implications for the pathophysiology and diagnosis of narcolepsy. *Curr Opin Neurol* 2002, **15**:739–745.

Paolicchi JM. The spectrum of nonepileptic events in children. *Epilepsia* 2002, **43** (Suppl. 3): 60–64.

Preblick–Salib C, Jagoda A. Spells. Differential diagnosis and management strategies. *Emerg Med Clin North America* 1997, **15**:637–648.

Rees MI, Lewis TM, Kwok JB, Mortier GR; Govaert P; Snell RG; Schofield PR, Owen MJ. Hyperekplexia associated with compound heterozygote mutations in the beta-subunit of the human inhibitory glycine receptor (GLRB). *Hum Mol Genet* 2002, **11**: 853–860.

Scheepers B, Clouth P, Pickles C. The misdiagnosis of epilepsy: findings of a population study. *Seizure* 1998, 7:403–406.

Schreier H. Munchausen by proxy. *Curr Probl Pediatr Adolesc Health Care* 2004, **34**:126–143.

Somijit S, Lee Y, Berkovic F, Harvey AS. Sandifer syndrome misdiagnosed as refractory partial seizures in an adult. *Epileptic Disord* 2004, **6**:49–50.

Tijssen MA, Vergouwe MN, van Dijk JG, Rees M, Frants RR, Brown P. Major and minor form of hereditary hyperekplexia. *Mov Dis* 2002, **17**:826–830.

Uldall P, Alving J, Hansen LK, Kibaek M, Buchholt J. The misdiagnosis of epilepsy in children admitted to a tertiary epilepsy centre with paroxysmal events. *Arch Dis Child* 2006, **91**:219–221.

Vanasse M, Bedard P, Andermann F. Shuddering attacks in children: an early clinical manifestation of essential tremor. *Neurology* 1976, **26**:1027–1030.

Vidaillhet M. Paroxysmal dyskinesias as a paradigm of paroxysmal movement disorders. *Curr Opin Neurol* 2000, **13**: 457–462.

Yang ML, Fullwood E, Goldstein J, Mink JW. Masturbation in infancy and early childhood presenting as a movement disorder: 12 cases and a review of the literature. *Pediatrics* 2005, **116**:1427–1432.

Zhou L, Chillag KL, Nigro MA. Hyperekplexia: a treatable neurogenetic disease. *Brain Dev* 2002, **24**:669–674.

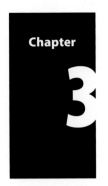

Chapter 3

Syncope

Florian Weissinger and Thomas Lempert

Definition

Syncope is defined as transient loss of consciousness and of postural control. Pathophysiologically, it is based on global cerebral hypoxia as a result of transient hypoperfusion of the brain. Recovery usually occurs spontaneously.

Syncope is not a disorder of its own but a symptom. A variety of different causes may underlie it. Syncope can be classified according to its etiology. Above all, the differentiation between potentially life-threatening cardiac syncope and rather harmless circulatory syncope is clinically relevant. Besides the etiological classification, syncope can be differentiated based on its clinical presentation. Convulsive syncope is accompanied by tonic or clonic muscle activity while the patient is unconscious. It occurs regardless of the respective etiology of the syncope. The term *presyncope* characterizes a precondition of syncope but without complete loss of consciousness.

Epidemiology

More than one third of the population at least experiences syncope once in their lives. In the general population, the incidence of syncope amounts to approximately 6 per 1000 person-years. Incidence rates are comparable for men and women; however, they increase significantly with advancing age (Soteriades et al. 2002).

In the industrial nations, syncope accounts for 3% to 5% of diagnoses in Emergency Departments, and 1% to 6% of hospital admissions take place due to syncope.

Diagnosis

"Fainting" as symptom

Patients with widely differing forms of reduced states of consciousness consult a doctor and report they have been "fainting." It is the treating physician's task to assign this "fainting" a diagnosis. In most cases, the cause of fainting is syncope, in particular when there was a complete loss of consciousness. However, it is essential for the further diagnostic and therapeutic approach to exclude other paroxysmal events which are associated with impaired consciousness and falls. Therefore, whenever a patient who experienced a transient state of reduced consciousness consults a doctor or presents in an emergency room, the first question to answer is whether the event was due to syncope in the proper sense or whether it was caused by something different. Misdiagnoses are not only made because patients and their relatives sometimes provide imprecise information but also because physicians may have a mistaken idea of the course of syncope. Reasons for that are the lack of opportunity to observe syncope first-hand and the impressive stereotype of the melodramatic "Hollywood syncope": the patient, or actress, respectively, sighs, sinks to the ground or, even better, into the arms of her male hero, lies motionless with closed eyes on the ground and finally starts blinking while regaining consciousness, asking "Where am I?"

Clinical phenomenology of syncope

This chapter describes the clinical characteristics of syncope and its distinction from generalized tonic-clonic seizures, which cause the most difficulties

The Paroxysmal Disorders, ed. Bettina Schmitz, Barbara Tettenborn and Donald L. Schomer. Published by Cambridge University Press. © Cambridge University Press 2010.

in daily clinical practice. The latter distinction is important as the underlying processes are pathophysiologically completely different, especially convulsive syncope which is associated with tonic or myoclonic phenomena and sometimes difficult to distinguish from generalized tonic-clonic seizures (Gastaut and Fischer-Williams 1957; Lempert et al. 1994).

Precipitants and precedents

Syncope is provoked by specific actions or circumstances, whereas epileptic seizures occur almost always spontaneously. Such provoking factors can be revealed by taking a careful history in about half of the cases. Among the more common precipitants are prolonged standing, especially in warm surroundings, violent and persistent coughing, micturition, exertion, intake of antihypertensive drugs, nitrates, or alcohol, loss of blood, venipuncture or any other invasive medical procedure, and aversive stimuli, such as the sight of blood and even attending rock concerts, a risk-factor especially for female teenagers.

Characteristic precedents of syncope are a bilateral tinnitus, frequently described as "buzzing" or "ringing in the ears," or reduced hearing which might culminate in closing of both ears "with a snap." Another typical premonitory symptom is "blacking out," a transient amaurosis while consciousness is still preserved. It is caused by the early hypoperfusion of retinal capillaries. In many patients, this blacking out is misunderstood as unconsciousness and, thus, it is necessary to ask specifically for a brief loss of vision prior to the loss of consciousness.

Descriptions such as dizziness, lightheadedness, warmth, general malaise and faintness are equally common. However, these terms are used in a similar manner by patients to describe an epileptic aura or the sensation which precedes a psychogenic non-epileptic seizure.

On the other hand, typical phenomena of an epileptic aura do not occur as precedents of syncope and include the sensation of a specific taste or smell, déjà vu and jamais vu, speech impairment or unilateral paresthesia (Benke et al. 1997). Preceding palpitations are also not specific for syncope although they may be a sign for tachycardia with reduced cardiac output.

Phenomena during syncope

Patients with syncope usually fall to the ground at the onset of unconsciousness. About half of them collapse atonically and flaccidly, whereas the other half falls stiffly with extended knees and hips (Lempert et al. 1994). Thus, a stiff fall – as in generalized tonic-clonic seizures – cannot be used as an unequivocal criterion for differential diagnosis. Falls during syncope can be directed backward, to the side or forward. The latter are occasionally associated with facial injuries.

In experimental studies, the frequency of tonic or myoclonic muscle activity during syncope ranges between 12% and 100%, with most of the studies finding the frequency between 70% and 90%. Thus, convulsive syncope is the rule rather than the exception, which can be explained by the fact that convulsions are an intrinsic component of the brain's response to hypoxia. The high variability of frequencies at which convulsions in syncope were observed is explained by their highly variable presentation. In daily clinical routine, a single myoclonic jerk of facial muscles, for instance, is frequently missed, whereas massive, repetitive myoclonic jerks of the entire body are often too easily attributed to an epileptic seizure. When reports from random observers of syncope were analyzed in clinical case series, convulsions were documented in 5% to 15% of patients (Alboni et al. 2001; Graham and Kenny 2001; Sheldon et al. 2002).

The most important criterion to differentiate syncopal and epileptic convulsions is their specific phenomenology. In contrast to epileptic muscle activity, syncopal myoclonic movements are arrhythmic. Mostly, they are multifocal rather than generalized; that is, they occur asynchronously in different regions of the body. Only in rare cases do they last longer than 30 seconds. Tonic phenomena are significantly less frequent in syncope and are usually less pronounced. Thus, they can be easily distinguished from the forced opisthotonus of generalized tonic-clonic seizures. A tonic extension of the body with flexion of the arms is more common in profound cerebral hypoxia, for example, due to prolonged asystole, or in syncope in children, such as breath-holding spells.

Automatisms can also be found in up to 80% of syncope. Typically, they are complex, involuntary movements such as licking of the lips, chewing, fumbling, lifting a hand to the head, sitting up or even standing up, which occur mostly in the second half of the syncope. They are usually singular movements, and for that reason they can easily be distinguished from the repetitive automatisms in complex-partial seizures.

As a rule, the eyes stay open during syncope as well as during an epileptic seizure. Upward turning of the eyes and lateral eye deviations can be observed in either case. However, in contrast to epileptic seizures, eye movements during syncope are usually transient and only last for a few seconds.

Hallucinations as an additional feature are frequently missed in daily clinical practice as physicians usually do not inquire about them and patients do not report them spontaneously. Visual and auditory hallucinations – often with a pleasant content – toward the end of syncope can be elicited with amazing regularity, which in rare cases can be confused with a preceding aura in partial epileptic seizures.

Postictal phase

For the differentiation of syncope and epileptic seizures, postictal phenomena are of particular importance. It is widely acknowledged that the single most powerful distinctive feature is the duration of postictal confusion as observed by an eye witness. After syncope, patients are fully re-orientated within very few seconds, and even after prolonged attacks lasting 1 to 2 minutes the postictal confusion or drowsiness lasts rarely longer than 30 seconds. Any longer-lasting disorientation suggests an epileptic seizure. However, it must be kept in mind that partial seizures of frontal lobe origin are frequently associated with a fast re-orientation. So, even this feature is not unequivocal, and additional criteria are necessary to distinguish an epileptic seizure from syncope.

After generalized tonic-clonic seizures, tongue bites can be found in about one third of the cases, whereas they occur only on rare occasions in syncope. Therefore, if present they are a quite reliable indicator for an epileptic seizure. On the other hand, urinary incontinence and head injuries occur about just as frequently in syncope as in generalized epileptic seizures. General symptoms such as exhaustion, fatigue, vomiting, headaches and muscle pain also occur after syncope; however, they are more frequent and pronounced after generalized tonic-clonic seizures.

Postictally, about two hours after a generalized tonic-clonic seizure there is an increase in serum creatine kinase (CK) levels over the basic level. Initial CK serum levels above 200 U/l point to an epileptic seizure. Furthermore, even a small increase of at least 15 U/l within 24 hours after the event is more indicative of an epileptic seizure. On the other hand, patients with syncope show only slightly increased CK serum levels immediately after the event and usually have no further increase over time (Neufeld et al. 1997).

The serum prolactin level increases one hour after a generalized tonic-clonic seizure, whereas after syncope it either increases or decreases. Therefore, assessment of serum prolactin levels is not useful for the distinction between syncope and epileptic seizure (Lusić et al. 1999). The most important features that differentiate syncope from epileptic seizures are summarized in Table 3.1.

Interaction between syncopal and epileptic mechanisms

In rare cases, there is an interaction between syncopal and epileptic mechanisms within a single attack. On one hand, this means that an epileptic seizure can emerge from syncope. This is documented in single case reports, mostly in children. Many other reports suggest that hypoxic convulsions during syncope have been misinterpreted as epileptic myoclonic movements. In certain forms of epileptic seizures, especially in complex-partial seizures of temporal lobe origin, cardiac arrhythmias can arise, which then can lead to syncope. If the medical history suggests epileptic and syncopal phenomena within the same attack, the diagnosis can only be made by means of ictal EEG and ECG recordings.

Presyncope

Presyncope is the prodromal stage of syncope in which there is only a less pronounced hypoperfusion of the brain and therefore no complete loss of consciousness. When reported, in addition to lightheadedness the following symptoms may suggest presyncope: sweating, nausea, impaired vision, blacking out, fading away, palpitations or hyperventilation. Occasionally, patients can fall even when consciousness is partially preserved. When patients with presyncope never experience a complete syncope with fall and loss of consciousness, the differentiation from metabolic and psychiatric disorders remains difficult.

Causes of syncope

In the previous section, the phenomenology of syncope in distinction from generalized tonic-clonic seizures was described. In the following, the second step of diagnosis will be introduced, that is, the etiological classification of syncope.

Table 3.1 Differential diagnostic signs of syncope and epileptic seizures

	Syncope	Generalized tonic-clonic seizure
Pre-ictal		
Immediate triggers	ca. 50% e.g., standing for a long time, vein puncture, urination, defecation	none
Subjective signs	presyncope dizziness, buzzing in the ears, black-out	epileptic aura e.g., nausea, déjà-vu experience, smell
Objective signs	sweating, paleness	focal motor initiation (optional)
Ictal		
Fall	limp or rigid	rigid
Motor phenomena	ca. 80% mild to severe arrhythmic multifocal or generalized mostly <30 s	100% mostly severe rhythmic generalized 1–2 min
Eyes	opened, deviation	opened, deviation
Urine incontinence	frequent	frequent
Biting of the tongue	very rare, every localisation	frequent, lateral
Duration	mostly <30 s	1–3 min
Post-ictal		
Reorientation phase	<30 s	4–45 min
Neurological focal symptoms	never	Todd's phenomena (6%)
Headache	frequent	frequent
Creatine kinase	>200 U/l (12%) slight increase or decrease within 24 h	>200 U/l (56%) further increase within 24 h
Prolactin	normal or increased	increased

Reflex-mediated syncope

Neurally mediated or neurocardiogenic, vasovagal syncope

By far, the most frequent form of syncope is the neurally mediated syncope, which accounts for about 18% (8% to 37%; Kapoor 2000) of all syncope and is responsible for the majority of etiologically unexplained syncope. Patients of all age groups can be affected by neurally mediated syncope. They are the most frequent cause for transient loss of consciousness, especially in young and otherwise healthy people.

Older terms are *vasovagal* or *vasodepressive* syncope. The well-established term "neurally mediated syncope" is probably the most appropriate because neither the vagus nerve ("vasovagal") nor reflexes originating from the heart ("neurocardiogenic") play an essential role. Pathophysiologically, there is a decrease in peripheral vascular resistance with a sudden and rapidly progressing hypotension, which can not be counterbalanced by an increase in cardiac output. Concomitantly, instead of a compensatory increase in pulse rate there is often a vagally mediated bradycardia. This bradycardia is not very relevant for the syncopal episode. The mechanisms underlying acute vasodilatation and bradycardia have not yet been explained. It has been assumed that the syncopal reaction is triggered by stimulation of cardiac mechanoreceptors due to an elevated tonus of the sympathetic system; however, as cardiac transplanted patients with completely denervated hearts are capable of developing this type of syncope, the significance of cardiac mechanoreceptors is rather doubtful.

Neurally mediated syncope can be triggered by all different kinds of unpleasant experiences, especially by physical pain or a trauma such as venipuncture. Also, in emotionally stressful situations with fear or terror, sometimes even at the sight of blood, such a vascular reaction can occur (also called "psychogenic fainting"). In addition, prolonged standing, dehydration, overtiredness, and a warm and stifling environment can facilitate the development of neurally mediated syncope.

Glossopharyngeal or trigeminal neuralgia can also cause a neurally mediated syncope. It is assumed that the syncopal reaction can be triggered by the intense, stabbing neuropathic pain on one hand but also by direct reflex-based mechanisms in the brainstem on the other.

Situational syncope

Situational syncope, also called reflex syncope, accounts for about 5% of all syncope. In this form, the syncopal reaction is an immediate consequence of certain situations or actions. Typical triggers of such syncope are micturition, swallowing, coughing, defecation, sneezing, screaming or lifting heavy weights.

This group comprises syncope with a different underlying pathogenesis. For instance, in micturition and swallowing syncope, just like in neurally mediated syncope, a reflex-mediated vasodilatation with or without bradycardia occurs so that these two forms of syncope blend into each other. On the other hand, some authors regard syncope after prolonged standing or associated with neuralgia as situational syncope.

Syncope can also appear after eating a carbohydrate-rich meal, particularly in elderly patients. These so-called "postprandial syncope" is caused by a redistribution of the blood volume to the abdomen while the peripheral vasoconstriction necessary to compensate for it is missing. An entirely different pathophysiology underlies syncope induced by coughing, screaming or weight-lifting. Here, pressing causes a sudden increase in intrathoracic pressure, which consequently results in a decrease in cardiac output and a drop in blood pressure.

This latter mechanism can be reproduced experimentally by the Valsalva maneuver (Duvoisin 1962). Intense pressing against the closed epiglottis increases the intrathoracic pressure. As the pressure gradient between the final part of the venous system in the peripheral capillaries and the right atrium of the heart is small, this increase in thoracic pressure results in a relevant decrease of venous backflow to the heart. An eventual drop of the mean arterial blood pressure below 60 mmHg causes syncope (Stucki 1958). The self-induction of syncope, popular in school-age children, is based on this mechanism combined with hyperventilation and orthostasis, which causes cerebral vasoconstriction.

Carotid sinus syndrome

Another form of reflex-mediated syncope occurs in the carotid sinus syndrome. In healthy individuals, firm pressure on the carotid sinus causes a slight drop in blood pressure and a transient decrease of heart rate. However, in rare cases the carotid sinus is hypersensitive, and even slight pressure on the posterior cervical triangle is sufficient to cause an extreme decrease in heart rate up to a brief asystole and a concomitant drop in blood pressure. In patients with such a hypersensitive carotid sinus, syncope might be elicited even by shaving or a turn of the head. Predominantly, elderly patients are affected, mostly men who often have accompanying atherosclerosis. However, evidence of carotid sinus hypersensitivity does not necessarily prove that previous syncope was also triggered by this mechanism. Carotid sinus syndrome is responsible for only about 1% of syncope.

Orthostatic syncope

Syncope is called orthostatic when it appears within a short time after rising, that is, when changing from a lying or sitting to a standing position. Before fainting, patients often notice presyncopal symptoms such as dizziness or lightheadedness. Orthostatic disorders are responsible for about 8% of syncope.

Based on their different clinical characteristics, two subtypes of pathological orthostatic reactions are distinguished: the hypoadrenergic orthostatic hypotension and the postural tachycardia syndrome.

Hypoadrenergic orthostatic hypotension

This condition is defined as the sustained decrease of systolic blood pressure by at least 20 mmHg or of diastolic blood pressure by at least 10 mmHg within three minutes after standing up or after passive head-up tilt on a tilt-table with an angle of at least 60°.

In healthy individuals, a change from a supine to a standing position results in redistribution of the circulating blood volume to the capacitance vessels of the lower body. This is compensated by a sympathetically mediated vasoconstriction and a reflex-based increase in heart rate. Blood pressure is usually restored to its initial value within 30 seconds. An insufficiency of these compensatory mechanisms results in an overshooting and sustained drop in blood pressure, which eventually leads to syncope.

The most frequent causes for such a regulatory disorder are fever, dehydration, prolonged bedrest and most commonly side-effects of drugs, including nitrates, antihypertensives, diuretics, tricyclic antidepressants, L-dopa and dopamine agonists. Furthermore, underlying medical and neurological primary diseases must be considered. From an internist's point of view, disorders such as Addison's disease or hypothyroidism should be excluded. Possible neurological primary diseases can be identified by a fixed heart rate which does not increase even as blood pressure drops and other autonomic abnormalities. Central parts of the autonomic nervous system can be affected, for example, in diseases such as multiple sclerosis or multiple system atrophy. Peripheral parts of the autonomic system can be affected by Guillain-Barré syndrome or polyneuropathy. When a transient

Fig. 3.1. Behavior of blood pressure and heart rate during the physiological orthostasis reaction, in hypoadrenergic orthostatic hypotension with (A) and without (B) cardiac denervation, and in the postural tachycardia syndrome. The vertical dashed line indicates the change from supine to upright position in each panel.

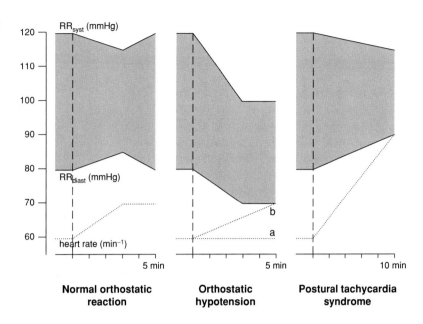

loss of consciousness occurs in a patient with diabetes mellitus, it can be caused among other things by hypoglycemia or by an orthostatic syncope as a consequence of diabetic polyneuropathy affecting the autonomic nervous system. When orthostatic hypotension occurs in the context of an isolated dysfunction of the autonomic nervous system, it is classified as pure autonomic failure.

Postural tachycardia syndrome

The postural tachycardia syndrome (synonyms: orthostatic tachycardia, hypersympathetic tone orthostatic intolerance, hyperadrenergic dysfunction) is probably the most frequent form of orthostatic dysregulation and can be found especially in younger, otherwise healthy patients with orthostatic syncope.

Its most prominent feature is the overshoot in orthostatic tachycardia. Within 10 minutes after changing to a standing position, the heart rate increases by at least 30 beats per minute or reaches a maximum of at least 120 beats per minute. In distinction from the hypoadrenergic orthostatic hypotension, there is no or only a very slight drop in systemic blood pressure, whereas the diastolic arterial pressure can even be significantly increased. Despite the stable blood pressure situation, the cerebral blood flow decreases excessively due to an increase in cerebrovascular resistance. Clinically, affected individuals experience increasing presyncopal symptoms when standing, and finally have complete syncope.

Symptomatic postural tachycardia can basically occur in all forms of hypovolemia, for example, in dehydration or due to loss of blood. In these cases, the tachycardia is regarded as a physiological reaction of the body to an additionally decreased volume of circulating blood while standing (Fig. 3.1). The etiology of the idiopathic postural tachycardia syndrome has not been entirely explained yet. Hypersensitivity of cardiac beta-receptors and an increased venous pooling in the legs due to dysfunctional venous constriction have been discussed as possible mechanisms. Usually, there are no further neurological or medical disorders to be found (Diehl and Linden 1999).

Hyperventilation syncope

Hyperventilation with hypocapnia can cause impaired consciousness and even a complete loss of consciousness. However, long before patients with hyperventilation experience impairment of consciousness, they present the typical signs of a tetanic attack, beginning with paresthesias followed by symmetrical, painful, tonic muscle cramps including the characteristic carpal pedal spasms. In a proportion of patients with postural tachycardia syndrome, hyperventilation also seems to play a role in triggering syncope.

Cardiac syncope

About 18% of syncope is due to cardiac causes. Cardiac syncope is associated with an increased mortality and is often treatable. Therefore, it is absolutely necessary to identify them. Etiologically, structural heart diseases and cardiac arrhythmias have to be considered.

Structural heart diseases with reduced cardiac output

All diseases in which the cardiac outflow channel is narrowed or venous return to the heart is impaired are associated with an increased risk for syncope. They account for approximately 4% of all syncope. In case of a decreased volume of circulating blood, caused for instance by reduction of peripheral vascular resistance, increasing the cardiac output per minute is not sufficient for compensation.

Syncope that occurs during physical exertion is strongly suggestive of a cardiac cause, as structural heart diseases with fixed cardiac output do not allow an adaption of the circulatory situation to the increased need of the body during stress. Structural heart diseases which frequently lead to syncope include coronary heart disease, heart failure, diseases of the valves, cardiomyopathies and congenital heart diseases.

In elderly patients, syncope can be a symptom of acute myocardial infarction. In rare cases, syncope occurs in association with aortic dissections. Also, obstructions of pulmonary circulation, for example, in pulmonary hypertension or in pulmonary arterial embolism, can result in a decreased output volume of the left ventricle, which eventually leads to syncope.

Arrhythmias

Approximately 14% of syncope is caused by cardiac arrhythmias and conduction disturbances in the heart. In general, any kind of cardiac arrhythmia can cause syncope. It is essential that the arrhythmia results in hemodynamic changes with a consecutive decrease in cerebral perfusion. Important bradycardic arrhythmias which are associated with syncope are the sick sinus syndrome, a second- or third-degree AV block and pacemaker dysfunctions.

Clinically, a diagnosis of syncope due to brady-arrhythmia is suggested when loss of consciousness sets in abruptly without typical prodromes. In contrast, patients frequently experience palpitations prior to tachycardic syncope, regardless of whether the tachycardia is supraventricular or ventricular. Diagnostic uncertainties can arise when distinguishing tachycardic arrhythmias from tachycardia associated with the postural tachycardia syndrome. The most important distinguishing feature is history and the reproducible occurrence of tachycardia after changing to an upright position.

The long Q-T syndrome is a disorder of the heart's electrical rhythm which is associated with torsades-de-pointes tachyarrhythmias, and clinically often manifests as syncope. Patients with long Q-T syndrome have an increased risk of sudden cardiac death; therefore, an electrocardiogram (ECG) should be recorded from all patients with syncope.

The clinical observations that suggest the presence of cardiac syncope are presyncopal palpitations, syncope in supine position, exertion induced syncope, first clinical manifestation in older patients, known cardiac disease and a pathological ECG.

Drug-induced syncope

Different medications can induce syncope, either by exceeding the required drug effect or as an unwanted side-effect of the treatment. According to the mode of action of the respective substances, the following symptoms are frequently observed: hypotension, bradycardia and/or hypovolemia. Examples of drugs associated with syncope are vasodilators such as nitrates, all kinds of antihypertensives, antidepressants and antiarrhythmic drugs.

Syncope in neurological disorders

Sometimes, syncope can occur as complication of neurological disorders. For instance, in the rare subclavian steal syndrome a transient hypoperfusion of the brainstem occurs due to subclavian artery stenosis proximal to the origin of the vertebral artery. On exercising the arm on the affected side, for example, when hanging up the laundry, the resulting hypoperfusion in the arm is compensated by reversed flow in the vertebral and basilar arteries, draining blood from the posterior cerebral circulation.

Syncope associated with migraine is particularly frequent in basilar migraine. This form of migraine occurs mostly in adolescent girls and young women. It is characterized by brainstem syndromes such as vertigo, double vision, dysarthria, tinnitus, hyperacusis and paresthesias at the onset of the attack.

During the attack, patients may experience loss of consciousness, which is generated centrally by involvement of the brainstem. As in other forms of migraine, headaches are not an obligatory symptom in basilar migraine. Other migraine patients may develop orthostatic syncope, which is caused by peripheral vasodilatation during the headache phase.

Disorders of the autonomic nervous system, for example, the Shy-Drager type, multiple system atrophy or the diabetic autonomic neuropathy, can cause orthostatic circulatory syncope as described previously in the section "Hypoadrenergic orthostatic hypotension."

Syncope in psychiatric disorders

Psychiatric co-morbidity in patients with syncope is frequently reported in the literature. It is occasionally implied that the psychiatric disorder itself can lead to syncope. However, other mechanisms of interaction between psychiatric disorders and transient impairment of consciousness seem to be more plausible, such as a secondary anxiety disorder following syncope of any etiology, pseudosyncope in the sense of psychogenic seizures, syncope induced by hyperventilation in the context of panic attacks, or drug-related orthostatic hypotonia, for instance, induced by tricyclic antidepressants.

Syncope of unknown etiology

Despite extensive diagnostic investigations, about one third of all syncope can not unequivocally be assigned to a specific etiology. The majority of these cases are probably neurocardiogenic syncope, which can either be diagnosed by following the patient over a longer clinical course or sometimes not at all. Without specific clues suggesting cardiac syncope, the prognosis quo ad vitam is usually good. In elderly patients, a clear diagnostic assignment can also be more difficult: Different disorders which can lead to syncope are simultaneously present, and drugs are taken which may also facilitate syncope.

Specific examination techniques

As described previously, the diagnosis of syncope is made in two steps. First, distinguish it from other paroxysmal events with impaired consciousness and/or fall. Second, assign the syncope to an etiology and work from there to prove or disprove its causality. How this diagnosis is made, and which diagnostic procedures are used, is explained in the following.

Diagnostics of syncope

Figure 3.2 shows an algorithm for the systematic evaluation of patients with transiently reduced state of consciousness. During the daily clinical routine, it can be

a helpful tool. However, the single steps in this algorithm can only be suggestions for the diagnostic evaluations. The great clinical variability of syncope may require modification of the diagnostic strategy on an individual basis.

Initial evaluation

The initial evaluation of a patient presenting after loss of consciousness includes a thorough history, a physical examination, supine and upright measurement of blood pressure and pulse rate, and an ECG.

Blood tests are only indicated either to distinguish syncope from non-syncopal attacks, for example, blood glucose levels in hypoglycemia or creatine kinase levels after a tonic-clonic epileptic seizure, or for cardiac enzyme markers in myocardial infarction or D-dimer levels in pulmonary embolism. Blood tests are usually of minor importance and are therefore not recommended as a standard procedure.

Usually, the initial evaluation suffices to distinguish syncope from other causes of impaired consciousness. The diagnostic steps necessary for more specific etiological causes for syncope can be approached in the following manner.

In the initial evaluation, patients with syncope can be divided into two groups: The first group includes patients with a clinically likely diagnosis or with a relatively certain pathogenetic mechanism for the syncope. The second group of patients with syncope are those of an unknown etiology. Patients with a certain or highly suspected diagnosis often require no further diagnostics but only few specific tests to either confirm or disprove the presumption.

Neurocardiogenic syncope has a distinctive history, so there are usually no further diagnostic steps necessary. In cases of doubt, a tilt-table test can help to increase the probability of the diagnosis. This test is positive if a drop in blood pressure with or without bradycardia can be induced while symptoms of syncope occur. A positive test result suggests that the earlier syncope was also caused by an easily inducible hypotensive reaction of the cardiovascular system, but does not prove it.

Usually, situational syncope is also diagnostically clear. If necessary, an attempt can be made to provoke the situation which led to syncope while monitoring blood pressure and ECG.

For the diagnosis of orthostatic syncope, history and measurements of blood pressure and pulse rate are essential. To determine if an underlying autonomic

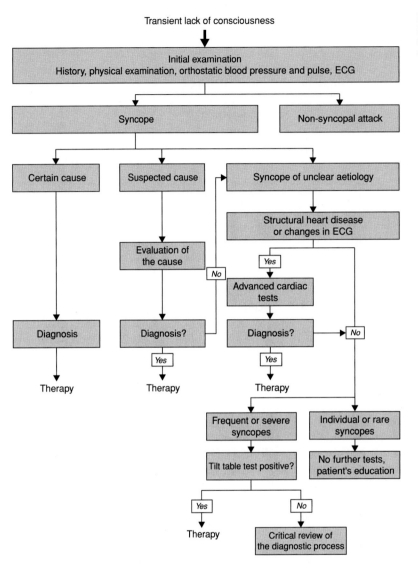

Fig. 3.2. Algorithm for the evaluation of patients with transient impairment of consciousness. (Modified from Brignole et al. 2004)

disorder exists, a simple function test such as the Valsalva maneuver can be helpful. If a disorder of circulatory regulation is suspected, further diagnostic steps are necessary to exclude an underlying neurological or medical primary disease. When orthostatic blood pressure is measured in patients where there is little clinical suspicion for syncope (especially the elderly), patients often show false-positive results, that is, orthostatic drops in blood pressure without any clinical relevance. Therefore, orthostatic complaints should always be inquired about prior to and during the blood pressure measurements.

Carotid sinus syndrome as the cause of syncope can also be suspected based on the patient's history. The presumed diagnosis can be corroborated by the carotid sinus pressure test. A positive test with hemodynamic changes and syncopal symptoms is suggestive when no other mechanisms of syncope is evident.

The causes of cardiac syncope can often be deduced from the initial evaluation. They comprise both pre-existing structural heart diseases, for example, aortic stenosis, disorders of the heart valves, or myocardial infarction; and arrhythmias such as a complete AV block or ventricular and supraventricular tachycardias. If one of these diagnoses is suspected, echocardiography and stress ECG (ergometry) should be performed to confirm it.

The diagnosis of drug-induced syncope can be suspected when the patient's history suggests a close temporal relationship between onset or change of pharmacotherapy and the occurrence of syncope.

Further diagnostic approach to syncope of unknown etiology

In the group of patients with syncope of unknown etiology, the further diagnostic approach is determined by individual risk factors. In patients with structural heart disease or conspicuous results in the ECG, arrhythmias are the most frequent cause of syncope. Therefore, following echocardiography and stress-ECG extended cardiac diagnostics should be performed in these patients. Continuous ECG monitoring with 24-hour (Holter) ECG monitors or loop recorders can confirm or exclude that syncopal symptoms are correlated to cardiac arrhythmias. If this is not successful, invasive procedures such as intracardial electrophysiological study or coronary angiography can be considered.

If the patient's history does not provide any indication of cardiac symptoms and if the results of ECG, ergometry and echocardiography are unremarkable, a diagnosis of organic heart disease or cardiac arrhythmia is very unlikely. This patient is more likely to have neurocardiogenic syncope. The examination of choice for this group of patients is the tilt-table test, which often allows confirmation of the latter diagnosis.

Treatment is not necessarily indicated in patients with infrequent neurocardiogenic syncope. The tilt-table test to confirm the diagnosis is also not required in these cases as it would not have any relevant consequences with regard to therapy. However, these patients should be followed and eventually re-evaluated if syncope occurs more frequently.

In elderly patients, assigning syncope to only one single etiology is even more challenging because different possible causes may co-exist. Also, the aim of the diagnostics should be to identify the one principle cause of syncope. If this is not possible, the most likely cause or the potentially most dangerous etiology for the syncope should be treated. After clinical evaluation and all tests are completed, if the etiology of syncope can not be unequivocally identified all diagnostic steps should be critically re-evaluated. Especially, re-appraisal of the patient's history and a physical re-examination can be helpful in the search for potential causes of syncope.

Examination methods

Medical history

As in all episodically occurring disorders, the historical information given by the patient and by any eyewitness is of vital importance for the diagnosis. Syncope has to be distinguished from other forms of transient loss of consciousness. Details from the medical history can give the first hint at the underlying cause of syncope. Table 3.2 lists some diagnostically relevant indicators of the etiology of syncope.

It is essential to get an accurate description of the event itself and its circumstances. Therefore, the information about position of the body, physical activity, potential predisposing factors, emotions and sensations at the onset and after the episode should be specifically addressed. If an eyewitness is available, specific questions about the type of fall, the complexion of the skin, the duration of unconsciousness, and myoclonus should be asked.

Irregularities in the patient's autonomic history, for example, dysfunction of urination or constipation, can indicate an underlying autonomic disorder. Pre-existing medical conditions are of special importance; however, earlier neurological and psychiatric disorders should also be specifically inquired. In any case, the medication taken and their dosage have to be ascertained. Furthermore, it must be clarified whether the current event was the first of its kind or if similar or identical episodes had occurred in the past. In addition, the question about heart diseases in the patient's family should not be omitted.

Physical examination

The physical examination of a patient after syncope involves first and foremost the screening of cardiopulmonary functions; the medical examination should especially focus on the following features: pathological heart sounds, cardiac arrhythmias, signs of heart failure and cervical (carotid) bruits.

The neurological examination is supposed to be normal in patients with syncope. Focal neurological symptoms may indicate an alternative diagnosis, such as cerebral ischemia or symptomatic epilepsy.

Measurements of blood pressure and heart rate

Nowadays, orthostatic blood pressure measurement is performed in a short version lasting 3 minutes, which is sufficient to evaluate orthostatic tolerance. After a five-minute rest in the supine position, the resting

Table 3.2 Diagnostic clues for the etiology of syncope

Triggers and accompanying symptoms	Probable etiology
Sudden onset without first signs or in supine position; injury when falling	Cardiac arrhythmia
Onset under physical strain	Cardiac or pulmonary obstruction
Presyncopal palpitations	Cardiac arrhythmia
Presyncopal dyspnea or chest pain	Acute myocardial infarction, pulmonary embolism
Presyncopal neurological focal symptoms	Basilaris-migraine, migraine with aura
Presyncopal symptoms seconds or minutes after sitting/standing up	Orthostatic syncope
Occurrence after standing for a long time, during unpleasant experiences, in emotionally stressful situations, during invasive medical operations, glossopharyngeal or trigeminal neuralgia	Neurocardiogenic syncope
Occurrence during urination, defecation, swallowing	Reflex neurocardiogenic syncope
Occurrence when coughing, screaming, lifting weights, orgasm	Pressure (Valsalva-induced) syncope
Occurrence after a meal	Postprandial hypotensive syncope
Occurrence when turning the head, pressure on the neck	Carotid sinus syndrome
Intake of alcohol or antihypertensive drugs	Orthostatic syncope
Family history of sudden cardiac death; peculiarities in the ECG, especially sinus bradycardia <40/min, sinus breaks >3s; AV-block of the 2nd or 3rd degree, alternating bundle branch block images; fast supraventricular or ventricular tachycardia; pacemaker dysfunction with breaks	Cardiac arrhythmia
Coincidence with onset of medication or dose change; intake of vasodilatant, antihypertensive, antidepressant or anti-arrhythmic drugs	Drug-induced syncope
Repeated episodes over several years with inconspicuous cardiac findings	Mostly neurocardiogenic or orthostatic syncope

blood pressure is measured. Then, the patient stands up and further measurements at intervals of 1, 2 and 3 minutes are performed. A sustained drop of systolic blood pressure by more than 20 mmHg or of diastolic blood pressure by at least 10 mmHg thereby suggests hypoadrenergic orthostatic hypotension, which may be a potential cause for syncope. The specificity of the test is significantly greater when the patient experiences typical symptoms during the test. An increase in pulse rate by up to 15 beats per minute after standing up is normal, and a reduced or missing increase is a sign of autonomic cardiac denervation. To detect a postural tachycardia syndrome, the pulse must be monitored over 10 minutes. The diagnosis can be made if a sustained increase in pulse rate by at least 30 beats per minute occurs.

ECG

Relevant ECG abnormalities are bradycardic or tachycardic arrhythmias, atrioventricular conduction defects or intraventricular conduction blocks, and signs of acute myocardial infarction or of cardiac hypertrophy.

Carotid sinus pressure test

For this test, the carotid sinus above the bifurcation of the carotid artery is massaged separately on each side for 5 to 10 seconds while ECG and blood pressure are recorded continuously. The test is considered positive if carotid sinus massage produces syncopal symptoms associated with asystole of at least 3 seconds duration or with a drop in systolic blood pressure of at least 50 mmHg.

Tilt-table test

The tilt-table test is a vital component for the diagnosis of those neurocardiogenic syncopes which cannot be diagnosed based on the medical history alone. The test should be reserved for patients with recurrent unexplained syncope in whom a structural heart disease or cardiac arrhythmias have been excluded as cause of the syncope.

To take the test, the patient is strapped to a tilt-table with a foot plate. After a resting period of 20 to 45 minutes in the horizontal position, the table is tilted at an angle of 60° to 80° for another 20 to 45 minutes, exposing the patient to passive orthostasis. ECG and blood pressure are continuously recorded through-out the investigation. If this procedure alone does not induce syncope, additional pharmacological provocation can be achieved by isoproterenol or nitrates. However, this may increase the number of false-positive results. The test result is only considered positive if the patient's typical symptoms of syncope can be induced.

EEG

The EEG during syncope shows generalized high-amplitude slow-wave activity at the onset of unconsciousness, followed by flattening of the EEG, and subsequently slow waves again before the normal background activity returns (Brenner 1997). This sequence is independent of the mechanism of syncope and of the clinical presentation as convulsive or non-convulsive syncope as it represents the common final path in terms of global cerebral hypoxia.

The significance of the EEG in the diagnosis of syncope is often overestimated. It could be shown that in unselected patients with syncope the recording of a postictal EEG was not helpful. Epileptiform patterns in an interictal EEG recording can indeed corroborate a diagnosis of epilepsy. However, additional syncopal attacks are not excluded. On the other hand, even in chronic epilepsy epileptiform patterns can be absent during interictal EEG recordings, thus also preventing a definite classification of the attacks. Also, episodic seizures induced by alcohol or benzodiazepine withdrawal are usually not associated with epileptiform patterns in the interictal EEG. Therefore, EEG recordings are not recommended as standard tests after syncope and should be reserved for patients with a positive history for epileptic seizures.

Cardiologic diagnostic procedures

Besides a twelve-channel ECG recording, the following cardiologic examination methods are relevant in extended diagnostics: stress-ECG (ergometry), echocardiography, long-term (Holter) ECG, intra-cardial electrophysiological studies and coronary angiography. All of these are specific cardiologic examinations which are beyond the scope of this text. Relatively new are the so-called loop recorders, which register the ECG over months on an infinite loop. In case of syncope, the current data can be stored and analyzed.

Differential diagnosis

Other epileptic seizures

Usually, the distinction between syncope and complex-partial seizures or absence seizures does not cause any problems as the two seizure types are not associated with falls. Complex-partial seizures often manifest with automatisms which can be similar to those in syncope (see previous sections). However, the seizure-related automatisms are usually more pronounced and prolonged. Also, the duration of complex-partial seizures of 2 to 3 minutes and a postictal state with altered consciousness are helpful to distinguish them from syncope. The differentiation of syncope and generalized tonic-clonic seizures has been discussed previously in the section about clinical phenomenology of syncope.

Falls, drop attacks and cataplexy

Sometimes even simple falls can be misinterpreted as fainting, especially when they occur suddenly and without an obvious accident to cause them such as stumbling. In these cases, an early differentiation based on the patient's history is essential as falls, especially in elderly people, are caused by sensorimotor and orthopedic problems which require a different diagnostic approach than cardiovascular syncope. During drop attacks, which are yet another category, a sudden loss of body tone with subsequent fall occurs, sometimes caused by vertebrobasilar hypoperfusion. Consciousness is never impaired in drop attacks. Therefore, they can be distinguished unequivocally from syncope when the medical history is taken thoroughly.

Cataplexy is also associated with attacks of abrupt loss of muscle tone in the entire body while consciousness is completely preserved. Cataplexies are usually triggered emotionally, for example, by joy, anger or surprise. They are one of the main symptoms of the narcolepsy-cataplexy syndrome.

Transient ischemic attacks

Transient ischemic attacks (TIA) which affect the vertebral basilar system are associated with a transient loss of consciousness in about 10% of cases (Grad and Baloh 1989). The underlying pathophysiology is a local decrease in cerebral perfusion of the mesencephalic reticular formation, which causes the loss of consciousness. However, a global cerebral hypoxia is usually absent. Additional neurological symptoms generated in the vertebral basilar system are indicative for the diagnosis.

Hypoglycemia

Metabolic disorders can also be associated with a progressive impairment of consciousness and eventually a complete loss of consciousness. The most prominent example is hypoglycemia. After a prodromal phase with hunger, increased salivation, sweating, tremor and progressive confusion, a complete loss of consciousness is not infrequent. The mostly prolonged course of the condition, the measurement of blood glucose levels, and the immediate response to administration of glucose are crucial factors for the diagnosis.

Psychogenic non-epileptic seizures

The most frequent non-epileptic differential diagnosis of syncope is psychogenic non-epileptic seizure (PNES). Both conditions can be triggered by emotional stress, may be accompanied by convulsions and carry a risk of injuries due to an abrupt fall. However, there are numerous features which make the differentiation from syncope easy. Psychogenic seizures are indeed frequently triggered by suggestion, their duration can amount from minutes to hours, the patient's eyes are typically closed and long-lasting tonic, clonic or complex movements can occur. Non-verbal reactions during the seizure and a partial memory of ictal events are signs of preserved consciousness.

Therapy

As a matter of principle, in the treatment of syncope preference should be given to causal therapy of an underlying condition rather than to mere symptomatic therapy. Treatment of recurrent neurocardiogenic and situational syncope consists primarily of educating a patient regarding individual triggering factors and how to avoid them. Furthermore, the patient should learn to recognize the premonitory symptoms of syncope to react to them in a timely manner, for example, by lying down in a supine position to prevent a fall with severe consequences. Leg-crossing and isometric tensing of leg, abdominal and gluteal muscles can also antagonize the peripheral vasodilatation, thus averting an impending syncope.

An improvement of orthostatic tolerance may be achieved by repeating the tilt-table maneuver several times. An easier and very effective way is through orthostasis training. Typically, this consists of the patient leaning forcibly with his back against a wall twice daily for 15 to 30 minutes each time. The feet stand close together, about 15 cm away from the wall. This training is repeated over the course of four weeks. Another important treatment option is increased dietary salt intake by an additional 3 to 5 g/day with plenty of fluids (2–3 l/day). If these measures are not sufficient to prevent frequent syncope, drug treatment should be attempted. First of all, the use of fludrocortisone (0.1–0.2 mg/day) or midodrine (2.5–10 mg t.i.d.) should be considered. Paroxetine (20–40 mg/day) or beta-blockers (e.g., metoprolol 50–100 mg b.i.d.) may also be used but the evidence is weak. The use of pacemakers in the treatment of neurocardiogenic syncope is controversial (Brignole et al. 2004).

Patients with orthostatic syncope benefit from an increased intake of fluids and salt. Sleeping with an elevated (more than 10°) upper body can improve the condition as well. Patients with orthostatic syncope should also learn to avoid triggering events and to take countermeasures. In some cases, wearing waist-high compression stockings or abdominal compression bandages may be indicated. However, this treatment is often poorly tolerated and leads to low compliance from the patients. Medications which can cause hypotension should be reduced or discontinued. If pharmacological treatment is necessary, fludrocortisone and midodrine can be used.

Cardiac syncope can sometimes be treated causally, for instance, by surgical correction of a valvular defect or of other obstructions of cardiac output or by catheter ablation of arrhythmogenic tissue. Treatment of cardiac arrhythmias consists first and foremost of medication. Beyond that, pacemakers and implantable defibrillators are available.

Prognosis

Approximately 35% of patients with syncope have a recurrent episode within one year (Kapoor 1990). Cardiac syncope is associated with a greater risk of sudden cardiac death and cardiovascular events such as myocardial infarctions. On the other hand, in patients with neurocardiogenic or orthostatic syncope neither cardiac nor overall mortality is increased in comparison to patients without syncope (Soteriades et al. 2002). Complications of syncope are first and foremost injuries due to unprotected falls and traffic accidents.

References

Alboni P, Brignole M, Menozzi C, Raviele A, Del Rosso A, Dinelli M, Solano A, Bottoni N. Diagnostic value of history in patients with syncope with or without heart disease. *J Am Coll Cardiol* 2001, **37**: 1921–1928.

Benke T, Hochleitner M, Bauer G. Aura phenomena during syncope. *Eur Neurol* 1997, **37**:28–32.

Brenner RP. Electroencephalography in syncope. *J Clin Neurophysiol* 1997, **14**;197–209.

Brignole M, Alboni P, Benditt DG, Bergfeldt L, Blanc J–J, Bloch Thomsen PE, van Dijk JG, Fitzpatrick A, Hohnloser S, Janousek J, Kapoor W, Kenny RA, Kulakowski P, Masotti G, Moya A, Raviele A, Sutton R, Theodorakis G, Ungar A, Wieling W; Task Force on Syncope, European Society of Cardiology. Guidelines on management (diagnosis and treatment) of syncope – update 2004. *Europace* 2004, **6**:467–537.

Diehl RR, Linden D. Differential diagnose der orthostatischen Dysregulation. *Nervenarzt* 1999, **70**:1044–1051.

Duvoisin RC. Convulsive syncope induced by the Weber maneuver. *Arch Neurol* 1962, 7:65–72

Gastaut H, Fischer-Williams M. Electro-encephalographic study of syncope; its differentiation from epilepsy. *Lancet* 1957, **273**;1018–1025.

Grad A, Baloh RW. Vertigo of vascular origin. Clinical and electronystagmographic features in 84 cases. *Arch Neurol* 1989, **46**:281–284.

Graham LA, Kenny RA. Clinical characteristics of patients with vasovagal reactions presenting as unexplained syncope. *Europace* 2001, **3**:141–146.

Kapoor W. Evaluation and outcome of patients with syncope. *Medicine* 1990, **69**:169–175.

Kapoor WN. Syncope. *N Engl J Med* 2000, **343**:1865–1862.

Lempert T, Bauer M, Schmidt D. Syncope: a videometric analysis of 56 episodes of transient cerebral hypoxia. *Ann Neurol* 1994, **36**:233–237.

Lusić I, Pintarić I, Hozo I, Boić L, Capkun V. Serum prolactin levels after seizure and syncopal attacks. *Seizure* 1999, **8**:218–222.

Neufeld MY, Treves TA, Chistik V, Korczyn AD. Sequential serum creatine kinase determination differentiates vaso-vagal syncope from generalized tonic-clonic seizures. *Acta Neurol Scand* 1997, **95**:137–139.

Sheldon R, Rose S, Ritchie D, Connolly SJ, Koshman ML, Lee MA, Frenneaux M, Fisher M, Murphy W. Historical criteria that distinguish syncope from seizures. *J Am Coll Cardiol* 2002, **40**:142–148.

Soteriades ES, Evans JC, Larson MG, Chen MH, Chen L, Benjamin EJ, Levy D. Incidence and prognosis of syncope. *N Engl J Med* 2002, **347**:878–885.

Stucki P. Der Kreislauf bei pressorischen Anstrengungen. *Archiv für Kreislaufforschung* 1958, **28**;242–317.

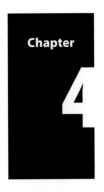

Chapter

4

Sudden falls

Ian Mothersill, Thomas Grunwald and Günter Krämer

Overview

The control of posture, stance and motion is highly demanding of the peripheral and central nervous system of a creature, especially if this creature is a relatively fast-moving bipedal one with a high center of gravity. A multitude of external and internal factors can disturb this balance and lead to a loss of equilibrium. This observation is supported by the fact that gait and stance have to be learned at the beginning of life, and that both can again pose particular problems later with age. Falls are a frequent medical problem in advanced age, not only due to age-associated changes in the control of gait and stance but also due to the greater incidence of neurological diseases such as Parkinson's disease or neuropathic and cerebrovascular disorders. About 30% of the people aged over 65 years fall at least once per year, and this number increases with each decade by 10%. Hence, it seems advisable to always regard each fall in that age group as being symptomatic until proven otherwise.

A comprehensive discussion of all causes of falling is not feasible here. The mere number of neurological disorders and syndromes that can cause falls, like pareses, disturbances of sensibility or coordination and acute impairment of consciousness of any etiology, is too extensive for a single chapter. However, the differential diagnosis of falls is a common task in a neurologist's practice, especially if we have to determine whether a manifest or a suspected neurological problem is the result or the cause of a fall. To define the most common paroxysmal causes of a fall resulting in a neurological visit, we first want to sum up the physiological requirements for the control of upright posture and balance. We then want to focus on those paroxysmal causes of a fall which are relevant, though not necessarily easily diagnosed, in daily clinical routine. Thus, we are not going to consider those causes of falls that are

not paroxysmal and relatively easy to detect by taking the history and performing a clinical examination, that is, pareses and sensory syndromes. Moreover, other paroxysmal disturbances like vestibular or cerebrovascular falls often have characteristic additional symptoms and are discussed in other chapters of this book.

At first glance, it may be helpful to classify the etiological possibilities according to whether the fall occurred with or without loss of consciousness. Although this approach appears obvious, it has its pitfalls. For example, a fall can lead to head injury, resulting in amnesia for its occurrence. On the other hand, there are proven epileptic seizures that lead to drops but are so short that consciousness is not impaired, or only so brief that the impact is experienced in full awareness and is remembered. The distinction of whether a fall occurs with or without initial loss of consciousness is thus of undisputed theoretical relevance in the daily clinical routine. However, it is often a difficult task to solve. We therefore want to approach the differential diagnoses of falls of unclear cause by a more physiological route.

The control of balance and upright posture covers three main tasks:

- The head and body have to be stabilized against gravity and external forces.
- The center of gravity has to be balanced above its (narrow) point of stance.
- The body has to be stabilized so that it is not unbalanced by its own intentional movements.

To accomplish these tasks, there has to be an interaction of a number of factors, whose disturbance can be the cause of falls (Massion 1997):

1) A multisensory input has to provide enough vestibular, proprioceptive and visual data about the three-dimensional position of the head, the

The Paroxysmal Disorders, ed. Bettina Schmitz, Barbara Tettenborn and Donald L. Schomer. Published by Cambridge University Press. © Cambridge University Press 2010.

body and the body parts. Missing or faulty information, due to impairments of peripheral sensory mechanisms or of central sensory processes, can disturb the control of stance and movement to such an extent that the body loses its balance. Therefore, disturbances of vision as well as polyneuropathies have to be considered for differential diagnosis just as vestibular drop attacks do. In the later cases, false information caused by endolymphatic pressure changes leads to unilateral stimulation of the otolith organs (utriculus or sacculus; see Chapter 6). Likewise, disturbances of central processing and integration of the multimodal sensory input can lead to falls, for example, due to lesions or seizures of parietal or temporal cortical areas. These areas contribute to the processing of vestibular stimuli, and seizure activity in these locations can clinically be associated with severe attacks of vertigo. In addition, central-processing disorders like Pusher syndrome caused by ischemic lesions of the postero-lateral thalamus can impair the perception of one's body in three-dimensional space.

2) To balance the center of gravity above one's point of stance both in motion and at rest, fast compensatory reactions to all disturbances of equilibrium as well as anticipating mechanisms are required, which enable motor programs to react to expected disturbances even before these have occurred at all, for example, to stabilize the body before and during intentional movements of a limb. The working of these "feedback" and "feed-forward mechanisms" (Ghez 1991) requires the integrity of excitatory and inhibitory descending pathways through which muscle tone is controlled subconsciously. Thus, all disturbances interfering with the initiation and control of motor programs and associated with a rise or decline of muscle tone can lead to falls, as for example, in acute or chronic pareses, as do impairments of the fine tuning of posture, balance and motion, such as extrapyramidal or cerebellar movement disorders, hyperekplexia and startle diseases, and so on.

3) Finally, although not all impairments of consciousness necessarily result in a fall, reduced conscious control implies a greater risk to do so. By principle, this applies to almost all generalized or complex focal seizures. Therefore, traumas

Table 4.1 Neurological causes of falls

1. *Sensory input:*
   1.1 Disturbances of vision
   1.2 Disturbances of equilibrium (vestibular drop attacks)
   1.3 Polyneuropathies
2. *Central processing and integration of the sensory input*
   2.1 Central visual disturbances (e.g., hemianopsia)
   2.2 Central disturbances of equilibrium (e.g., vertigo as a symptom of temporo-lateral seizures)
   2.3 Disturbances of graviception (e.g., Pusher syndrome with lesions of the postero-lateral thalamus)
   2.4 Disturbances of multimodal sensory input integration (e.g., disturbances of the body representation or neglect in right-sided parietal lesions)
3. *Motor systems to support body posture*
   3.1 Lesions of the pyramidal tracts (pareses)
   3.2 Extra-pyramidal motor disturbances (e.g., Parkinson's disease, hyperkinesias, L-dopa sensitive dystonia)
   3.3 Cerebellar disturbances (e.g., paroxysmal ataxia)
   3.4 Disinhibition of reflex systems (e.g., hyperekplexia, startle diseases)
   3.5 Atonic brain stem seizures (e.g., inflammatory or cancerous lesions of the reticular formation)
   3.6 Age-related disturbances of locomotion
   3.7 Syndrome des genoux bleus (of the blue knees) = drop attacks of elderly females
4. *Conscious control*
   4.1 Syncope (vasovagal, cardiovascular, orthostatic, impaired liquor circulation, e.g., hydrocephalus, syringobulbia, etc.)
   4.2 (Non-epileptic) drop attacks
   4.3 Cataplexia (and other disorders of sleep-wake regulation)
   4.4 Non-epileptic psychogenic seizures
   4.5 Epileptic seizures
   4.6 Other causes (e.g., metabolic (hypoglycemia, hypothyreosis), tumors in the area of the posterior base of the skull, etc.)

caused by falls can occur in most forms of epilepsy, a risk not to be taken lightly. However, we want to stress the fact that most seizures of this kind are not associated with falls. On the other hand, there are types of seizures that are defined precisely by the obligatory falls themselves.

Thus, a multitude of diseases has to be taken into account for the differential diagnosis of the cause of a fall. Table 4.1 gives an incomplete overview of important examples of neurological reasons causing a fall.

Many of the possible underlying diseases may be detected for the first time during the evaluation of a fall but are basically chronic illnesses in which falls are associated with objective findings verified during the neurological examination. Other life-threatening events, like a sudden fall due to a massive intracerebral hemorrhage, will rarely cause differential diagnostic problems. By contrast, patients presenting with a first fall or repeated paroxysmal falls and in whom neurological examinations do not yield any objective findings are a common challenge in clinical practice. In this context, it is important to consider the following diagnoses:

- Syncope
- Drop attacks
- Cataplexia
- Startle diseases
- Extrapyramidal movement disorders
- Normal-pressure hydrocephalus
- Non-epileptic (psychogenic) seizures
- Epileptic seizures and epilepsies

Syncope

Syncope is dealt with in length in Chapter 2. However, here we must emphasize again that they are an important cause of unexplained falls, not least because they occur much more often than epileptic seizures. On the other hand, they quite often do cause diagnostic problems due to their manifold symptoms. Their semiology can, at times, be very complex and is not explainable by the symptoms of "going black before the eyes" or "rushing or roaring in the ears" or by the possibly accompanying paleness, vertigo and nausea, to which history-taking sometimes is limited.

In fact, oro-alimentary and manual automatisms, vocalizations, visual or auditory hallucinations can occur during syncope, and when they do it is indeed possible to mistake them for focal epileptic seizures (Lempert et al. 1994). With a sustained cerebral hypoxia/anoxia, a tonic phase with or without myoclonia, that is, convulsive syncope, appears. Such cases lead to the false diagnosis of a generalized tonic-clonic seizure. In addition, falls during syncope can be associated both with a loss and with an increase of muscle tone. Therefore, syncope has to be taken into account during the evaluation of falls of uncertain cause, even when their symptoms may seem unusual at the first glance.

Drop attacks

Drop attacks are non-epileptic events that lead to falls and can be associated with disturbances localized either in brain areas supplied with blood by the posterior circulation of the vertebro-basilar artery but also by the anterior circulation of the right and left internal carotid arteries and their branches. Most drop attacks are probably vascular events, but they can also be caused by a multitude of other reasons (Hacke et al. 1991) such as tumors in the area of the third ventricle or in the posterior base of the skull (Lee et al. 1994).

Drop attacks occur without warning and without recognizable trigger while standing or walking. Consciousness remains unimpaired or is only affected for a short time. There is no accompanying vertigo, and sensory functions as well as the strength of the leg muscles return to normal immediately after or within a very short time after the fall. Drop attacks are not accompanied by movements of the head, change of posture or other focal neurological signs.

Drop attacks of the vertebro-basal circulation are caused by a transient ischemia of the cortical spinal pathways or the paramedian reticular formation. The patient's history most often contains other symptoms like vertigo, diplopia or ataxia. By contrast, drop attacks of the anterior circulation are based on an ischemic disturbance of the parasagittal pre-motor or motor cortex (Meisner et al. 1986).

Drop attacks usually are a diagnosis by exclusion. In our view, the so-called cryptogenic falls of elderly females, sometimes called "syndrome des genoux bleus" or syndrome of the blue knees, also belong to this category. There is no effective medical treatment.

Cataplexia

An important differential diagnosis of recurring falls is cataplectic attacks in the course of narcolepsy. The prevalence of narcolepsy is between 0.02% and 0.05% (Hublin et al. 1994). Its four cardinal symptoms are irresistible attacks of sleepiness, sleep pareses, hypnagogic or hypnapompic hallucinations which appear at the beginning or end of sleep, and finally cataplexia. Only few patients present with all symptoms. Patients usually suffer most from excessive daytime sleepiness in the form of imperative sleep attacks, which can almost always be ascertained and which are obligatory for a positive diagnosis and from the cataplectic attacks, which occur in 60% to 100% of cases (Bassetti and Aldrich 2000).

Cataplexia is defined by a paresis of the skeletal muscles due to a sudden emotion. The triggering emotions are usually of a positive nature. Cataplectic attacks are most commonly triggered by sudden laughter. However, surprise, agitation or, more rarely, negative emotions like fear or anger can be a trigger, too. The resulting pareses are usually not so pronounced as to result in a fall. Often only the cranial muscles are involved, resulting in symptoms that have even found their place in common language, for example, when someone stands with "mouth agape" or "drops his jaw" with surprise. However, the pareses can spread caudally and incorporate the muscles of the legs, which make a fall unavoidable. Again the everyday language knows the phenomenon as "to be paralyzed by fear." Consciousness is retained during the fall itself and can be associated with paroxysmal difficulties breathing or with vegetative symptoms. Attacks usually do not last longer than 60 seconds. However, prolonged attacks can rarely persist for up to 20 minutes (Honda 1988).

Pathophysiologically, the loss of tonus during a cataplectic seizure, similar to that in REM sleep, is associated with reduced activity of the locus coeruleus localized in the brainstem. As discussed, this can be indirectly attributed to a lesion of hypothalamic neurons producing the hypocretin peptide. A disturbance in the hypothalamic hypocretin system seems to be associated with sleep attacks and the appearance of cataplectic symptoms both in a dog model and in humans (for an overview, see Siegel et al. 2001).

Whenever typical emotional triggers can be found in falls with unimpaired consciousness, cataplectic seizures have to be suspected as a differential diagnosis if other symptoms of the narcoleptic tetrad are present. Further diagnostic evaluation demands polysomnographic recordings, including a multiple sleep latency test (MSLT) and, if necessary, a screening for the human antigens for leukocytes HLA-DR 15 and DQ6. However, a negative antigen study does not exclude the diagnosis of narcolepsy (Bassetti and Aldrich 2000).

Startle diseases

In startle diseases, the physiological startle reaction is pathologically increased and leads, among others things, to a paroxysmal loss of control of the body posture. If a startle reaction triggers consecutive epileptic seizures, they are called "startle-induced seizures" and establish the diagnosis of "startle epilepsy" (see "Startle epilepsies").

Affected children show an abnormal startle reaction immediately after birth. During the startle reaction, in contrast to the Moro reflex, a flexion pattern occurs. A postnatal elevation of muscle tone in the extremities, reminiscent of para- or even tetraplegia, disappears within the first six months. With the beginning of walking the impairment increases, as the children stiffen when noise or a sudden touching occurs. Then falls occur more often, in which the normal defense reaction is impaired by the flexion pattern of the arms. In severe cases, the danger of falls remains a lifelong feature.

Hyperekplexia constitutes an increased startle reaction, which is autosomal-dominantly inherited and whose underlying cause has been proven to be a disorder of the alpha1 sub-unit of the inhibitory glycerine receptor on chromosome 5 (Zhou et al. 2002). Previous authors have suggested differentiating between familial and sporadic forms of hyperexplexia, but this has not been widely accepted.

Clinically a "minor" and a "major" form of hyperekplexia can be distinguished (Andermann et al. 1980). Whereas the minor form is characterized by an excessive and prolonged startle reaction, the major form has additional symptoms with a general increase of muscle tone and loss of the postural control. In the minor form, falls are caused by the massive and violent startle reaction itself, where in the major form they are a result of the loss of postural control. Especially with the major form, this can lead to diagnostic problems in differentiating hyperekplexia from startle-induced epileptic drop seizures. In these cases, a clear differentiation is only possible with simultaneous EEG and EMG recording during such an event.

The normal startle response has been precisely defined (Gogan 1970). The initial reaction to a startle begins 20 to 40 ms after the stimulus and has a duration of 150 to 200 ms. After that, a phase of relative inactivity occurs for 250 to 300 ms, followed by a phase of reorientation which lasts 3 to 10s. With our own ictal polygraphic recordings, we found the following pathological results (Mothersill et al. 2000):

- Hyperekplexias are distinguished by an increased initial startle reaction of up to 1 second duration. This is then followed in the minor form by a reorientation phase or an akinetic phase, in which the patient is fixed in the posture taken during the startle.
- In startle-induced seizures, the duration of the initial startle reaction does not or only minimally exceeds the normal 20 to 40 ms. However, instead of the phase of reorientation it is followed by an epileptic seizure, either as axial spasms, or tonic or atonic seizures.
- In rare cases, a combination of pathologically increased startle reaction plus consecutive

31

epileptic seizure can be found (discussed later).

As a therapy in hyperekplexias, small doses of clonazepam have been described as effective (0.1 mg/kg of bodyweight). However, our own experiences with this treatment have not been convincing.

Extrapyramidal movement disorders

Extrapyramidal movement disorders are dealt with in other chapters of this book. It is not uncommon for patients with a Parkinsonian disease or syndrome to suffer from falls, especially during bradykinetic or akinetic phases, and also during motor fluctuations induced by dopamine where there are peak-dose dyskinesias and off-periods. Patients may show a pronounced postural instability and often fall backward. Patients with progressive supranuclear palsies (Remler and Daroff 1996) or multisystem atrophies also have an increased inclination to fall.

In subcortical vascular encephalopathy (SVE, Binswanger syndrome, an extrapyramidal gait disorder), reoccurring falls are frequently an early symptom. In comparison to the idiopathic Parkinson's disease, a forward shifting of the body's center of gravity is less frequently seen. More often, a slight flexion in the hips and knees can be observed. Etiologically, a progressive disconnection of frontal and parietal supplementary motor areas responsible for the planning and initiating of movements is the assumed etiology (Bäzner et al. 2003).

Normal-pressure hydrocephalus

Apart from a gait disorder with frequent falls, the so-called normal-pressure hydrocephalus is clinically characterized by urinary incontinence and by progressive neuropsychological defects up to dementia. The pathogenesis of gait disorder and falls has not yet been completely clarified. Most likely, there is a disturbance of the integrative locomotor centers in the frontal lobes due to an antero-lateral expansion of the lateral ventricles. Early diagnosis is especially important with a subgroup of patients who might profit from a shunt operation. Evidence for this is a clear clinical change for the better after a lumbar puncture, where one drains off a significant volume of spinal fluid (30–50 ml).

Non-epileptic seizures

Non-epileptic seizures will be discussed more extensively in Chapter 12; however, they will be also briefly addressed here, as they are an important differential diagnosis of unclear, reoccurring drop events. Most of the times, non-epileptic seizures consist of a number of symptoms, which taken by themselves are not a proof but can help to support the diagnosis when such attacks are suspected.

Among these signs are closed eyes during the event, rapid to-and-fro head movements from one side to across the midline, apical (instead of lateral) biting of the tongue and uncontrolled trashing about of the limbs, which can also sometimes be seen with hypermotor phenomena of fronto-mesial seizures. Just like the semiology, the duration of psychogenic seizures can also be very variable. However, in most cases they clearly exceed the length of epileptic seizures.

Falls often occur with non-epileptic seizures. If the falls are followed by violent jerks or of high-frequency shaking of the body and limbs, the untrained observer often believes these to be generalized tonic-clonic (grand mal) seizures. An exact observation or, even better, an analysis of a slow-motion video recording of a fall event quite often shows that protective movements are taken during the fall itself to reduce the impact, which is rarely if ever seen in epileptic seizures. On the other hand, these signs do not apply to all non-epileptic seizures. Psychogenic seizures can indeed lead to injuries which can be much more serious than mere grazes or lacerations. There are documented cases of fractures, even as severe as basal skull fractures, as a result of non-epileptic seizures.

The diagnosis of non-epileptic seizures is based initially on a history of typical symptoms. However, only recording a typical attack can provide final proof. To this end, the gold standard is the simultaneous video/EEG recording in the context of a long-term monitoring. If there is no possibility for a video documentation, a mobile long-term inpatient EEG might be sufficient. However, this presupposes the presence of staff trained in the observation and description of epileptic seizures. In contrast, ambulatory long-term EEG recordings are problematic because the EEG signal is often contaminated by artifacts, and it cannot be assured in each case that the recorded event was typical for the patient's seizures. Ideally, a video/EEG recording of critical events should therefore be seen and evaluated together with the patient and relatives who have witnessed previous falls.

However, the positive diagnosis of non-epileptic seizures does not exclude the concomitance of epileptic seizures, as both forms can be present in the same patient. In these cases, it is advisable to taper off any anti-epileptic drugs, which due to safety reasons is best done under in-patient conditions, and to observe the patient for another week after all medication has been stopped. If during this time there is no clinical or encephalographic evidence of epilepsy, then the diagnosis of non-epileptic seizures is justified.

Epileptic seizures and epilepsies

Seizures that may result in falls

Absences

Typical absences (Table 4.2) are characterized by a loss of consciousness beginning and ending abruptly, accompanied by rhythmic generalized spike and wave complexes with a frequency of 3 Hz in the EEG. The main clinical feature is the sudden discontinuation of all motor and cognitive activities, which sometimes can only be detected if adequately tested for. Typical is the motionless staring into space. However, there also may be slight motor phenomena like a tonic upward deviation of the eyes, rhythmic eyelid movements or oral automatisms. These concomitant phenomena or changes of posture are often more predominant in so-called atypical absences, in which focal signs can also be observed. The ictal EEG shows a bilateral spike and wave activity of usually lower (rarely higher) frequency than seen during typical absences and can also show focal components. In typical absence seizures, the semiology and EEG findings strongly indicate the diagnosis of idiopathic epilepsy. However, sometimes this diagnosis is complicated by so-called "complex absences" that are associated with motor automatisms or by so-called "myoclonic absences" with jerks, discussed in more detail later.

Falls are not a typical feature of absence seizures, which might be surprising in the face of the fall into the water by "Johnny Head-in-Air," with whom Heinrich Hoffman, the famous German author of "Shock-headed Peter" (Struwwelpeter), has given an image to absence epilepsy. In reality, most children stop if during walking they suffer an absence seizure instead of walking along uncontrolled. Although atonic components may occur, like a short sagging of head or body, with these too falls almost never occur. Although rare, falls can be a potential complication of absence seizures. Wirrel at al. (1996) found that 16 (27%) out of 59 explored patients with typical absence seizure had already been injured once during a seizure. Falls from

Table 4.2 Absence epilepsies

Definition	Idiopathic epilepsies with primary generalized seizures (absences)
Epidemiology	Childhood AE (CAE) about 12%, juvenile AE (JAE) about 4% of the epilepsies of childhood
Begin	CAE 2–12 years, JAE 10–17 years
Etiology	Polygenetic; no pathological findings in MRI
Seizures	Absences, sometimes additional generalized tonic clonic seizures; in JAE myoclonic seizures can occur
EEG	Generalized spike-waves (CAE: 3/s; JAE: 3,5–4/s) commonly provoked by hyperventilation, photosensitivity in up to 20%; normal background activity (in cases of atypical AE slowing of the background activity can at times be observed, then often with associated with pharmacoresistance)
Prognosis	Seizure freedom can be obtained in up to 60–65%
Therapy	Pharmacological: valproate or ethosuximide (CAE), if necessary lamotrigine; if therapeutic problems occur phenobarbital (low doses), clobazam, clonazepam
Special Forms	
Myoclonic Absence Epilepsy	Rare but more often associated with falls; often in combination with typical absences and tonic-clonic seizures; treated with valproate (if necessary in combination with lamotrigine or ethosuximide) in up to 50% long-term seizure-freedom can be achieved
Eyelid Myoclonia with Absences	Rare; absences always in combination with rhythmic eyelid myoclonia, which also can occur independently of absences. In the EEG polyspike-wave complexes, which can be triggered by eye-closure (in a brightly lit room). Therapy as above, seizure freedom however is less often achieved

bicycles turned out to be the most risky. Of course, such falls are not primarily due to the semiology affecting posture but are rather due to not being able to control the bicycle.

Myoclonic seizures

Myoclonia is short, shock-like contractions of single muscles or groups of muscles leading to involuntary movement. In principle, all muscles can be affected. However, in typical myoclonic seizures muscles of the neck, shoulder and arms are mostly involved. The expression of the myoclonia can be so subtle that they cannot be seen and, in fact, may be only experienced subjectively. On the other hand, they may be so distinct that objects held in the hands may be "thrown."

Table 4.3 Juvenile myoclonic epilepsy

Definition	Idiopathic epilepsy with myoclonic seizures
Epidemiology	Up to 10% of all epilepsies
Begin	Mostly in juveniles (up to 18), more rarely up to the age of 26 years
Etiology	Polygenetic; no pathological findings in MRI
Seizures	Myoclonic seizures, often additional generalized tonic-clonic seizures, and absences
EEG	Generalized polyspike-waves, photosensitivity in up to 30%
Prognosis	Seizure freedom can be obtained in up to 85%; high risk of reoccurrence if medication is discontinued
Therapy	Pharmacological: valproate, if necessary lamotrigine, topiramate, levetiracetam; if unsuccessful phenobarbital, clonazepam (myoclonia), ethosuximide (absences), zonisamide

Table 4.4 Progressive myoclonus epilepsies

Definition	Miscellaneous diseases with myoclonia, other seizure types, multiple (mostly cerebellar) neurological deficits and (mild or more pronounced) progressive dementia
Types	Unverricht-Lundborg (autosomal-recessive; relatively benign course); Lafora-type (autosomal-recessive; fast progression, lethal within 2 – 10 years); mitochondrial diseases (MERFF; maternal mitochondrial transmission; variable begin and course); more rare types: neuronal ceroidlipofuscinosis; sialidosis; Gaucher disease
Epidemiology	Rare in comparison to other epilepsies
Begin	Variable, mostly in childhood (MERFF up to 65 years)
Seizures	Myoclonia, often generalized tonic-clonic seizures, partly with absences, partly focal (occipital) seizures
EEG	Non-uniform
Prognosis	Poor, except for the Unverricht-Lundborg type
Therapy	Pharmacological: valproate, if necessary lamotrigine, topiramate, levetiracetam; if unsuccessful phenobarbital, clobazam; the myoclonia can sometimes be treated with high doses of piracetam (36–48 g/d); in some cases good results can be obtained with acetazolamide, (if necessary with potassium substitution); NB: phenytoin should not be used

Because most myoclonic seizures are associated with juvenile myoclonic epilepsy (Table 4.3), they typically occur in the morning after awakening. It is not rare that morning toilet objects, such as toothbrushes, are seemingly "thrown" out of the hands.

Myoclonic seizures rarely lead to falls. However, if they involve the muscles of the legs, it is conceivable that the patient may drop to his knees or fall abruptly. Typically, consciousness in these falls is not impaired, and the patient arises after the fall without help. However, myoclonic seizures can also occur in the context of other seizures, such as with other idiopathic generalized epilepsies or with the Lennox-Gastaut syndrome (see below). In addition, focal seizures of the primary motor cortex can be associated with myoclonic symptoms and thus impair the ability to stand or walk when leg muscles are affected. On the other hand, there are so-called negative motor areas, whose electrical stimulation during functional cortical mapping results in motor inhibition and thus in a loss of motor tone. This is especially the case after stimulation of the rostral part of the supplementary motor area and the stripe of cortex directly before the primary motor area (Lüders et al. 1987). Thus, so-called negative myoclonia can induce a sudden loss of tone in circumscribed muscle groups, have an impact on movement and finally lead to a fall (Capovilla et al. 2000).

Myoclonia can also be generated independently of seizure events by cortical, subcortical and spinal structures, however, mostly without directly leading to falls. On the other hand, in patients with progressive myoclonus epilepsies (Table 4.4) it is quite common that myoclonia can be severe enough to cause falls. Myoclonia of these patients is commonly provoked by voluntary movements and thus shows the characteristic feature of action or intentional myoclonia, which during the later course of the disease can lead to the patient being wheelchair-bound. In severe cases, massive action myoclonia may make it necessary to fixate a patient in the wheelchair, for example, to prevent them from being thrown to the ground while trying to shake a greeting hand. In contrast, in patients able to walk falls are more often caused by multiple negative myoclonia affecting the muscles of locomotion.

Generalized tonic-clonic seizures

The classic "grand mal seizure" can occur in the context of different epilepsy syndromes both as a primary and as a secondary event. Primary generalized seizures are characterized by both clinical and electroencephalographic evidence of involvement of both hemispheres at seizure onset. In contrast, secondary generalized tonic-clonic seizures (Table 4.5) are the

Table 4.5 Epilepsy with generalized tonic-clonic seizures

Definition	Idiopathic epilepsy with primary generalized tonic-clonic seizures (grand mal seizures)
Epidemiology	Approximately 5% of all epilepsies
Begin	6–35 years
Etiology	Polygenetic; no pathological findings in MRI
Seizures	Generalized tonic-clonic seizures (typically on awakening), at times additional absences and/or myoclonic seizures
EEG	Generalized spike-waves or polyspike-waves; partly (10%) provocation by hyperventilation; photosensitivity in up to 20%; mostly normal background activity, more rarely generalized slowing, at times focal (especially frontal) spikes possible
Prognosis	Seizure freedom can be obtained in up to 90%
Therapy	Pharmacological: valproate, if necessary lamotrigine, topiramate, levetiracetam; if unsuccessful phenobarbital

result of initial focal seizure activity in one hemisphere propagating to both hemispheres. This differentiation is not a mere academic question of classifying different types of seizures but has important consequences as to therapeutic options, to the choice of the medication and to the prognosis of the disease. Therefore, a precise description of the beginning of a seizure is of paramount importance. However, in many cases it cannot be obtained because either the beginning of a seizure was not seen or the observing people were so impressed by the seeming dramatics of the event that they were incapable of accurately describing it. Still, specific questioning of the observers should try to shed light onto the clinical symptoms of the seizure, especially its onset.

Primary generalized tonic-clonic seizures

During the course of their epilepsies, a number of patients learn to become aware of an impending seizure hours and even days before it occurs. These feelings, the so-called prodroma, should not be mistaken as part of the seizure in the sense of an aura. The neurophysiological substrate of these prodromal symptoms is as yet unexplained. However, it is surmised that they are an expression of heightened cortical excitability leading to a decrease in the seizure threshold. The seizure itself begins with a sudden loss of consciousness, which initially is accompanied by a short spasm of the axial flexor muscles as well as a short elevation and abduction of the arms and an adduction and flexion of the legs. The eyes are opened wide. There

is an upward deviation of the bulbi and frequently a mydriasis. Immediately afterward, the tonic phase of the seizure begins, which may lead to a fall if the patient is standing. At first, a tonic contraction of the muscles of the trunk often leads to a vocalization, the so-called initial cry. This is due to a forced expiration.

The tonic increase in muscle tone then spreads to involve the limbs. In this phase, the tonic contraction of the jaw muscles can lead to a tongue bite, which is usually lateral. Incidentally, because of the speed of this course of events it is illusory to think that the tongue biting can be avoided by inserting a rubber wedge between the teeth. Moreover, the massive increase in tone of the jaw muscles is so severe that the mouth cannot be opened, and it would demand quite an effort associated with a risk of injuring teeth if one would try to keep the patient's airway free by the use of force.

During the tonic phase respiration ceases due to the contraction of thoracic muscles, resulting in an increasing cyanosis. Vegetative symptoms, such as a marked rise of heart rate and blood pressure, as well as copious perspiration and an increase in tracheobronchial secretion, can be observed. After a few (maximum 20) seconds, the tonic phase ceases and is followed by a phase with tremoring of the muscles, the frequency of which quickly declines from initially 8 Hz to about 4 Hz. This then leads to the clonic phase of the seizure with repetitive cycles of massive tonic contraction and consecutive complete atonia, caused by neuronal inhibition. Clinical signs of the clonic phase are repetitive flexor spasms, whose rate slowly decreases. The whole seizure usually lasts approximately 1 to 2 minutes and ends with an atonia of all muscles. This atonia also includes the sphincter muscles with the possibility of enuresis or encopresis. After the seizure, spontaneous breathing starts at once. The patient either falls asleep or slowly returns to consciousness with initial disorientation. There is amnesia for the event itself, and patients usually become aware of having had a seizure due to its after-effects, like diffuse headaches and muscle pains or sometimes by a bite wound of the tongue or the cheek. Less commonly, injuries due to a fall or seizure-associated trauma such as a dislocation of the shoulder can occur. A cause of intense postictal back pain can even be a compression fracture of the vertebral bodies caused by the seizure itself.

An EEG recorded from the surface of the skull is generally less meaningful, as it is usually superimposed by massive muscle artefacts. At best, a generalized flattening can be discerned in the earliest phase of the seizure. Intracranial recordings from subdural electrodes, performed during invasive presurgical evaluations of patients with pharmacoresistant focal epilepsies, show that a flattening in the scalp EEG is not necessarily caused by a desynchronization but can also be caused by high-frequency spike activity, so-called "low-voltage fast activity." Such invasive recordings show during the tonic phase rhythmic spike activity of high frequency, which gradually decelerates. During the clonic phase rhythmic bursts of poly-spikes appear, which are always followed by slow waves which represent inhibition. The surface EEG in the postictal phase shows an initial diffuse flattening, which slowly evolves into diffuse delta activity. In spite of the massive superimposition of muscle artefacts, ictal EEG recordings of tonic-clonic seizures can be helpful in the differential diagnosis of a seizure. The typical pattern of the EMG artefact during the tonic then clonic phase can, for example, be helpful to differentiate between a generalized epileptic seizure or a hypermotoric non-epileptic, psychogenic seizure.

Secondary generalized tonic-clonic seizures

During the terminal (generalized) phase, these seizures present clinically and electroencephalographically the same as primary generalized tonic-clonic seizures. The differentiation is only possible if an initial focal seizure has been clinically observed or reported, or if a seizure recording with simultaneous EEG and video monitoring verifies a focal beginning. Typical symptoms of focal seizures are outlined further later. The phase of the secondary generalization can often give a clue to the lateralization of the primary epileptogenic area. If the propagation of the seizure activity takes place in the frontal lobe of the same hemisphere in which the focal seizures begins, quite often it results in a forced deviation of the eyes and head to the opposite side and in a tonic extension of the contralateral arm.

The correct differential diagnosis of primary and secondary generalized seizures has important therapeutic consequences. For example, carbamazepine, which belongs to the drugs of first choice in the treatment of focal seizures, may not only remain without effect in primary generalized seizures but even lead to an exacerbation of the seizure events. On the other hand, the prognosis of idiopathic epilepsy with primary generalized seizures is often much better than of focal epilepsy. However, only with the latter can a surgical intervention lead to permanent seizure freedom.

Focal seizures

Whereas in childhood 75% of the seizures initially diagnosed are primarily generalized, in adults about two thirds of newly diagnosed seizures are focal with or without secondary generalization (Camfield et al. 1996). Focal seizures can be symptoms of an idiopathic epilepsy, such as the benign focal seizures of childhood, or in adults with temporal lobe epilepsy. However, in adults this is so rare that it can, in practice, be neglected. The majority of focal seizures in adults are symptomatic or suspected symptomatic (cryptogenic) epilepsies, meaning that they are caused by a cortical lesion that has either been identified by imaging methods (symptomatic) or is very likely but could not (yet) be found.

The classification of seizures by the International League Against Epilepsy primarily differentiates between simple and complex focal seizures, depending on whether consciousness is impaired (complex focal) or not (simple focal). Of course, the exact semiology of focal seizures depends on the localization of both its onset and of the area responsible for the clinical symptoms, the so-called symptomatic zone. The analysis of seizure semiology is an important part of the presurgical evaluation of pharmacoresistant focal epilepsies, whose search for localizing and lateralizing signs has added much to our understanding of the pathophysiology of focal seizures. It has been shown that epilepsy surgical resection leads to seizure freedom in a minimum of 70% of all patients with mesial temporal lobe epilepsy secondary to hippocampus sclerosis. Also in patients with temporal-lateral lesions or extratemporal epilepsies, comparably good results can be obtained by epilepsy surgery (Grunwald et al. 1999).

Mesial temporal lobe epilepsy

In adults with focal seizures, the most frequent epilepsy syndrome is mesial temporal lobe epilepsy, in which a unilateral atrophy and sclerosis of the hippocampus constitutes the morphological correlate of the primary epileptogenic focus. In many cases, here focal seizures begin with an epigastric aura, that is, with a feeling of nausea in the area of the stomach. This feeling then often rises to the chest or head. This is followed by the classic semiology of complex focal mesio-temporal seizures, which frequently begin with oro-alimentary automatisms, mostly in the form of lip-smacking, swallowing or chewing, or more rarely, whistling or spitting. Vocalizations or incomprehensible or intelligible but nonsensical verbalizations can occur as well as manual automatisms, which also can help lateralize the seizure's origin. Patients often fumble with the ipsilateral hand, whereas the contralateral is dystonic. This is often accompanied by motionlessness and staring. The postictal phase of re-orientation usually takes some minutes but can be of shorter duration if the seizure event remains limited to the temporal lobe of the non-dominant hemisphere. Conversely, seizures of the dominant hemisphere not uncommonly lead to postictal aphasia, which can last for several minutes and which, with adequate testing, again can be used as a lateralizing sign.

Lateral temporal lobe epilepsy

Seizures from the lateral temporal lobe can also be associated with an epigastric aura. However, more often lateral temporal auras are unspecific or take the form of a feeling of déjà-vu, acoustic or visual hallucinations, or an acute rotatory vertigo. Rare seizure forms, whose only symptom consists of a Wernicke aphasia, can easily be attributed to the lateral temporal lobe. However, discriminating lateral temporal seizures from those originating within the mesio-temporal lobe can sometimes be difficult using non-invasive methods because seizure activity can propagate very quickly from lateral to medial temporal regions. A possible clue to a more lateral origin of the seizure is an early appearance of automatisms of the legs. If the patients are lying on their backs, this often takes the form of pedaling. However, this symptom should be interpreted with care as it can occur both with temporal and frontal seizures.

The interictal EEG in temporal lobe epilepsy often shows a uni- or bi-temporal slowing of background activity with spikes or sharp waves in one or both temporal lobes. Due to the interconnection of both mesial-temporal lobes, bi-temporal EEG findings do not necessarily argue against a unilateral focus. Typically, ictal surface EEG recordings show rhythmic temporal theta activity with postictal focal slowing in the same area.

Frontal lobe epilepsy

The second most common type of focal seizures in adults, albeit much rarer in comparison to temporal seizures, are the frontal lobe epilepsies. Due to the mere size of the frontal lobes, the semiology of frontal seizures is extremely variable. Seizures within the primary motor cortex lead to contralateral myoclonia, which in some cases takes the form of a so-called "Jacksonian march" and can spread to half of the body. The further away the seizure origin is situated from the primary motor cortex, the more complex the motor phenomena can be. For example, they can span from bilateral asymmetric tonic or dystonic posturing, as seen in seizures of the supplementary motor cortex, to a tonic deviation of the eyes and head to the opposite side, the so-called versive seizures with seizures in the area of the fronto-dorso-lateral eye area, or be associated with screaming and vehement hypermotoric movements, which can be so bizarre that they are not uncommonly misinterpreted to be psychogenic events. Such seizures arise from the fronto-orbital cortex or the anterior gyrus cinguli. In addition, the surface EEG is mostly not conclusive as it is either overlaid by movement artifacts or does not contain any clear focal signs.

Many areas of the frontal cortex are anatomically unfavorable for surface EEG recordings, so that focal seizure activity cannot be adequately recorded. However, typical for frontal in contrast to temporal seizures is that they start very abruptly, are shorter in duration (lasting around 30 seconds) and end with an immediate or almost immediate re-orientation. Frontal seizures occur more often during the night than temporal seizures, and then not uncommonly in series of several in a row, in rare cases up to 20 or 30 seizures per night.

Parietal or occipital lobe epilepsy

In clinical series, these are rarer than frontal seizures. Typical for a parietal seizure origin are focal sensory phenomenon with contralateral dysesthesia. Even more rarely are pain, grimacing seemingly due to pain or a change of the perception of the body. Occipital seizures are often characterized by simple or complex visual hallucinations, which cannot be assumed to be pathognomonic as similar phenomena can also be caused by seizure activity in the posterior temporo-lateral or temporo-basal cortex. However, clinically suggestive signs are ictal saccadic eye movements or an ictal nystagmus, symptoms which may occur even with full consciousness. Parietal and occipital seizures rarely remain confined to the area of their origin but propagate quickly into other brain areas. The paths of

37

propagation can vary such that parietal or occipital symptoms may occur at onset but either frontal or temporal semiology may develop. Even the side of propagation may change. Therefore, a presumptive diagnosis of multifocal seizures should always prompt us to consider unifocal seizures with different propagation modes as a differential diagnosis.

Falls in focal seizures

As mentioned previously, falls in the context of focal seizures are surprisingly rare. This is mainly due to the fact that temporal seizures constitute the majority of these events and that their semiology rarely is associated with falls. However, in temporal lobe seizures ictal or postictal ambulatory automatisms or flight tendencies are not rare, during which the patient may walk around disoriented or even run away. This implies that during a seizure, many of the reflex and control mechanisms responsible for balance and gait remain unimpaired. Falls can occur, especially if unexpected obstacles impede the way or the patient fails to perform corrective movements necessary to avoid tripping and losing balance.

A specific form of falls in temporal seizures has been discussed by Landolt (1960), who coined the term of "temporal syncope." This term does not denote complex partial seizures in which a fall occurs but seizures resembling falls caused by cerebrovascular malfunctioning. Gambardella et al. (1994) reported six patients with temporal lobe epilepsy in whom temporal syncope was seen during presurgical evaluations. Based on non-invasive and, in one case, invasive EEG recordings, the authors argued that temporal syncope can indeed occur in temporal lobe epilepsy, albeit mostly only over the course of many years. According to these findings, the underlying mechanism probably consists of spread using very fast propagation pathways to extra-temporal areas, especially those affecting the pontine reticular formation function, which then could be responsible for the fall. The fact that these patients remained seizure-free postoperatively would speak against additional contralateral or extra-temporal epileptogenic foci. However, in our own experience temporal syncope is extremely rare, if it exists at all. By contrast, falls are more common during focal seizures with the following semiologies:

1. **Akinetic postural**. Initially, patients are unresponsive and show a motionless stare. This is followed by a postural motor pattern often in combination with a versive movement leading to a shift of the body's center of gravity. Due to the persisting akinesia, no compensatory movements are possible, and inevitably a fall ensues. In combined video-controlled EEG-EMG recordings of 15 patients, we show that this postural phase occurs without a rise of muscle tone, which differentiates these from tonic or secondary generalized seizures (Mothersill et al. 2000). Akinetic postural falls carry a greater risk of injuries due to the akinesia and absence of protective or defensive movements. In most cases, the initial seizure semiology is indicative of a temporal seizure origin with a consecutive propagation to frontal structures. However, because the same symptoms can sometimes be observed in extra-temporal seizures, akinetic postural falls cannot be used for localization purposes.

2. **Hypermotor**. Seizures of fronto-mesial and fronto-orbital origin are often associated with violent movements of all limbs, sometimes involving rotatory movements along the body's longitudinal axis. These events usually arise out of sleep and thus rarely lead to falls. On the other hand, it is not uncommon that patients are "thrown" out of their beds by the violence of their ictal movements. Therefore, these patients often prefer to sleep on a mattress on the floor rather than in a normal bed to avoid the potential risk of injury. Of course, seizures with this semiology are indicative of an origin within the frontal lobes. However, note that parietal lobe seizures may exhibit a fast propagation to the fronto-mesial cortex and may produce clinical symptoms only when these structures become secondarily involved.

Secondary generalization

In principle, all focal seizures can generalize secondarily, although this is more frequent with neo-cortical than with temporo-mesial seizures. Initial clinical symptoms of the generalized phase can involve a frontally generated head deviation to the contralateral side, sometimes accompanied by a tonic extension of the contralateral arm. In itself this may lead to a fall, which certainly becomes more likely when the tonic phase affects trunk and legs in a standing patient.

Seizures defined by falls: epileptic drop attacks

Generalized tonic seizures

Tonic seizures, which are defined by falls and thus can be grouped under the so-called epileptic drop attacks, occur in three different forms.

Pure axial tonic seizures are characterized by a tonic contraction of the neck muscles, the head being slightly flexed or hyperextended and the eyes opened wide. In axorhizomelic tonic seizures, the muscles of the shoulders can also become involved, which causes elevation and abduction of both arms. As a rule, falls do not occur in axial or axorhizomelic tonic seizures. The third form of tonic seizures, classical tonic drop seizures, turned out to be the most frequent form of epileptic drop attacks in a study of epileptic falls we performed using combined video-EEG-EMG monitoring (Mothersill et al. 2000). These seizures are characterized by an abrupt and massive bilateral, either symmetric or asymmetric, increase of muscle tone with a duration of 400 to 800 ms. Clinically, a uniform movement pattern with a flexion of head, body and both hips develops. The latter is so fast that it inevitably results in a fall. In some cases, signs of a seizure may be present before the onset of the tonic phase. This occurs mostly in the form of an atypical absence, during which the EEG shows high-amplitude spike-and-wave or sharp-and-slow-wave activity. The onset of the tonic phase then usually correlates with the occurrence of the last spike-and-wave complex.

During the actual tonic seizure, the EEG shows a generalized flattening or electro-decremental response while the simultaneous EMG recording shows a massive rise of muscle tone with an abrupt beginning and end. The tonic phase can then be followed by an atypical absence. The generalized tonic seizures usually last between 5 and 20 seconds and show additional vegetative symptoms such as initial apnea, then a tachy- or bradycardia, hypersalivation, mydriasis, cyanosis or flush. In some cases, a tonic status can occur (Vigevano et al. 1997). Generalized tonic seizures may appear with different epilepsy syndromes but are characteristic of the Lennox-Gastaut syndrome (Table 4.6).

Atonic and myoclonic astatic seizures

Atonic seizures can affect only circumscribed muscle areas. Typically, this leads to a short nodding movement of the head or to a short loss of tone of a

Table 4.6 Lennox-Gastaut syndrome

Definition	Epilepsy with (1) multiple seizure types mostly however tonic; (2) typical EEG changes (see below) and (3) mental retardation and psychiatric disturbances
Epidemiology	Approx. 3 – 10% of the epilepsies of childhood
Begin	Mostly between 3–5 years, at times preceded by West's syndrome
Etiology	In up to 80% symptomatic (perinatal cerebral diseases, cerebral malformations, or tumors, etc.); in about 20% idiopathic
Seizures	Generalized atonic, tonic-clonic, myoclonic or myoclonic-astatic seizures, and in particular generalized tonic seizures occurring especially nocturnally as well as focal seizures
EEG	Often slowing of the background activity; generalized sharp-slow waves as well as paroxysms of 10–12/s rhythms in sleep
Prognosis	Mostly pharmacoresistant, in about 80% lasting cognitive deficits
Therapy	Pharmacological: valproate, lamotrigine, topiramate, levetiracetam, felbamate, clobazam; in some cases a curative epilepsy surgery can be tried, otherwise if necessary palliative epilepsy surgery (implantation of a vagal nerve stimulator; callosotomy)

limb. They can involve all skeletal muscles, which is why atonic seizures are grouped under the "epileptic drop attacks." In theory, such a generalized loss of tone inevitably ought to lead to a fall, during which the patients would slump down like a puppet whose strings had been suddenly severed. We tested this assumption empirically using simultaneous video-EEG/EMG recordings with which we were able to register atonic drop seizures in 67 patients.

Falls either occurred during pure atonic seizures ($n = 35$), during an atonia in connection with an atypical absence ($n = 17$) or during an atonia following a myoclonia in the context of a myoclonic-atonic or myoclonic-astatic seizure ($n = 15$). All recorded drop attacks had in common a phase of generalized atonia with a minimal duration of 250 ms. Myoclonic-atonic seizures began with a symmetric myoclonia of both arms accompanied by a flexion of the head. Theoretically and actually, as described in the literature (Dravet et al. 1997), these myoclonia in themselves could be the cause for falls. However, in 82 patients we recorded myoclonic-atonic seizures that in all respect fulfilled the criteria of myoclonic-astatic seizures (Doose 1992) without any of the patients falling down. In all these cases, the duration of the generalized atonia never

Table 4.7 Myoclonic-astatic epilepsy

Definition	According to ILAE classification cryptogenic (however, at least sometimes possibly idiopathic) epilepsy with myoclonic and other seizures
Epidemiology	1.7% of the epilepsies of childhood beginning before the sixth year of age
Begin	Before the age of five years
Etiology	Multifactorial, with significant genetic factors (positive family history in 37% of first and second grade relatives)
Seizures	Myoclonic, atonic, myoclonic-astatic, atypical absences, generalized tonic-clonic seizures, rarely tonic seizures
EEG	Theta activity with parietal maximum; generalized (poly-) spike-waves, often photosensitivity
Prognosis	Rarely good response to valproate and seizure-freedom after around three years, then normal cognitive development, however in some cases pharmacoresistance and lasting cognitive deficits
Therapy	Pharmacological: valproate, lamotrigine, topiramate, ethosuximide; in some cases phenobarbital, benzodiazepines

exceeded 100 to 150ms. Thus, the crucial criterion for the occurrence of a fall is the duration of the atonic phase. During an atonic episode of 100 ms, the distance covered in free-fall would be 5 cm. Whether in this time an impairment of consciousness occurs cannot be reliably ascertained. However, it seems that in each case, fast reflex movements can counterbalance the change of body posture so that a fall can be avoided. In contrast, during a generalized atonia of 250 ms the distance covered in free fall would be 31 cm. Even if consciousness is retained, this cannot be compensated for and thus inevitably leads to a fall. The EMG in our recordings of atonic drop seizures showed a complete atonia for 250 to 400 ms. In the EEG, we found a simultaneous, regular or irregular, spike-and-wave activity or an irregular generalized slowing.

Generalized atonic seizures usually occur in connection with the Lennox-Gastaut syndrome. However, myoclonic-astatic seizures resulting in falls are a symptom of the rare myoclonic-astatic epilepsy of early childhood, which constitutes about 1.7% of the epilepsies beginning before the age of 6 years (Table 4.7).

Startle epilepsies

As described previously, the startle reflex is a normal physiological phenomenon. Uncontrolled startle reflexes leading to excessive motor reactions emerge in the context of startle diseases and have to be differentiated from epileptic seizures. On the other hand, there are epilepsies in which seizures can be provoked by sudden stimuli like noises, touching and so on. Although these reflex seizures do not display a homogenous clinical picture, they are grouped together under the term startle epilepsy. In most cases, the seizures are symmetric or asymmetric tonic, or show a tonic postural semiology typical for a focal supplementary motor seizure. If these seizures occur while the patient is standing, they are often associated with falls.

Many of the patients with this type of seizure suffer from symptomatic epilepsy with generalized (or not classifiable) seizures and have multiple disabilities. For example startle epilepsy occurs most frequently in children with Down syndrome (Guerrini et al. 1990). The underlying brain damage is quite often diffuse.

On the other hand, some frontal lobe epilepsies that, in principle, can be treated by epilepsy surgery can also be associated with startle-induced seizures (Manford et al. 1996; Serles et al. 1999). In our own experience, this kind of seizure is not uncommonly found in hemiparetic patients with a porencephalic cyst after perinatal brain damage. Note that these are patients who may profit from a functional hemispherectomy (see Oguni et al. 1998).

Startle epilepsy usually begins in childhood or in young teenagers. If suspected, this diagnosis can usually be confirmed by simultaneous video-EEG monitoring during, in which a seizure is provoked by an unexpected presentation of the adequate stimulus. As these seizures quite often turn out to be pharmacoresistant, possible epilepsy surgical options should be clarified and magnetic resonance imaging (MRI) scans should be performed according to an epileptological protocol, if necessary under anesthesia. Although rarely used in the long-term treatment of epilepsy, clobazam can in some of these cases lead to seizure freedom.

Falls as a side-effect of anti-epileptic medication

It must be mentioned that taking anti-epileptic drugs has been shown to be a risk factor for the occurrence of falls, at least for women of older age. The same has been known for benzodiazepines.

More than 8000 female patients from four American centers, who previously had participated in a study of osteoporosis-associated fractures, entered a prospective cohort study of CNS-active medication, including in addition to benzodiazepines drugs such as hypnotics, antidepressants and anti-epileptic drugs. During an average follow-up time of a year, 28% of the women fell at least once, and almost half of them at least twice or even more often. The taking of anti-epileptic drugs was shown to be a significant risk factor (multivariate odd-ratio 2.56; 95% CI = 1.49–4.41) and was even greater than the corresponding risks for benzodiazepines (1.51; 95% CI = 1.14–2.01) or antidepressants (1.45; 95% CI = 1.14–2.07; Ensrud et al. 2002).

Treatment of epileptic drop attacks

Drug therapy

Epileptic drop seizures or seizures that can lead to a fall are primarily treated with pharmacotherapy. As for the medical therapy of specific epilepsy syndromes and potential side-effects of anti-epileptic medication, we have to refer to the corresponding literature. To summarize briefly, the choice among available anti-epileptic drugs will have to take into consideration whether the patient suffers from primary generalized or focal seizures. Among the well-established, older anti-epileptic drugs, valproate still is the first choice for the treatment of primary generalized seizures. In pure absences, ethosuximide can be successful. Of the newer anti-epileptic drugs both lamotrigine and topiramate, possibly even levetiracetam, are suitable. Phenobarbital is effective with primary generalized seizures but should only be used as an exception in long-term treatment because of its cognitive side-effects.

Benzodiazepines, especially clobazam or clonazepam, play an important role as a temporary measure in the therapy of exacerbating seizures or when seizure frequency increases while changing from one drug to another. Major drawbacks of this group of drugs are the development of tolerance and possible addiction. However, they can be indispensable in some patients with pharmacoresistant epilepsies, especially because in a small number of these patients habituation does not occur.

The first-choice drug for the treatment of focal seizures among the well-established anti-epileptic drugs is carbamazepine followed by valproate, which is only minimally less effective. Phenytoin is compa-rable to carbamazepine as far as effectiveness is concerned. However, because of its negative side-effects as well as the fact that it is more difficult to manage due to its nonlinear pharmacokinetics, phenytoin is used more reluctantly, at least in Europe. Nevertheless, this drug can be very effective in difficult-to-treat secondary generalized seizures. Phenobarbital also is effective. However, we mentioned its side-effects previously and note that because of them, this drug is used rather restrictively. All modern anti-epileptic drugs have proven to be effective against focal seizures. Thus, we have effective alternatives with the drugs that have been approved so far. They are listed here alphabetically: gabapentin, lamotrigine, levetiracetam, oxcarbazepine, tiagabine (only as add-on) and topiramate. Owing to possible side-effects, rarely used but in some cases important additions to the anti-epileptic drug repertoire are felbamate (with severe therapy-refractory epilepsy such as the Lennox-Gastaut syndrome) and vigabatrin (especially in treating West's syndrome). In individual cases, it may be helpful to consider an add-on therapy with bromide, acetazolamide, piracetam (especially with myoclonia), primidone or sultiam. The latter has proven especially effective in the treatment of the so-called benign focal epilepsies of childhood.

Resective epilepsy surgery

If a patient suffers from pharmacoresistant focal seizures, the feasibility of epilepsy surgery should always be considered. In these cases, resective surgery is meant to be curative, meaning that it aims at lasting seizure freedom, although in some patients they may need continued anti-epileptic medication. In some syndromes, such as mesial temporal lobe epilepsy with unilateral hippocampal sclerosis, the chances of success are known to be very good. The same holds true for some other focal epilepsy syndromes circumscribed extra-hippocampal or extra-temporal lesions like low grade gliomas, cavernomas and so on (Grunwald 1999), and this also applies to a number of focal epilepsies whose seizures can be associated with falls. Less commonly known is the fact that epilepsy surgery is also an option for children and some adults with severe, and in some cases catastrophic, epilepsies and drop attacks due to extensive unilateral hemispheric lesions such as large porencephalic cysts. In these cases, a functional hemispherectomy may lead to seizure freedom without inducing any additional neurological or neuropsychological deficits.

In each case, the decision for surgery should only be made after meticulous presurgical evaluation in a specialized epilepsy center. Also, a decision against epilepsy surgery should not be made without giving patients and relatives the chance to make an informed decision after an adequate presurgical workup.

Palliative epilepsy surgery

In quite a few pharmacoresistant epilepsies with drop attacks, there is no chance of potentially curative epileptic surgery. In these cases, the indication for palliative surgery should be considered and discussed with the patient and/or relatives. Palliative epilepsy surgery does not aim at complete seizure freedom. It either tries to reduce the frequency of seizures to improve the patient's quality of life or it aims to stop at least the severe and more injury-prone falls. Currently, there are two methods available: vagal nerve stimulation and the callosotomy.

Vagal nerve stimulation

The left vagal nerve is stimulated intermittently via an electrode that is connected subcutaneously to a generator implanted under the left clavicle. After implantation stimulation is performed, for example, for 30 seconds every 5 minutes. Although the exact physiological mechanisms are as yet unclear, this stimulation can influence the seizure threshold through an excitation of afferent fibers of the vagal nerve. While complete seizure cessation is rare, a number of clinical trials have shown that a significant reduction of seizure frequency can be achieved, for example, a reduction of more than 50% in 45 of 95 patients (Scherrman et al. 2001).

In patients with Lennox-Gastaut syndrome, significant improvements have been reported (Hornig and Murphy 1997, Murphy et al. 1995). Frequent side-effects are intermittent hoarseness during stimulation, paresthesia in the throat and, less frequently, impairment of breathing possibly due to pharyngeal constriction during stimulation. Overall, the vagal nerve stimulator is well tolerated by the patients. A re-implantation to change the batteries is necessary after approximately 3 to 5 years and is requested by most patients (Schmidt and Elger 2002).

The implantation of a vagal nerve stimulator should be considered in cases of proven pharmacoresistance if there is no possibility for resective epilepsy surgery or if previous surgery did not result in satisfactory seizure control. In our view, it should also be discussed if the patient declines surgery due to subjective or objective reasons or wishes to postpone it. Last but not least, it should be held in mind that the implantation of a vagal nerve stimulator is reversible; however, the resection of brain tissue is not.

Callosotomy

Callosotomy rarely leads to seizure freedom. Instead, its main goal is to reduce the severe drop attacks with multiple injuries by transecting the corpus callosum to prevent the spread of seizure activity to both hemispheres. A transection of the anterior two thirds of the corpus callosum is performed in most cases. A complete transaction is only carried out if the previous, more limited approach did not lead to the desired results. After callosotomy, postoperative deficits always have to be taken into account. Postoperative autism and an accentuation of already existing hemiparesis may occur but are usually reversible. The inevitable disconnection syndrome is usually well-tolerated and does not lead to a noticeable deterioration in quality of life. However, this is only true for patients in whom unilateral language dominance can be proven preoperatively. By contrast, patients with atypical language dominance and language functions represented in both hemispheres are at risk not only to suffer additional severe cognitive deficits but also to develop an alien-hand syndrome, which worsens the patient's quality of life considerably.

Nonetheless, callosotomy should be considered as palliative treatment in pharmacoresistant, catastrophic epilepsies that cannot be treated curatively with surgery or are associated with frequent and severe drop attacks. However, care should be taken prior to surgery to demonstrate distinct pre-existing cognitive deficits and confirmation of unilateral language dominance. In these cases, quite satisfactory therapeutic results can be achieved (Gates and DePaola 1996). Otherwise, an attempt to treat with vagal nerve stimulation certainly has to be favored.

References

Andermann F, Keene DL, Andermann E, Quesney LF. Startle disease or hyperekplexia: further delineation of the syndrome. *Brain* 1980, **103**:985–997.

Bäzner H, Daffertshofer M, Hennerici M. Subkortikale vaskuläre Enzephalopathie. *Aktuelle Neurologie* 2003, **30**:266–280.

Bassetti C, Aldrich MS. Narcolepsy, idiopathic hypersomnia, and periodic hypersomnias. In: Culebras A. (ed.) *Sleep disorders and neurological disease.* New York, Basel: Marcel Dekker, 2000, pp. 323–354.

Camfield PR, Camfield CS, Gordon K et al. Incidence of epilepsy in childhood and adolescence: a population-based study in Nova-Scotia from 1997–1985. *Epilepsia* 1996, **37**:19–23.

Capovilla G, Rubboli G, Beccaria F, Meregalli S, Veggiotti P, Giambelli PM, Meletti S, Tassinari CA. Intermittent falls and fecal incontinence as a manifestation of epileptic negative myoclonus in idiopathic partial epilepsy of childhood. *Neuropediatrics* 2000, **31**:273–275.

Doose H. Myoclonic astatic epilepsy of early childhood. In: Roger J, Bureau M, Dravet C, Dreifuss FE, Perret A, Wolf P. (eds.) *Epileptic syndromes in infancy, childhood and adolescence.* London: John Libey, 1992, pp. 103–114.

Dravet C, Guerrini R, Bureau M. Epileptic syndromes with drop seizures in children. In: Beaumanoir A, Andermann F, Avanzini G, Mira L. (eds.) *Falls in epileptic and non-epileptic seizures during childhood.* London: John Libbey, 1997, pp. 95–111.

Ensrud KE, Blackwell TL, Mangione CM, Bowman PJ, Whooley MA, Bauer DC, Schwartzt AV, Hanlon JT, Nevitt MC for the Study of Osteoporotic Fractures Research Group. Central nervous system-active medications and risk for falls in older women. *J Am Geriatr Soc* 2002, **50**:1629–1637.

Gambardella A, Reutens DC, Andermann F, Cendes F, Gloor P, Dubeau F, Olivier A. Late-onset drop attacks in temporal lobe epilepsy: a reevaluation of the concept of temporal lobe syncope. *Neurology* 1994, **44**:1074–1078.

Gates JR, DePaola L. Corpus callosum section. In: Shorvon S, Dreifuss F, Fisch D, Thomas D. (eds.) *The treatment of epilepsy.* Oxford: Blackwell Science, 1996, pp. 722–738.

Ghez C. Posture. In: Kandel ER, Schwartz JH, Jessell TM (Hrsg.) *Principles of neural science.* New York, Amsterdam, London, Tokyo: Elsevier, 1991, 3. Aufl., pp. 596–607.

Gogan P. The startle and orienting reactions in man. A study of their characteristics and habituation. *Brain Res* 1970, **18**:117–135.

Grunwald T, Kurthen M, Elger CE. Predicting surgical outcome in epilepsy, how good are we? In: Schmidt D, Schachter SC. (eds.) *Epilepsy, problem solving in clinical practice.* London: Martin Dunitz, 1999, pp. 399–410.

Guerrini R, Genton P, Bureau M, Dravet C, Roger J. Reflex seizures are frequent in patients with Down syndrome and epilepsy. *Epilepsia* 1990, **31**:406–417.

Hacke W, Hennerici M, Gelmers HJ, Krämer G. *Cerebral ischemia.* Berlin: Springer, 1991, p. 71.

Honda Y. Clinical features of narcolepsy: Japanese experiences. In: Honda Y, Juji T. (eds.) *HLA in narcolepsy.* Berlin: Springer, 1988, pp. 24–57.

Hornig GW, Murphy JV, Schallert G, Tilton C. Left vagus nerve stimulation in children with refractory epilepsy: an update. *Southern Med J* 1997, **90**: 484–488.

Hublin S, Kaprio J, Partinen M, Heikkila K, Kskimies S, Guillemiault C. The prevalence of narcolepsy: an epidemiological study of the Finnish twin cohort. *Annals of Neurology* 1994, **35**:709–716.

Landolt H. *Die Temporallappenepilepsie und ihre Psychopathologie. Ein Beitrag zur Kenntnis psychophysiologischer Korrelationen bei Epilepsie und Hirnläsionen.* (Bibliotheca Psychiatrica et Neurologica, Fasc. 112). Basel: Karger, 1960.

Lee MS, Choi YC, Heo JH, Choi IS. "Drop attacks" with stiffening of the right leg associated with posterior fossa arachnoid cyst. *Movement Disorders* 1994, **9**:377–378.

Lempert, Bauer M, Schmidt D. Syncope: a videometric analysis of 56 episodes of transient cerebral hypoxia. *Annals of Neurology* 1994, **36**:233–237.

Lüders H, Lesser RP, Morris HH, Dinner DS, Hahn J. Negative motor responses elicited by stimulation of the human cortex. In: Wolf P, Dam M, Dreisuss FE. (eds.) *Advances in epileptology.* New York: Raven Press, 1987, pp. 229–231.

Manford MR, Fish DR, Shorvon SD. Startle-provoked epileptic seizures: features in 19 patients. *J Neurol Neurosurg Psych* 1996, **61**:151–156.

Massion J. Physiological mechanisms involved in falling. In: Beaumanoir A, Andermann F, Avanzini G, Mira L. (eds.) *Falls in epileptic and non-epileptic seizures during childhood.* London: John Libbey, 1997, pp. 11–18.

Meisner I, Wiebers DO, Swanson JW, O'Fallon WM. The natural history of drop attacks. *Neurology* 1986, **36**:1029–1034.

Mothersill IW, Hilfiker P, Krämer G. Twenty years of ictal EEG-EMG. *Epilepsia* 2000, **41** (Suppl. 3):519–523.

Murphy JV, Hornig G, Schallert G. Left vagal nerve stimulation in children with refractory epilepsy.

Preliminary observations. *Arch Neurol* 1995, **52**:886–889.

Oguni H, Hayashi K, Usui N, Shimizu H. Startle epilepsy with infantile hemiplegia: report of two cases improved by surgery. *Epilepsia* 1998, **39**:93–98.

Remler BF, Daroff RB. Falls and drop attacks. In: Bradley WG, Daroff RB, Fenichel GM, Marsden CD. (eds.) *Neurology in clinical practice. Principles of diagnosis and management.* Volume I, 2nd edn. Boston: Butterworth-Heinemann, 1996, pp. 23–28.

Scherrmann J, Hoppe C, Kral T, Schramm J, Elger CE. Vagus nerve stimulation: clinical experience in a large patient series. *J Clin Neurophysiol* 2001, **18**:408–414.

Schmidt D, Elger CE. *Praktische Epilepsiebehandlung. Praxisorientierte Diagnose und Differenzialdiagnose, rationale Therapiestrategien und handlungsorientierte Leitlinien.* 2. Auflage. Stuttgart, New York: Thieme, 1999.

Serles W, Leutmezer F, Pataraia E, Obrich A, Groppel G, Czech T, Baumgartner C. A case of startle epilepsy and SSMA seizures documented with subdural recordings. *Epilepsia* 1999, **40**:1031–1035.

Siegel JM, Moore R, Thannickal T, Nienhuis R. A brief history of hypocretin/orexin and narcolepsy. *Neuropsychopharmacology* 2001, **25** (Suppl. 5):S14–20.

Vigevano F, Fusco L, Yagi K, Seino M. Tonic seizures. In: Engel Jr J, Pedley TA (eds.) *Epilepsy: a comprehensive textbook.* Philadelphia: Lippincott-Raven, 1997, pp. 617–625.

Wirrell EC, Camfield PR, Camfield CS, Dooley JM, Gordon KE. Accidental injury is a serious risk in children with typical absence epilepsy. *Arch Neurol* 1996, **53**:929–932.

Zhou L, Chillag KL, Nigro MA. Hyperekplexia: a treatable neurogenetic disease. *Brain & Dev* 2002, **24**:669–674.

Paroxysmal headaches

Hans-Christoph Diener and Marc Andre Slomke

Definition

According to the criteria of the International Headache Society (IHS), a migraine is defined as a disease with periodic occurring headache episodes, typically associated with autonomic symptoms, for example, nausea or vomiting and sensitivity to light and noise. The headache is aggravated by physical activity (International Headache Society 2004).

Epidemiology

In all Western industrialized countries including the United States, the incidence of migraines is 6% to 8% in men and 15% to 20% in women (Lipton and Stewart 1997; Lucas et al. 2005; Steiner et al. 1999). Only 50% of these patients ever consult a physician. The other 50% treat their headaches with over-the-counter medication (Lipton et al. 2007). In 10% of all migraine patients, the episodes are so frequent and severe that continuous care by a physician is necessary. Migraine prevalence is comparable across countries and continents. Only in China and Japan does the prevalence seem to be slightly lower.

The incidence of migraines in childhood is 3% to 5%. Before adolescence, migraine prevalence is the same in boys and girls. Most frequently, migraines begin between the ages of 10 and 20. Migraines can also begin later in life. First occurrence of migraine headaches after the age of 50 is extremely rare. If headache episodes occur for the first time at this age, a symptomatic headache must be excluded. Women who have a genetic risk for migraines (positive family history) and who are treated with hormone substitution after menopause can develop de novo migraines at that particular age.

After adolescence, the frequency and severity of migraine attacks is greater in women than in men.

This most probably has to do with female sex hormones (Massiou and Bousser 2000; Silberstein 1995). Migraine headaches reach their peak in terms of frequency and severity between the ages of 35 and 45 years. Thereafter, it declines both in women and men. However, some patients suffer from frequent and severe migraine attacks beyond the age of 65 years. Migraine headaches beginning in childhood will improve or disappear during adolescence in 50% of the patients, but still can recur later in life.

Diagnosis

Migraine without aura is defined as recurrent attacks of headaches, lasting between 4 and 72 hours, accompanied by pulsating hemicrania, nausea, sometimes vomiting and photo- and phonophobia, as well as a general feeling of malaise. The headaches are severe and are accentuated by physical activity. In some attacks, the headache can be all over the head.

Migraine with aura or former "classic migraine," migraine accompagnée, is accompanied by neurological deficits like visual field loss (flickering scotoma), perception of zig-zag lines (fortifications), hemihypesthesia and speech or language problems before or usually right at the beginning of a migraine headache (Kelman 2007). These neurological deficits progress gradually over 5 to 20 minutes and do not exceed 60 minutes. In migraine with prolonged aura, the aura symptoms can last up to one week, followed by total recovery (International Headache Society 2004).

Basilar migraine is a special type of migraine headache with aura. Besides visual field loss, patients might suffer from impaired vision, vertigo, tinnitus, hearing loss, diplopia, ataxia and paraparesis of the legs or even tetraparesis. Rare types of migraines are ophthalmoplegic migraine (with incomplete lesions of the

The Paroxysmal Disorders, ed. Bettina Schmitz, Barbara Tettenborn and Donald L. Schomer. Published by Cambridge University Press. © Cambridge University Press 2010.

III or VI nerve) and pure retinal migraine with transient monocular blindness.

In more than half of attacks, the pulsating-throbbing headaches are one-sided, although the side might switch between or during an attack. Migraine attacks often start in the early morning. Typical triggers are menstrual flow, previous alcohol consumption, changes in the sleeping-waking rhythm, previous or current stress, hunger or decrease of caffeine intake. Changing weather conditions can also cause a migraine attack (Kelman 2007). There is poor scientific evidence for many of the aforementioned triggers. Typical additional and premonitory phenomena are nausea, fluid retention, tiredness, depression, irritability and craving for sweets (Kelman 2004; Schoonman et al. 2006).

Migraines have a genetic disposition. Genetics play a more important role for migraine with aura than for migraine without aura (Wessman et al. 2007). Three different gene defects were described in patients with hemiplegic migraine (van de Ven et al. 2007).

Migraine is diagnosed by headache history and neurological examinations. Additional imaging (CT, MRI) is not required if the neurological examination is normal (Quality Standards Subcommittee of the American Academy of Neurology 1994). Magnetic resonance imaging (MRI) is potentially "dangerous" in patients with migraines because of misinterpretation of hyperdense white matter lesions in T2-weighted images, which are not due to disturbed blood flow or demyelinization. Referral to a neurologist is necessary when focal neurological deficits, cognitive dysfunction or seizures occur.

Diagnostic imaging or repeated examinations are necessary if:

- First occurrence of severe intolerable headaches, particularly after physical strain (cerebral or subarachnoidal hemorrhage)
- Pyrexia, meningism (abscess, severe paranasal sinusitis)
- Atypical headaches with focal neurological signs
- Focal neurological signs (beyond migraine aura) like motor weakness, hyperreflexia or neuropsychological deficits
- Signs of increased intracranial pressure or papilledema
- Continuous worsening of headaches despite adequate treatment and after exclusion of medication overuse headache

- Additional occurrence of epileptic seizures
- Psychopathological symptoms in combination with headaches
- Changes of the pain characteristics of long-lasting existing primary headaches
- Tumor phobia

Differential diagnosis

The basic differential diagnostic considerations are presented in Table 5.1.

Pathophysiology

Doctors of antique times already knew that only few structures of the brain, particularly the meninges, blood vessels and some of the greater veins, are pain sensitive. For 60 years, vascular mechanisms have been assumed as decisive mechanisms in the origin of migraine pain (Graham and Wolff 1938). According to the vascular theory, initial vasodilatation of cerebral and particularly meningeal blood vessels leads to a headache. This would explain why the intake of vasoconstrictive drugs such as ergotamine ease pain (Graham and Wolff 1938). At the beginning of the 1980s, immunohistological examinations in animals showed that meningeal vessels are encircled by bipolar C-fibers, originating from the ipsilateral trigeminal ganglion (Edvinsson and Uddman 1982). These fibers transmit the actual pain stimulus to the trigeminal ganglion and further on via nociceptive brainstem nuclei to the thalamus and cortex. These C-fibers contain vasoactive neuropeptides such as substance P, calcitonin gene-related peptide (CGRP) or neurokinin A and presumably other peptides, which are unknown so far. The release of these peptides leads to specific vessel changes, more than just simple caliber fluctuations: increase of endothelial permeability, plasma extravasation, aggregation and degranulation of mast cells are the consequences (Moskowitz 1984). These data gained in animal experiments were reproduced in humans during acute migraine attacks. Increased concentrations of CGRP in the venous blood of patients during a migraine attack were found. A dramatic decrease of CGRP was seen after intake a triptan (Edvinsson et al. 1991). Therefore, the release of neuropeptides plays a central role in the development of head pain. CGRP antagonists are effective in the treatment of migraine attacks (Olesen et al. 2004) and are presently in clinical development in Phase 3.

Table 5.1 Differential diagnosis of headaches

Entity	Localization	Age/Gender	Time	Duration	Characteristics	Trigger	Additional symptoms
Migraine without aura	temporal, frontal, hemicrania	adolescence, women > men	morning	12–72 h	pulsating, throbbing	alcohol, stress, weekend, menstruation	nausea, vomiting, photophobia, seeking silence
Migraine with aura	temporal, frontal hemicrania	as above	morning	12–36 h	pulsating throbbing	as above	visual field loss, sensory disturbances, speech disturbances, nausea, vomiting
Cluster headache	unilateral, retro-orbital	>30 years of age, 80% men	mostly at night	30–120 min	intolerable, stabbing	alcohol, nitrates	ptosis, miosis, lacrimation, rhinorrhea, motor. agitation
Tension type headache	diffuse, frontal, parietal	women > men	during daytime	12–16 h	dull oppressive	alcohol, stress	sleep disturbances, dizziness
Medication overuse headache	diffuse or migraine features	women > men (10:1)	morning	daily	dull or daily migraine attacks	drug withdrawal	paleness, anemia, ergotism, kidney dysfunction
Post-traumatic headache	diffuse	all age groups	all day long	daily, weeks, months	dull, oppressive	bending down, pressing	frequent use of analgesics
Post puncture headache	diffuse, occipital	not in children or > 65 years	all day long	3–7 days	dull throbbing	upright position	tinnitus, vertigo, hearing loss, nausea, double vision
Arteritis temporalis	bitemporal, frontal	> 60 years	all day	weeks, months	dull, stinging	chewing	increased sedimentation rate and CRP, pyrexia, leukocytosis, joint and muscle pain
Trigeminal neuralgia	unilateral, V2 > V3	older age, women > men	during daytime	seconds	severe, stinging, burning	eating, chewing, swallowing	weight loss
Idiopathic facial pain	unilateral, cheek	30–40 years, women > men	during daytime	all day long, daily	dull, oppressive	none	tumor phobia, sleep disturbance, depression

The release of neuropeptides explains the actual origin of pain but not how and why the attack begins so abruptly in humans. Two recent observations gave a better possible understanding of this problem. A French group demonstrated that a special form of migraine, familial hemiplegic migraine (FMH), is due to a gene defect on chromosome 19. A Dutch group found that this gene encodes a neuronal P/Q-calcium channel. Later, two other genetic defects were identified causing familial hemiplegic migraine (Wessman et al. 2007). Therefore, it seems likely that migraines are an ion-channel disease.

The second important finding was the result of a positron-emission tomography (PET) study by a group in Essen (Weiller et al. 1995). This study demonstrated activation of specific anti-nociceptive brainstem areas (region of the periaqueductal gyrus, locus coeruleus, raphe nucleus) during migraine attacks. Whether this activity reflects the so-called migraine generator or shows a structure that aims to terminate the attack is yet unknown. Interestingly, the brainstem activation still existed after successful treatment of the migraine attack with sumatriptan.

Therapy

Therapy of a migraine attack

5-HT 1B/1D-agonists (triptans)

The serotonin-($5\text{-HT}_{1B/1D}$) receptor agonists suma-triptan, zolmitriptan, naratriptan, rizatriptan,

Table 5.2 Therapy of acute migraine attacks with 5-HT 1B/1D-agonists (in order of the year of approval)

Substance	Dose	Contraindications/remarks
Sumatriptan	25, 50 and100 mg p.o., 25 mg suppository, 10 and 20 mg nasal spray, 6 mg s.c. (auto-injector)	hypertension, coronary heart disease, angina pectoris, myocardial infarction, M. Raynaud, peripheral artery disease, TIA or stroke, pregnancy, lactation, children, severe liver or kidney insufficiency, multiple vascular risk factors
Zolmitriptan	2.5 and 5 mg p.o., melt tablet, 5 mg nasal spray	see sumatriptan
Naratriptan	2.5 mg p.o.	see sumatriptan
Rizatriptan	10 mg p.o. or melt tablet	see sumatriptan, 5 mg dose in patients who use propranolol
Almotriptan	12.5 mg p.o.	see sumatriptan
Eletriptan	20, 40 and 80 mg p.o.	see sumatriptan
Frovatriptan	2.5 mg p.o.	see sumatriptan

almotriptan, eletriptan and frovatriptan (Table 5.2) are specific migraine treatments that are ineffective in tension-type headaches. The efficacy of all triptans has been shown in large placebo-controlled studies (Ferrari et al. 2001). Comparative trials investigating triptans versus aspirin or non-steroidal anti-inflammatory drugs (NSAID) have to date failed to show a superiority of triptans for pain relief after two hours. However, triptans achieved a greater pain-free rate and were effective in patients who were non-responders to NSAIDs.

In an emergency room setting, sumatriptan 6 mg s.c. was slightly more effective than 1000 mg acetyl-salicylic acid (ASA) i.v. but had more side-effects. In comparative studies, ergotamine was less effective than sumatriptan, zolmitriptan, almotriptan and eletriptan (Diener et al. 2002). Triptans are effective at any time within an attack. They are more effective when taken early in the attack when the headache is still mild (Mathew et al. 2007). Triptans will also improve the typical additional symptoms like nausea or vomiting, photo- and photophobia, and improve the ability to return to work.

If a migraine attack lasts longer than 8 hours, migraine symptoms might recur after the end of the pharmacological effect of a migraine treatment, the so-called "headache recurrence." This is defined as a worsening of headache intensity from being pain-free or suffering from mild headaches to moderate or severe headache in a time period of 2 to 24 hours after the first effective intake of drugs. Recurrence is more common among triptans than among ergotamine tartrate or NSAIDs. Migraine recurrence is observed in 15% to 40% of patients after oral intake of triptans, whereas the second intake of the same drug is effec-tive again. If the first triptan dose is ineffective, it is not recommended to administer a second dose during the same migraine attack.

Taken too frequently, all triptans can lead to an increase in the frequency of attacks and finally to chronic migraine and medication overuse headache (Diener and Limmroth 2004). Therefore, triptans should not be taken more than 10 days a month. Life-threatening adverse events, such as myocardial infarction, severe cardiac arrhythmia and stroke, were found in a frequency of 1 : 1,000,000 persons who used sumatriptan (Welch et al. 2000). In almost all of these cases, contraindications were not observed, for example, pre-existing coronary heart disease, or the diagnosis of migraine was wrong. The same good safety profile holds for the other triptans. Some trip-tans, such as naratriptan, 50 mg sumatriptan, are already available as over-the-counter medication in some European countries. Patients suffering from migraine with aura should take a triptan after the aura symptoms have resolved. Triptans are not effec-tive when taken prophylactically during the aura phase. Triptans are not approved for the treatment of migraines in children and adolescents (the only excep-tion is sumatriptan nasal spray). The efficacy rates of triptans in children approached those of adults, but the placebo effect was much greater than in adults.

The side-effects of triptans are a feeling of tight-ness in the chest and neck, paraesthesia of the extremities, sensation of cold, fatigue, dizziness and drowsiness. Contraindications are shown in Table 5.2.

Comparison of triptans

Sumatriptan s.c. has the shortest time of onset of effec-tive action, about 10 minutes (Ferrari et al. 2001). Oral sumatriptan, almotriptan and zolmitriptan are effective after 45 to 60 minutes. Rizatriptan and eletriptan have a quicker onset of action compared to naratriptan and frovatriptan, up to 4 hours. Improvement of headache after 2 hours, the most important parameter in clinical studies for the effectiveness of migraine drugs, is best after the subcutaneous application of sumatriptan at a rate from 70% to 80%. Sumatriptan nasal spray and sumatriptan suppository have a similar effect (60%). Oral sumatriptan 25 mg is less effective than 50 and 100 g (approximately 50–60%) but shows fewer side-effects. Naratriptan and frovatriptan (each 2.5 mg) are less effective than sumatriptan but also show fewer side-effects and a lower rate of headache recurrence. A similar efficacy can be seen with rizatriptan 5 mg, zolmitriptan 2.5 mg and almotriptan 12.5 mg. Rizatriptan 10 mg is slightly more effective than 100 mg of sumatriptan. The most effective oral triptan is eletriptan in a dose of 2×40 mg, but it also has the greatest rate of adverse events. The frequency of recurrent headache is between 15% and 40% with the different triptans. An initial combination of a triptan with a long-acting NSAID is more effective than each drug as monotherapy and leads to fewer recurrences (Brandes et al. 2007).

Ergot alkaloids

Ergotamine and dihydroergotamine (DHE) have been available for a long time. The standard dose of oral ergotamine is 1 to 2 mg. Ergotamine is also available in some countries at a dose of 2 mg as a suppository. DHE is available as a tablet and in some countries as a nasal spray or for s.c. or i.v. injection. The number of good clinical trials incorporating ergotamine is rather small. Tfelt-Hansen et al. provided a summary of 18 controlled double-blind trials of oral ergotamine, or oral ergotamine plus caffeine (Tfelt-Hansen et al. 2000).

In ten of these trials, ergotamine was compared with placebo, whereas ergotamine served as the standard comparative drug in eight other trials without placebo-control. The dose of ergotamine varied from 1 to 5 mg with a median of 2 mg, and in several trials repeated intake of ergotamine was used. The reported parameters for efficacy were not all validated and varied considerably from benefit based on a clinical interview to use of changes on a verbal headache scale. Other methodological flaws in these trials include the lack of clearly stated inclusion criteria, no reporting of baseline criteria and the randomization procedure, unusual design of some of the crossover trials with a variable number of attacks per patient and superiority claims without appropriate statistics (Tfelt-Hansen et al. 2000). Despite the limited number of studies with contemporary methodology that involve ergotamine, there is evidence for the efficacy of ergotamine, which is summarized briefly here.

- Ergotamine (1–5 mg) was superior to placebo for some parameters in seven trials and no better than placebo in three studies using a dose of 2 to 3 mg (Dahlöf 1993).
- In two comparative trials, there was no significant difference in measures of pain relief at 2 hours between oral ergotamine 2 mg plus 200 mg caffeine and oral diclofenac-potassium 50 or 100 mg (McNeely and Goa 1999). However, diclofenac-potassium reduced pain more effectively than ergotamine plus caffeine at 1 hour after treatment and, in contrast to the comparator, was also significantly different compared with placebo.
- Drugs such as ergocristine, tolfenamic acid, dextropropoxyphene, naproxen sodium and pirprofen were generally found comparable to ergotamine.
- The combination of lysine-acetylsalicylate, equivalent to 900 mg aspirin, plus metoclopramide (10 mg) was superior to the combination of ergotamine and caffeine (2 mg ergotamine and 200 mg caffeine) for most of the outcome parameters assessed (Titus et al. 1999).

As mentioned previously, triptans were superior to ergotamine in all head-to-head trials. Ergots are used in patients who report good efficacy in the past. They should be considered in patients with early recurrence after the use of a triptan.

Antiemetics and simple analgesics

During a migraine attack, most patients suffer from gastrointestinal symptoms. Antiemetics like metoclopramide or domperidone (Table 5.3) will not only improve nausea but will also promote peristaltic movement of the GI tract and thereby speed absorption of oral drugs.

Analgesics (NSAIDs)

Acetylsalicylic acid (ASA; Diener et al. 2006), ibuprofen, diclofenac-potassium and paracetamol are analgesics of first choice for non-severe migraine headaches (Table 5.4). Older studies of analgesics

Table 5.3 Antiemetics in migraine therapy

Substance	Dose	Adverse effects	Contraindications
Metoclopramide	10–20 mg p.o. 20 mg rectal 10 mg i.m., i.v., s.c.	early dyskinesia syndrome, agitation	children under 14 years of age, hyperkinesia, epilepsy, pregnancy, prolactinoma
Domperidone (Motilium®)	20–30 mg p.o.	fewer and milder than with metoclopramide	children under 10 years of age

Table 5.4 Analgesics for the treatment of a migraine attack

Substance	Dose	Adverse events	Contraindications
Acetylsalicylic acid, ASA-lysinate	1000 mg p.o. i.v.	GI upset, bleeding	ulcer, asthma, hemorrhagic diathesis, pregnancy month 1–3
Ibuprofen	400–600 mg	like ASA	like ASA (lower rate of bleeding complications)
Naproxen	500–1000 mg	like ASA	like ASA
Diclofenac	50–100 mg	like ASA	like ASA
Metamizol	1000 mg	allergic reaction, neutropenia	neutropenia, kidney failure
Paracetamol (acetaminophen)	1000 mg	hepatotoxicity	liver diseases, kidney insufficiency
ASA plus paracetamol plus caffeine	2 × 250 mg + 200 mg + 50 mg	see ASA and paracetamol	

did not meet the requirements for modern study designs. The combination of ASA, paracetamol and caffeine is more effective than the monosubstances or the combination of two compounds (Diener et al. 2005). The optimal dose for an initial dose to treat an acute migraine attack is 1000 mg for ASA and paracetamol, 400 to 600 mg for ibuprofen and 50 to 100 mg for diclofenac-potassium. Metamizol (dipyrone) is also effective for migraines. Analgesics should be given as an effervescent or chewable tablet. Lysined ASA in combination with metoclopramide is almost as effective as sumatriptan and zolmitriptan. NSAIDs such as naproxen and tolfenamic acid are also effective.

Preventive treatment of migraine

If migraine attacks are too frequent, intake of acute medication is not the solution. In these cases, migraine preventive therapy should be considered. Other reasons to initiate migraine prevention are:

- Suffering from three or more migraine attacks per month that do not response to attack treatment, or if side-effects of the acute therapy are not tolerated.
- Increase in the frequency of attacks and intake of pain or migraine drugs more than 10 days a month.

- High disability and frequent absence from work or inability to perform homework.

The aim of migraine prophylaxis is a reduction of frequency, severity and duration of migraine attacks and the prevention of medication overuse headache. Optimal migraine prophylaxis leads to a reduction of attack frequency, severity and duration of at least 50%. Patients should be asked to keep a headache diary and document the frequency of attacks and success or failure of the particular attack medication.

Substances for preventive migraine therapy

Effective for preventive migraine therapy are the non-selective beta-blocker propranolol and the beta-1-selective beta-blocker metoprolol (Table 5.5). Bisoprolol is presumably also effective but has been examined in only a few studies. From the group of calcium antagonists, only flunarizine is effective. Pure calcium channel blockers such as nimodipine and nifedipine are not effective. Typical side-effects of flunarizine are fatigue, weight gain, depression and dizziness and, in very rare cases in elderly patients, movement disorders like Parkinson's disease or dyskinesia.

Neuromodulators (antiepileptic drugs) have proven to be effective in migraine prophylaxis

Table 5.5 Migraine prophylaxis: Effective substances in the order of therapeutic choice

First choice: Beta-receptor-blockers

Substance	Dosage (mg/day)	Remarks/Mechanism of action	Side-effects	Contraindications
Metoprolol	initially 50, later 150–200	beta-1-selective	fatigue, hypotonia disturbances of sleep,	AV-block, bradycardia,
Propranolol	initially 40, later 160–200	non selective	bronchospasm bradycardia	asthma, diabetes

Second choice: Neuromodulators and calcium-antagonists

Substance	Dosage (mg/day)	Remarks/Mechanism of action	Side-effects	Contraindications
Topiramate	50–100 mg	unknown	paraesthesia, cognitive impairment, weight loss	kidney stones, glaucoma
Valproic acid	500–600 mg	GABAergic acting drug	tremor, hair loss, weight gain	liver dysfunction, pregnancy
Flunarizine	initially 5 mg, later 10 mg in men, 5 mg in women	long half-life calcium-channel antagonists	fatigue, weight gain, depression, Parkinsonism, tremor	depression, obesity extrapyramidal disorders

Third choice: ASA, NSAIDs and serotonin-antagonists

Substance	Dosage (mg/day)	Remarks/Mechanism of action	Side-effects	Contraindications
Acetylsalicylic acid	300 mg	inhibitor of prostaglandin synthesis	GI problems, asthma, tinnitus	asthma, pregnancy
Naproxen	3 × 250 mg	inhibitor of prostaglandin synthesis	GI problems neutropenia	GI ulcers, thrombocytopenia
Methysergide	2–8 mg	not >6 months (retroperitoneal fibrosis) serotonin-antagonist (5-HT2)	muscle pain, dizziness, edema, weight gain	hypertension, hepatic disease, coronary artery disease, pregnancy
Pizotifen	3 × 0.5 mg	serotonin-antagonist (5-HT2)	fatigue, weight gain, anticholinergic effects	pregnancy, glaucoma
Lisuride	3 × 0.025 mg	dopamine-agonist	headache, nausea	CHD, PVD

(Table 5.5). Valproic acid used in a daily dose is 500 to 600 mg (Klapper 1997). Sometimes higher doses are necessary. Topiramate is effective with a daily dose of 50 to 100 mg (Bussone et al. 2005). Topiramate is also effective in chronic migraine with and without medication overuse headache (Diener et al. 2007; Silberstein et al. 2007). Lamotrigine is not effective in reducing the frequency of migraine attacks but did reduce the frequency of migraine auras. ASA in a dose of 300 mg per day does have a small migraine preventive effect (Table 5.5). The serotonin antagonists pizotifen and methysergide are also effective as preventive therapy but are no longer available in many countries. The effect of magnesium is debated; if effective at all, the reduction of frequency of attacks is not very distinctive.

Amitriptyline, a tricyclic antidepressant, is popular in the United States despite weak scientific evidence (Silberstein 2000). Tricyclic antidepressants should be considered in patients with migraine and tension-type headache and in migraine patients with comorbid depression. NSAIDs like naproxen and ASA are also effective in migraine prevention. Their limitations are due to side-effects like nausea, vomiting, stomach pain, tinnitus, vertigo, gastrointestinal ulcer and bleedings.

Menstrual migraines can be treated with 2 × 500 mg naproxen for four days before and three days after the period. Estrogen replacement will reduce migraine days during menstruation but will lead to a rebound in migraine attacks afterwards (MacGregor et al. 2006). A similar phenomenon was observed with a short-term prophylaxis of naratriptan (Mannix et al. 2007).

Only beta-blockers are permitted as preventive medication during pregnancy. All other migraine prophylactic drugs, except for magnesium, are contraindicated.

Non-medical migraine prophylaxis

Behavioral therapy

Patients suffering from highly frequent migraines – defined as three or more attacks per month – should receive additional psychological treatment. Most psychological treatments used in migraine therapy are behavior therapies. There are enough studies available to evaluate the evidence of therapies like these. Other therapies fail to show an evaluation of their concepts. The most important unimodal concepts are thermal and EMG biofeedback training and progressive muscle relaxation. Multimodal methods are cognitive-behavioral pain-coping trainings or stress management. As well as unimodal, multimodal therapy concepts are not used specifically for pain treatment in migraine therapy but aim for unspecific variables like "strengthening of self-control competence" (unimodal) or "minimization of impairment or improved stress management" (multimodal). All behavioral therapies are more effective than placebo treatment and comparably effective as a preventive medication. Additional effects are only seen in the combination of biofeedback plus progressive muscle relaxation (PMR).

Approximately 50% of all migraineurs benefit from behavior therapies. PMR is especially appropriate for younger patients with a shorter duration of the disease where a good outcome is noted if the duration is less than two years. There is also a lower functional impairment as well as reduced pain frequency.

Cognitive-behavioral concepts are very important if patients have a lot of stress in everyday life, distinctive depressive symptoms and a maladaptive coping behavior. Minimal contact of 7 to 10 sessions is needed, and standard treatment sessions should number between 12 and 16. Group- and single-therapies show the same effectiveness. Before starting pain treatment, patients suffering from manifest panic/anxiety attacks or depression must be treated medically or by psychotherapeutics.

Cluster headaches

Definition and epidemiology

Cluster headache is a non-symptomatic paroxysmal strictly one-sided headache with additional autonomous symptoms (Massiou and Bousser 2000). Cluster headaches are rare (1 : 200). In 90% of patients, headaches occur in spring or autumn in so-called "clusters" with an episode lasting between one week and three months in duration. In 10% of cases, there is a chronic cluster headache with no pain-free intervals lasting more than 14 days a year as a minimum. Men are overrepresented with a 4 : 1 ratio.

Clinical symptoms

The attacks are strictly one-sided, with the most severe pain seen periorbitally, retro-orbitally and temporally. There are ipsilateral peripheral vegetative symptoms such as conjunctival injections, lacrimation, swollen nasal mucosa, rhinorrhea, miosis, ptosis and edema of the ipsilateral eyelid also noted very characteristically. These severe pain attacks in cluster patients last between 15 to 60 minutes, rarely longer. They occur several times in 24 hours, mostly at night. Every single attack can be provoked by alcohol, nitroglycerine or histamine. Patients suffering from a cluster headache attack are agitated and can neither sit still nor lay down relaxed.

Differential diagnosis

Malignant tumors infiltrating the cavernous sinus must be excluded as a potential differential diagnosis. Rare differential diagnoses are Tolosa-Hunt syndrome, aseptic inflammation of the cavernous sinus with hypesthesia in the first trigeminal nerve, and a fistula of the cavernous sinus where there is usually permanent eye redness. Cranial imaging is indicated for exclusion of symptomatic reasons and for initial diagnosis of the disease.

Pathophysiology

Aseptic inflammation and vasodilatation in the cavernous sinus seem to play an important role. During an attack, a significant increase of CGRP and vasoactive-intestinal peptide (VIP) could be demonstrated. This means that similar to a migraine, a sudden release of vasoactive neuropeptides plays a key role.

Therapy

Oral drugs are useless in attacks lasting up to 20 minutes because of their late effect (Kelman 2007). Few substances and treatments are known to be effective:

- Inhalation of 100% oxygen (7 l per minute, facial mask, sitting position)

- Subcutaneous injection of sumatriptan 6 mg
- Zolmitriptan 5 mg nasal spray

Preventive therapy of cluster headaches is indicated if the attacks occur mostly at night and cannot be managed by any acute treatment and if the cluster lasts more than two weeks (Lucas et al. 2005).

The medication of first choice to interrupt a phase of cluster headaches is prednisone 100 mg per day over 3 to 5 days followed by decreasing dosage in the next days, as well as the subcutaneous injection of sumatriptan 6 mg. This therapy can be extended with verapamil (Isoptin®) 3 × 120 mg per day. Some patients profit by prophylactic intake of lithium carbonate with plasma blood levels between 0.3 and 1.2 mmol/l. But in this case, side-effects like polyuria, abdominal problems, tremor, sleeping disorders and vomiting are limiting.

In few studies, valproate in a dosage up to 2000 mg per day had a preventive effect. In particular cases, topiramate (Topamax®) showed a positive effect. Verapamil especially can be combined with other medications if a single-treatment regimen fails. In cases of resistance to therapy, cryo-coagulation or high-frequent-rhizotomia of the Gasserian ganglion can be tried. Peripheral or central effective analgetic, anticonvulsive, thymoleptic or neuroleptic and antihistaminic drugs are non-effective. Psychological therapy concepts are also non-effective. Acupuncture is contraindicated and often triggers attacks.

Chronic paroxysmal hemicrania

This headache disorder has a prevalence of approximately 0.5 to 1 per 100,000 (Kelman 2004). It is characterized by an intensive stinging, strictly one-sided and mostly retro-orbital pain located in the forehead and the ear region. Additional symptoms such as lacrimation, rhinorrhea, miosis and conjunctival injection located at the side of the pain are possible. The only therapeutic effective drug is indomethacin. Interestingly, non-steroidal antirheumatics are not effective. The effectiveness can be used as diagnostic criteria.

Other paroxysmal headaches

Consumption of ice-cream, spices or flavor enhancer (glutamate) or the application of coldness (ice water, ice pack) can also trigger headaches. Benign cough headache, headaches during physical exertion (weight lifting) and coital headache also belong in this cat-

egory. The therapy is primarily with beta receptor blockers. The differential diagnosis is primarily subarachnoid hemorrhage.

Hypnic headache leads to holocranial nightly headaches in older women, occurring out of sleep and not responding to analgetics or migraine treatment. These headaches respond to caffeine immediately. Lithium given in the evening is effective.

Trigeminal neuralgia

Definition, epidemiology and clinical symptoms

Paroxysmal pain of short duration (seconds) located in a region of one of the trigeminus nerves is very characteristic for the trigeminal neuralgia. There are idiopathic forms that are the most frequently encountered but there also exist non-idiopathic neuralgia caused by structural lesions, for example, immunological processes like multiple sclerosis, or tumors. Trigeminal neuralgia is relatively frequent with a prevalence of 1 : 3000, and it is a disease of the older age.

There are paroxysmal (lasting seconds), stinging, most-severe pain attacks in the region of one or more of the trigeminal nerves, less frequent in the region of the glossopharyngeal nerve, intermediate nerve, superior laryngeal nerve and greater occipital nerve. Typical triggers are eating, chewing, swallowing or brushing one's teeth. Between each single attack, the patient is pain-free most of the time.

Pathophysiology

In idiopathic trigeminal neuralgia, there seems to be a trigemino-vascular mechanism with a narrowed spatial association of a small vascular loop, mostly of the inferior cerebellar artery with a nerve trunk of the trigeminal nerve in the posterior cranial fossa. An irritation of the nerve over years and the dismantling of the myelin sheath lead to kind of a short-circuit between parallel going C-fibers and A-delta-fibers, so that single touches or sensible stimuli are experienced as pain.

Symptomatic trigeminal neuralgia and also long-lasting pain in the area of the trigeminal nerve occurs because of demyelinization in multiple sclerosis, zoster (post-zoster neuralgia) and Tolosa-Hunt syndrome or inflammation of the cavernous sinus. Schwann-cell tumors of the trigeminal nerve are rare and go along with pain plus paraesthesia and an atrophy of the masticatory muscles.

Table 5.6 Medication prophylaxis of trigeminal neuralgia and other neuralgia

Substance	Medium Dosage	Side-effects
Carbamazepine	600–1500 mg	fatigue, skin rash, vertigo, ataxia, nausea, headache, leukopenia, elevated liver enzymes, diplopic images
Gabapentin	160–3200 mg	fatigue, vertigo, tremor
Phenytoin	300–400 mg	skin rash, nausea, ataxia, fatigue, elevated liver enzymes, gingiva-hyperplasia, hirsutism
Oxcarbazepine	600–2400 mg	like carbamazepine but milder, hyponatremia

Drug therapy

An acute attack only lasts seconds, and because of this it is not responding to acute therapy. Preventive therapy is shown in Table 5.6. Non-responders can try a combination of carbamazepine and amitriptyline. Regular intake of drugs with constant blood levels is very important.

Other peripheral or central acting analgetics are not effective in typical neuralgia. Surgical interventions should only be performed in cases of absolute resistance to therapy. Microvascular decompression (Janetta procedure) is effective in younger patients. After a suboccipital trepanation and using a microscope, the trigeminal nerve is separated from small associated arteries.

The death rate of this intervention is approximately 1% and the morbidity up to 5%, with the most frequent complication being hearing loss and peripheral facial paresis. Thermocoagulation or cryocoagulation should be performed in older patients by using short-term anesthesia. The rate of relapse is 15% to 25% within seven years. Unfortunately, most patients still undergo teeth extractions or surgeries because of assumed sinusitis.

References

Brandes JL, Kudrow D, Stark SR, O'Carroll CP, Adelman JU, O'Donnell FJ, Alexander WJ, Spruill SE, Barrett PS, Lener SE. Sumatriptan-naproxen for acute treatment of migraine: a randomized trial. *Jama* 2007, **297**(13):1443–54.

Bussone G, Diener H, Pfeil J, Schwalen S. Topiramate 100 mg/day in migraine prevention: a pooled analysis of double-blind randomised controlled trials. *Int J Clin Pract* 2005, **59**:961–968.

Dahlöf C. Placebo-controlled clinical trials with ergotamine in the acute treatment of migraine. *Cephalalgia* 1993, **13**:166–171.

Diener HC, Reches A, Pascual J, Jansen J-P, Pitei D, Steiner T, on behalf of the Eletriptan and Cafergot Comparative Study Group. Efficacy, tolerability and safety of oral eletriptan and ergotamine plus caffeine (Cafergot) in the acute treatment of migraine: a multicentre, randomised, double-blind, placebo-controlled comparison. *Eur Neurol* 2002, **47**:99–107.

Diener HC, Limmroth V. Medication-overuse headache: a worldwide problem. *Lancet Neurology* 2004, **3**:475–483.

Diener H, Pfaffenrath V, Pageler L, Peil H, Aicher B. The fixed combination of acetylsalicylic acid, paracetamol and caffeine is more effective than single substances and dual combination for the treatment of headache: a multi-centre, randomized, double-blind, single-dose, placebo-controlled parallel group study. *Cephalalgia* 2005, **25**:776–778.

Diener HC, Lampl C, Reimnitz P, Voelker M. Aspirin in the treatment of acute migraine attacks. *Expert Rev Neurother* 2006, **6**(4):563–73.

Diener HC, Bussone G, Van Oene J, Lahaye M, Schwalen S, Goadsby PJ. Topiramate reduces headache days in chronic migraine: a randomized, double-blind, placebo-controlled study. *Cephalalgia* 2007, **27**:814–823.

Edvinsson L, Ekman R, Jansen I, McCulloch J, Mortensen A, Uddman R. Reduced levels of calcitonin gene-related peptide-like immunoreactivity in human brain after subarachnoid haemorrhage. *Neurosci Lett* 1991, **121**:151–154.

Edvinsson L, Uddman R. Immunohistochemical localization and dilatory effect of substance P on human cerebral vessels. *Brain Res* 1982, **232**:466–471.

Ferrari MD, Roon KI, Lipton RB, Goadsby PJ. Oral triptans (serotonin 5-HT1B/1D agonists) in acute migraine treatment: a meta-analysis of 53 trials. *Lancet* 2001, **358**:1668–1675.

Graham JR, Wolff HG. Mechanism of migraine headache and action of ergotamine tartrate. *Arch Neurol Psych* 1938, **39**:737–763.

International Headache Society. The international classification of headache disorders. 2nd edn. *Cephalalgia* 2004, **24** (Suppl. 1):9–160.

Kelman L. The premonitory symptoms (prodrome): a tertiary care study of 893 migraineurs. *Headache* 2004, **44**:865–872.

Kelman L. The triggers or precipitants of the acute migraine attack. *Cephalalgia* 2007, **27**(5):394–402.

Klapper J, on behalf of the Divalproex Sodium in Migraine Prophylaxis Study Group. Divalproex sodium in migraine prophylaxis: a dose-controlled study. *Cephalalgia* 1997, **17**(2):103–108.

Lipton RB, Stewart WF. Epidemiology and comorbidity of migraine. In: Goadsby PJ, Silberstein SD. (eds.). *Headache*. Boston: Butterworth-Heinemann, 1997, p. 75–97.

Lipton RB, Bigal ME, Diamond M, Freitag F, Reed ML, Stewart WF. Migraine prevalence, disease burden, and the need for preventive therapy. *Neurology* 2007, **68**(5):343–9.

Lucas C, Chaffaut C, Artaz MA, Lanteri-Minet M. FRAMIG 2000: medical and therapeutic management of migraine in France. *Cephalalgia* 2005, **25**(4): 267–79.

MacGregor EA, Frith A, Ellis J, Aspinall L, Hackshaw A. Prevention of menstrual attacks of migraine: a double-blind placebo-controlled crossover study. *Neurology* 2006, **67**(12):2159–63.

Mannix LK, Savani N, Landy S, Valade D, Shackelford S, Ames MH, Jones MW. Efficacy and tolerability of naratriptan for short-term prevention of menstrually related migraine: data from two randomized, double-blind, placebo-controlled studies. *Headache* 2007, **47**(7):1037–49.

Massiou H, Bousser M-G. Influence of female hormones on migraine. In: Olesen J, Tfelt-Hansen P, Welch KMA. (eds.). *The headaches.* 2nd edn. Philadelphia: Lippincott, Williams & Wilkins, 2000, p. 261–267.

Mathew NT, Finlayson G, Smith TR, Cady RK, Adelman J, Mao L, Wright P, Greenberg SJ. Early intervention with almotriptan: results of the AEGIS trial (AXERT Early Migraine Intervention Study). *Headache* 2007, **47**(2):189–98.

McNeely W, Goa KL. Diclofenac-potassium in migraine. *Drugs* 1999, **57**:991–1003.

Moskowitz MA. The neurobiology of vascular head pain. *Ann Neurol* 1984, **16**:157–168.

Olesen J, Diener H, Husstedt IW, Goadsby PJ, Hall D, Meier U, Pollentier S, Lesko LM, for the BIBN 4096 BS Clinical Proof of Concept Study Group. Calcitonin gene-related peptide (CGRP) receptor antagonist BIBN4096BS is effective in the treatment of migraine attacks. *N Engl J Med* 2004, **350**:1104–1110.

Quality Standards Subcommittee of the American Academy of Neurology. Practice parameter: the utility of neuroimaging in the evaluation of headache in patients with normal neurologic examinations. *Neurology* 1994, **44**:1353–1354.

Schoonman GG, Evers DJ, Terwindt GM, van Dijk JG, Ferrari MD. The prevalence of premonitory symptoms in migraine: a questionnaire study in 461 patients. *Cephalalgia* 2006, **26**(10):1209–13.

Silberstein SD. Migraine and women. The link between headache and hormones. *Postgrad Med* 1995, **97**:147–153.

Silberstein SD. Practice parameter: evidence-based guidelines for migraine headache (an evidence-based review): report of the Quality Standards Subcommittee of the American Academy of Neurology. *Neurology* 2000, **55**:754–762.

Silberstein SD, Lipton RB, Dodick DW, Freitag FG, Ramadan N, Mathew N, Brandes JL, Bigal M, Saper J, Ascher S, Jordan DM, Greenberg SJ, Hulihan J. Efficacy and safety of topiramate for the treatment of chronic migraine: a randomized, double-blind, placebo-controlled trial. *Headache* 2007, **47**(2):170–80.

Steiner TJ, Stewart WF, Kolodner K, Liberman J, Lipton RB. Epidemiology of migraine in the England. *Cephalalgia* 1999, **19**:305–306.

Tfelt-Hansen P, Saxena PR, Dahlöf C, Pascual J, Lainez M, Henry P, Diener HC, Schoenen J, Ferrari MD, Goadsby PJ. Ergotamine in the acute treatment of migraine. A review and European consensus. *Brain* 2000, **123**:9–18.

Titus F, Lainez J, Leira R, Diez E, Monteiro P, Dexeus I. Double-blind, multicentric, comparative study of lysin acetylsalicylate (1620 mg equivalent to 900 mg aspirin) + metoclopramide (10 mg) versus ergotamine (2 mg) + caffeine (200 mg) in the treatment of migraine. *Cephalalgia* 1999, **19**:371.

van de Ven RC, Kaja S, Plomp JJ, Frants RR, Van Den Maagdenberg AM, Ferrari MD. Genetic models of migraine. *Arch Neurol* 2007, **64**(5):643–6.

Weiller C, May A, Limmroth V, Jüptner M, Kaube H, van Schayck R, Coenen HH, Diener HC. Brain stem activation in spontaneous human migraine attacks. *Nature Med* 1995, **1**:658–660.

Welch KMA, Mathew MT, Stone P, Rosamond W, Saiers J, Gutterman D. Tolerability of sumatriptan: clinical trials and post-marketing experience. *Cephalalgia* 2000, **20**:687–695.

Wessman M, Terwindt GM, Kaunisto MA, Palotie A, Ophoff RA. Migraine: a complex genetic disorder. *Lancet Neurol* 2007, **6**(6):521–32.

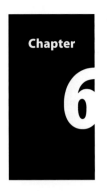

Paroxysmal vertigo attacks

Marianne Dieterich

Paroxysmal attacks of vertigo and dizziness are not considered to be unique disease entities. For example, sometimes vertigo is attributed to vestibular disorders, whereas dizziness is not (Brandt et al. 2005). The two terms actually cover a number of multisensory and sensorimotor syndromes of various etiologies and pathogeneses. Thus, they can only be elucidated by taking an interdisciplinary approach.

After headaches, vertigo and dizziness are among the most frequent presenting symptoms of patients, not only in neurology departments. According to a survey of over 30,000 persons, the prevalence of vertigo as a function of age lies around 17%. It rises to 39% in those over 80 years of age. Paroxysmal vertigo attacks can be caused by a dysfunction or a lesion of the peripheral or central vestibular system, resulting in an association with either "ear signs" such as tinnitus and hearing loss or signs of a brainstem or cerebellar dysfunction. Such signs and symptoms must be considered when taking the patient's history, for they are essential for making a correct diagnosis. This chapter will focus on the most frequent vertigo syndromes (Table 6.1; Brandt et al. 2005; Brandt 1999).

Peripheral vestibular vertigo syndromes

Benign paroxysmal positioning vertigo (BPPV)

Definition

Benign paroxysmal positioning vertigo (BPPV) is the most common cause of vertigo, not only in the elderly (Table 6.1). It is so frequent that about one third of all over 70 have experienced BPPV at least once if not more often. This condition is characterized by brief attacks of rotatory vertigo, which can be accompanied by nausea. BPPV is elicited by extending the head or positioning the head or body toward the affected ear. Both rotatory vertigo and rotatory-linear nystagmus toward the undermost ear can occur after such positioning. There is a short latency of seconds in the form of a crescendo/decrescendo course of maximally 30 to 60 seconds.

Epidemiology

BPPV can appear at any time from childhood to old age, but at least the idiopathic form is typically a disease of the elderly, peaking in the sixth and seventh decades. Approximately half of all cases have to be classified as degenerative or idiopathic (women:men = 2:1), whereas the symptomatic cases (women:men = 1:1) are most frequently caused by head injury (17%) or vestibular neuritis (15%) (Baloh et al. 1987). BPPV also occurs strikingly often in cases of extensive bed rest in connection with other illnesses or after operations. About 10% of the spontaneous cases and 20% of the trauma cases show a pronounced BPPV that is bilateral and generally asymmetrical.

The condition is considered benign because it usually resolves spontaneously within weeks to months. However, in some cases it can last for years. We found that in 50% of our patients, the history of the disorder until its diagnosis had lasted more than four weeks, and in 10% more than six months. If not treated, BPPV persisted in about 30% of our patients; another 20% to 30% had relapses within months or years (with a recurrence risk of 15% per year).

Diagnosis

Characteristic symptoms of BPPV include brief, in part, severe attacks of rotatory vertigo with and without nausea, which are caused by rapid changes in head

The Paroxysmal Disorders, ed. Bettina Schmitz, Barbara Tettenborn and Donald L. Schomer. Published by Cambridge University Press. © Cambridge University Press 2010.

Table 6.1 Frequency of different vertigo syndromes in 3036 out-clinic patients of dizziness unit (1989–1999)

Vertigo Syndrome	N	%
1. BPPV	533	17.6
2. Phobic postural vertigo	434	14.3
3. Central vestibular vertigo	364	12.0
4. Peripheral vestibulopathy	263	8.7
5. Basilar, vestibular migraine	241	7.9
6. Menière's disease	200	6.6
7. Bilateral vestibulopathy	89	2.9
8. Psychogenic vertigo (without Brandt 1999)	89	2.9
9. Vestibular paroxysmia	63	2.1
10. Labyrinthine fistula	8	0.3
Other vertigo syndromes [st]	109	3.6
Vertigo of unknown origin	132	4.3
Other central vestibular syndromes [st st] (without vertigo)	396	13.0
Other diseases	115	3.8
Total	3036	

*Non-vestibular ocular motor disorders in myasthenia, peripheral eye muscle paresis or imbalance of gait in dementia or polyneuropathy.
**Brain stem syndromes with ocular motor disorders without vertigo (e.g., infarctions)

position relative to gravity. Typical triggers include lying down or sitting up in bed, turning over in bed, bending over to tie one's shoelaces or extending the head to look up or do something above one's head. If BPPV is elicited while the patient is upright, there is a danger of falling. However, it is in part quite unpredictable whether attacks of vertigo are triggered or not. They frequently occur in the morning and are most pronounced during the first change in position after sleep. Repeated changes in position cause a transient lessening of the attacks. The complaints are so typical that a diagnosis can be made solely on the basis of the patient history. Occasionally, even the side or affected ear can be identified because rotatory vertigo occurs when the patient lies down on one specific side.

The beating direction of the nystagmus depends on the direction of the gaze. It is primarily rotating when the gaze is to the undermost ear and mostly vertical (to the forehead) during the gaze to the uppermost ear. The nystagmus corresponds to an ampullifugal-based excitation of the posterior vertical canal of the undermost ear.

If the typical positioning nystagmus can be elicited without any additional central signs and symptoms, further testing is not necessary. The next step is then to observe the patient's response to treatment.

Differential diagnosis

Despite correct positioning exercises (physical liberatory maneuvers) and especially in cases of therapy-refractory rotatory vertigo, the following syndromes should be considered along with unilateral BPPV in the differential diagnosis: central positional nystagmus, bilateral BPPV particularly post-traumatic (10%), BPPV of the horizontal canal (too rarely diagnosed), vestibular paroxysmia, and central infratentorial lesions that imitate BPPV (very rare).

Pathophysiology

There are two models that explain how nystagmus and vertigo arise. According to the histologically based "cupulolithiasis" model of Schuknecht (Schuknecht 1969), heavy, inorganic particles (otoconia) of specific weight become detached from the utricular otoliths of the cupula as a result of trauma or spontaneous degeneration. They settle in the underlying ampulla of the posterior canal. Whereas the cupula normally has the same specific weight as the endolymph, it is now heavier with these particles, that is, the canal is transformed from a sensor of rotatory acceleration into a transducer of linear or angular acceleration. This hypothesis was generally accepted for many years despite its inability to explain many of the typical criteria of nystagmus in cases of positioning vertigo.

In contrast, the canalolithiasis hypothesis (Brandt et al. 1994; Parnes and McClure 1991) can explain all symptoms of positioning nystagmus. According to this hypothesis, the particles float freely within the endolymph of the canal instead of being firmly attached to the cupula, and the "heavy conglomerate," which almost fills the canal, is assumed to be the cause of the positioning vertigo. The movement of the conglomerate causes either an ampullifugal or ampullipetal deflection of the endolymph, depending on the direction of the sedimentation. A valid model of the pathomechanism of BPPV must be able to predict the direction, latency, duration and fatigability of the typical nystagmus as well as changes in these parameters due to other head maneuvers (Fig. 6.1). All of this is explained by the canalolithiasis model.

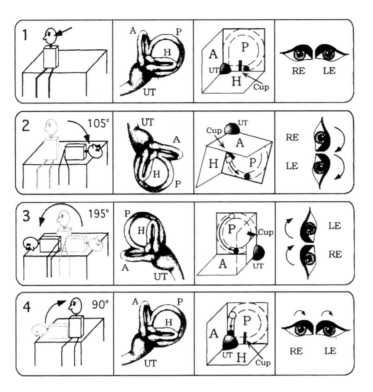

Fig. 6.1. Schematic drawing of the Semont liberatory maneuver of a patient with typical BPPV of the left ear. Panels from left to right: position of body and head, position of labyrinth in space, position and movement of the clot in the posterior canal (which causes cupula deflection) and the direction of the rotatory nystagmus. The clot is depicted as an open circle within the canal; a black circle represents the final resting position of the clot (Brandt et al. 2005). In the sitting position, the head is turned horizontally 45° to the unaffected ear. The clot, which is heavier than endolymph, settles at the base of the left posterior semicircular canal (Brandt 1999). The patient is tilted approximately 105° to the left (affected) ear. The change in head position, relative to gravity, causes the clot to gravitate to the lowermost part of the canal and the cupula to deflect downward, inducing BPPV with rotatory nystagmus beating toward the undermost ear. The patient maintains this position for 3 min (Schuknecht 1969). The patient is turned approximately 195° with the nose down, causing the clot to move toward the exit of the canal. The endolymphatic flow again deflects the cupula so that the nystagmus beats toward the left ear, now uppermost. The patient remains in this position for 3 min (Parnes and McClure 1991). The patient is slowly moved into the sitting position; this causes the clot to enter the utricular cavity (reproduced with permission from Brandt et al. 1994) (A, P and H = anterior, posterior, horizontal semicircular canals; CUP = cupula; UT = utricular cavity; RE = right eye; LE = left eye).

Therapy

Physical liberatory maneuvers

When correctly performed, all three physical liberatory maneuvers of Semont or Epley (Fig. 6.1) are successful in almost 90% of patients (Fife et al. 2008; Herdman et al. 1993).

As the therapy of first choice, we recommend the physical liberatory maneuver depicted in Figure 6.1 (e.g., BPPV of the left posterior semicircular canal; Brandt et al. 1994). It is important that the head of the sitting patient is turned by 45° to the healthy ear to put the responsible posterior canal into a position parallel to the plane of movement during the positioning. Relief is thus achieved in about 50% of the cases with one single maneuver. The positioning nystagmus toward the uppermost ear indicates that the plug has left the canal, that is, the therapy was successful. Positioning nystagmus toward the undermost healthy ear indicates that the liberatory maneuver failed and must be repeated. These maneuvers should be repeated five times a day until the patient is symptom-free.

The alternative liberatory maneuver of Epley requires that the patient's head and trunk be rotated after being tilted backward into a slightly head-hanging position (Fig. 6.2). This maneuver is as effective as the other. However, if the plug is not dislodged during the outpatient visit, the patient can be quickly instructed how to proceed on their own at home. As a rule, almost all patients are free of complaints after several days or sometimes a few weeks (Levat et al. 2003). Despite successful liberatory maneuvers, many patients later complain of transient attacks of postural vertigo and dizziness for a few days. This can be attributed to the partial repositioning of the otoconia toward the otolith organs, that is, most likely an otolithic vertigo. Patients should be informed in advance about this side-effect of the maneuvers, which goes away within a few days.

Surgery

According to our experience with more than 1000 BPPV patients, only one proved to be refractory

Fig. 6.2. Schematic drawing of modified Epley liberatory maneuver in a patient with BPPV of the left posterior semicircular canal. Abbreviations as in Fig. 6.1.

(1) In the sitting position, the head is turned horizontally 45° to the affected (left) ear.

(2) The patient is tilted approximately 105° backward into a slightly head-hanging position, causing the clot to move in the canal, deflecting the cupula downward, and inducing the BPPV attack. The patient remains in this position for 1 minute.

(3a) The head is turned 90° to the unaffected ear, now undermost.

(3b) The head and trunk continue turning another 90° to the right, causing the clot to move toward the exit of the canal. The patient remains in this position for 1 min. The positioning nystagmus beating toward the affected (uppermost) ear in positions 3a and 3b indicates effective therapy.

(4) The patient is moved into the sitting position (reproduced with permission from Brandt et al. 1994).

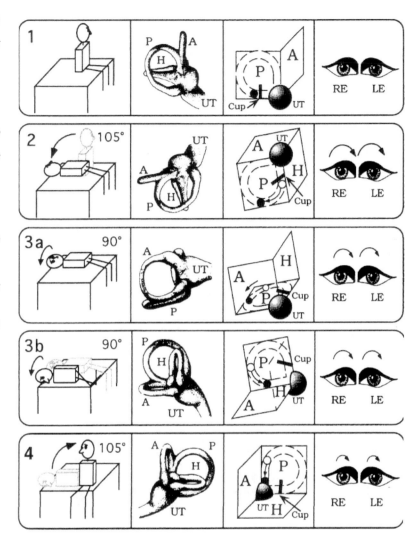

to therapy and required operative sectioning of the posterior canal nerves. Such selective neurectomy is difficult, and there is a risk of a permanent hearing loss. Neurectomy has now been replaced by plugging of the posterior canal. It is evidently a safer and more effective measure than sectioning of the nerve; however, in our opinion it is used too often in some centers, that is, before the possibilities of the simple, effective physical therapy have been exhausted.

BPPV of the horizontal canal

The cardinal features of the less frequent, but still too seldom diagnosed horizontal canal BPPV (hBPPV; Baloh et al. 1993) are as follows:

- Turning the head along the longitudinal axis of the supine body (either to the right or to the left) can induce it. This results in an ampullipetal deflection of the cupula, with more severe vertigo and nystagmus when the head is turned to the side of the affected ear.
- The beating direction of nystagmus corresponds to the stimulation or inhibition of the horizontal canal, that is, it beats linear and horizontal to the undermost ear.
- Repeated positioning maneuvers cause hardly any fatigue of the positioning nystagmus.
- The duration of both the attacks and the nystagmus is longer because of the so-called central storage mechanism of velocity in the horizontal canal. Positioning nystagmus

frequently shows a reversal of direction during the attacks; this corresponds to post-rotatory nystagmus phases I and II.

The typical case of horizontal BPPV can also only be explained by canalolithiasis, although it has occasionally been observed that the mechanism switches from canalolithiasis to cupulolithiasis (Brandt 1999; Brandt et al. 2005). In the rare form of horizontal BPPV due to cupulolithiasis, characterized by nystagmus beating horizontally to the uppermost ear, the "zero point" of positioning nystagmus beyond which the direction changes can be determined by turning the patient's head 10° to 20° around the longitudinal axis while in a supine position. This is possible because the cupula of the ipsilateral horizontal canal is then parallel to the gravity vector. In this way one can determine which side is affected by horizontal BPPV.

There is some evidence that persistent horizontal BPPV occurs if the canal narrows toward its exit in an ampullifugal direction. Then the congealed clump cannot leave the canal because of its size. Otherwise, one could assume that the particles would independently and inevitably leave the canal with every accidental rotation around the longitudinal axis of the body, for example, in bed. The striking feature of horizontal BPPV is that it does not fatigue. Likewise, it is general experience that horizontal BPPV is difficult to treat by a single positioning maneuver.

Therapy

Simple 270° rotations toward the unaffected ear around the longitudinal axis while the patient is supine have been successful (Fife et al. 2008; Lempert and Tiel-Wilck 1996). Bed rest with positioning of the head to the side of the unaffected ear (for 12 hours) is also effective (Vanucchi et al. 1997). Serial and alternating positioning according to the method of Brandt and Daroff (Brandt and Daroff 1980) are more likely to lead to success (Herdman et al. 1993) because the repeated bilateral head positioning evidently causes the disintegration of the conglomerate and wash-out of the particles from the canal.

Menière's disease

Definition

Menière's disease develops from endolymphatic labyrinthine hydrops, which are characterized by periodical rupturing of the membrane separating the endolymph space from the perilymph space. This triggers attacks that generally last at least 20 minutes, most often several hours. Patients present with rotational vertigo, nausea and vomiting as well as tinnitus, hearing loss and aural fullness in the affected ear. Monosymptomatic attacks that are purely cochlear or vestibular can occur above all at the beginning of the disease. During the course of the disease, most patients develop a persistent hypoacusis of the affected ear.

Epidemiology

Menière's disease is without doubt diagnosed too often. In dizziness units, it is somewhat more frequent than vestibular neuritis, with a frequency of around 7% to 9%. Its onset is usually between the fourth and the sixth decades. It seldom occurs in childhood or after the eighth decade. Men are affected somewhat more often than women (Brandt et al. 2005). The disease begins in one ear; there is a very irregular, at first generally increasing and then in the course of several years decreasing, frequency of attacks. The patients are at first free of complaints in the attack-free interval, but then they develop increasing deficits such as unilateral peripheral vestibular hypofunction, unilateral tinnitus and hearing loss, usually the deeper tones. Although the onset of the disease is unilateral, the other ear can also become affected with time. The longer one follows patients with Menière's disease, the more often one sees bilateral illnesses. In an early stage up to two years' duration, about 15% of the cases are bilateral; 30% to 60% of patients develop a bilateral illness after one or two decades. In the meantime, it has been generally acknowledged that the course of Menière's disease is on the whole relatively benign, having a remission rate of the episodes but not of chronic hearing loss of about 80% within 5 to 10 years.

Diagnosis

Menière's disease is typically a combination of abruptly occurring attacks with vestibular and/or cochlear symptoms, fluctuating, slowly progressive hearing loss and, in the course of time, tinnitus. During the attack, there is first a unilateral short vestibular excitation, then a temporary vestibular deficit with the following clinical findings:

- During the initial vestibular excitation, the patient has ipsiversive rotatory vertigo and ipsiversive nystagmus;
- During the vestibular deficit, there are contraversive rotatory vertigo and contraversive nystagmus;
- There are cochlear symptoms in the form of tinnitus, reduced hearing of the affected ear, as well as pressure and a feeling of fullness in the ear; and
- Deviation of gait and a tendency to fall.

The diagnosis of monosymptomatic forms is frequently difficult or uncertain. The attacks generally last several hours, during which time the vertigo changes from an acute rotatory vertigo into a postural vertigo that later leads to a worsening of gait instability. In rare cases, the first phase of the acute attacks can also be characterized by a brief, severe rotatory vertigo or a sudden drop attack due to the hydrops and shifting of the otoliths, Tumarkin's otolithic crisis.

The American Academy of Ophthalmology and Otolaryngology, Head and Neck Surgery (American Academy of Ophthalmology and Otolaryngology 1995) has formulated the following diagnostic criteria:

Certain Menière's disease:

- Histopathological confirmation of endolymphatic hydrops
- Symptoms as in "Definite Menière's disease" criteria

Definite Menière's disease:

- Two or more attacks of vertigo each lasting more than 20 min
- Audiometrically documented hearing loss in at least one examination
- Tinnitus or aural fullness in the affected ear
- Other causes excluded

Probable Menière's disease:

- At least one of vertigo episode
- Audiometrically documented hearing loss in at least one examination
- Tinnitus or aural fullness in the affected ear
- Other causes excluded

Possible Menière's disease:

- Episodic vertigo but without documented hearing loss
- Sensorineural hearing loss, fluctuating or fixed, with disequilibrium but without definite episodes of vertigo
- Other causes excluded

Differential diagnosis

The first attacks of Menière's disease must be differentiated from an acute unilateral vestibular deficit which, for example, occurs in connection with vestibular neuritis. Here the duration of the attacks is helpful. In Menière's disease, they generally last several hours and maximally one day, whereas in vestibular neuritis the attacks last several days. The accompanying symptoms are also helpful for the diagnosis, for example, "ear symptoms" in Menière's disease and inflamed eye signs and hearing disturbances in Cogan's syndrome or hearing disorders and possibly central signs of infarctions of the AICA/A. labyrinthi. Central disorders of the oculomotor system or central vestibular function also occur after lacunar infarctions or multiple sclerosis plaques in the area of the entry zone of the VIIIth cranial nerve. Because a caloric hyporeactivity occurs in all of the aforementioned diseases, caloric testing cannot be used in the differential diagnosis.

Rare, sudden, recurrent falls, so-called vestibular drop attacks or Tumarkin's otolithic crisis which occur in the early or late stages of Menière's disease without definite triggers, antecedent signs, or disturbances of consciousness, are difficult to differentiate from drop attacks due to vertebrobasilar ischemia. Such attacks apparently result from fluctuations in endolymphatic pressure caused by unilateral exacerbation of the otoliths and inadequate vestibulospinal postural reaction.

Another important differential diagnosis is basilar/vestibular migraine, which can manifest not only in the form of short attacks but also as attacks lasting several hours. Vestibular paroxysmia, which is caused by neurovascular compression, is also characterized by recurrent attacks with vertigo and/or occasionally other ear symptoms. Contrary to Menière's disease, these attacks typically last only seconds to minutes.

Pathophysiology

Menière's disease develops from endolymphatic labyrinthine hydrops characterized by periodical rupturing of the membrane separating the endolymph space from the perilymph space. The cause of hydrops is an impaired resorption in the endolymphatic sac due to perisaccular fibrosis or an obliteration of the endolymphatic duct which interrupts the longitudinal endolymph flow. Despite various indications that an inflammatory genesis or an auto-immunological process is involved, no prospective studies on immune-blocking medications have to date been performed. In reviews of the literature covering a large number of therapy studies, only betahistine and diuretics (Claes and van de Heyning 1997; James and Thorp 2001) have been confirmed to have positive effects on the frequency of attacks. For this reason, H1 agonist and H3 antagonist betahistine is currently recommended as the prophylactic therapy of first choice. At the beginning it should be given in a high dosage of 3 times 48 mg per day (Strupp et al. 2008). The microcirculation is improved by the drug's action on the precapillary sphincters of the stria vascularis and at the same time it exercises a regulating influence by means of the H3 receptors on the vestibular nuclei (Van Cauwenberge and De Moor 1997; Yabe et al. 1993). This possibly leads to reduced production and increased resorption of the endolymph. A placebo-controlled, double-blind study has shown that it has a significant influence on the natural course of the disease, especially on the vestibular symptoms. The production of endolymph can also be reduced by the method suggested by Schuknecht, that is, "switching off the inner ear" by instillation and diffusion of ototoxic antibiotics, such as gentamycin, which mainly cause destruction of the hair cells. In the meantime, this method has been so refined that it is possible to selectively affect the secretory epithelium while largely sparing the vestibular and cochlear sensory cells.

Therapy

Treatment of attacks

The acute attack is itself limited. Vertigo and nausea can be reduced by antivertiginous drugs used in other acute disorders of labyrinthine function, for example, dimenhydrinate 100 mg as suppository or benzodiazepine.

Prophylactic therapy

The goal of prophylactic treatment is to reduce the endolymphatic hydrops. Therefore in cases of repeating attacks of rotatory vertigo, possibly with fluctuat-

ing loss of inner-ear hearing, tinnitus, or pressure in the ear, the following treatment is indicated:

- Betahistine, 3×2 tablets/day containing 20 to 24 mg for 4 to 12 months, dose can be tapered depending on course (the patient should keep a vertigo diary to document the effects of therapy);
- If improvement is insufficient, hydrochlorothiazide plus triamterene ($\frac{1}{2}$ to 1 tablet mornings) can be administered in addition to betahistine;
- ENT specialists recommend administration of steroids; however, no studies have yet proven their efficacy.

In rare cases of frequent Menière's attacks with or without inner ear hearing loss which are intractable to drug treatment, intratympanal instillations of ototoxic antibiotics are indicated, for example, 1 to 2 ml gentamycin at concentrations of 20 to 40 mg/ml at interims of two or, better, more weeks. Instillations used to be done on a daily basis until Magnusson et al. (Magnusson et al. 1991) observed that the onset of ototoxic effects was delayed. Nowadays, only single instillations are recommended at interims of several weeks. However, there is still no consensus on the dose and the duration of the interims (Blakley 2000).

At first, endolymphatic sac operations used to be performed everywhere and were considered a type of shunt operation. However, it was realized that they had only a placebo effect (Brandt et al. 2005). Nowadays, they are considered obsolete. Currently, less than 1% to 3% of patients are considered for operative measures.

Besides preventing any further attacks of Menière's disease and treating an acute attack, another important principle of treatment is to promote central compensation of the peripheral vestibular deficits by means of physical therapy.

Treatment of vestibular drop attacks

Recurrent vestibular drop attacks or Tumarkin's otolithic crisis constitute an extreme impairment for patients in their everyday life. Moreover, they are dangerous because of the high rate of injuries. Depending on the severity of the disorder, intratympanic gentamicin treatment can be administered with success. The prerequisite for such treatment is that the causative ear can be definitely identified.

Perilymph fistulas

Definition and epidemiology

The underlying cause of all perilymph fistulas is pressure that is pathologically transmitted between the perilymphatic space and the middle ear (round or oval window) or between the perilymphatic space and the intracranial space. The pressure is caused by a defect or an abnormal elasticity of the bony labyrinth. Episodic dizziness or rotatory vertigo of various intensity and duration lasting from seconds to days, oscillopsia, imbalance and hearing loss elicited by changes in pressure, for example, by coughing, pressing, sneezing, lifting or loud noises, result. The dizziness or vertigo often occurs during changes in head position, for example, when bending over and when surmounting great differences in altitude, such as mountain tours and flights.

The incidence and prevalence of perilymph fistulas are not known due to the uncertain diagnosis but it appears that they are relatively greater in childhood. However, perilymph fistulas can occur at any time in life, and there is no obvious preference for either gender. The course of the illness varies, and sometimes the attacks are rare or frequent; as a rule, they resolve spontaneously and there are symptom-free periods of varying duration. However, the fistula can be reactivated by new traumas.

Diagnosis

The clinical spectrum of complaints is characterized by a wide range of symptoms: episodic dizziness or rotatory vertigo of various intensity and duration lasting from seconds to days, oscillopsia, imbalance and hearing loss (Brandt et al. 2005). This variability depends on the site of the fistula, so that either canal or otolith symptoms dominate. Consequently, it is difficult to establish the diagnosis. Rotatory vertigo suggests more the canal type, whereas unsteadiness and gait ataxia suggests more the otolith type. Linear and rotatory nystagmus, oscillopsia and a tendency to fall in a certain direction can occur in both forms.

When taking the patient history, it is important to ask about traumas that could cause or trigger such attacks, for example, barotrauma, head trauma, ear trauma including operations on the ear, or excessive Valsalva maneuvers due to lifting heavy weights.

A very important new variant of the perilymph fistula, is the dehiscence of the superior semicircular canal (Minor et al. 1998; Minor et al. 2001). It is probably the most frequent and the most overlooked one. The main symptoms are loud-sound induced rotatory or postural vertigo with oscillopsia. In more than half of the patients, these complaints first occur after slight head concussion or barotrauma. Observance and apparative analysis of the eye movements reveal rotating vertical nystagmus. The diagnosis can be confirmed by thin-slice CT of the petrous bone, which shows a bony apical defect of the anterior canal, and by three-dimensional analysis of eye movements induced by changes in pressure. The "vestibulo-collic reflex" clearly shows an electrophysiologically reduced sensory threshold in the affected ear.

The Tullio phenomenon is characterized by the occurrence of vestibular otolith or canal symptoms due to loud sounds. In such cases, one should try to trigger vertigo and eye movements by exposing each ear of the patient separately to loud sounds of different frequencies.

The diagnosis can be established by provocation tests. With these tests, one tries to trigger attacks while simultaneously observing using Frenzel's glasses or recording the resulting eye movements. Such tests include the Valsalva maneuver, the tragal pressure test, examination with a Politzer balloon and positional maneuvers, such as the head-hanging position. The affected side can also be identified with the pressure test by means of the Politzer balloon or the tragal pressure test: a feeling of increased pressure in the ear, tinnitus, reduced hearing or autophonia. All of these symptoms can also indicate the affected ear. A fistula of the horizontal canal is indicated by a linear horizontal nystagmus, whereas a fistula of the vertical canal is characterized by a vertical rotatory nystagmus.

The imaging techniques of MRI and CT, in the form of high-resolution, thin-slice CT, can be helpful, especially to prove congenital labyrinth dysplasias and the presence of an internal perilymph fistula of the anterior semicircular canal. ENT specialists use exploratory tympanoscopy when fistulas of the round and oval windows are strongly suspected. However, some specialists consider this examination rather insensitive and unspecific.

Differential diagnosis

The differential diagnosis of perilymph fistulas includes the following illnesses: benign paroxysmal positioning vertigo, positional vertigo of central origin, Menière's disease, vestibular paroxysmia, somatoform phobic postural vertigo, labyrinthine trauma and bilateral vestibulopathy.

Therapy

The therapy of first choice for "external fistulas" is conservative because most fistulas close spontaneously.

Conservative therapy

Conservative therapy consists of 1 to 3 weeks of absolute bed rest with moderate elevation of the head, if necessary a mild sedative, the administration of laxatives (to avoid pressing during bowel movements) and several weeks of limited physical activity that avoids all heavy lifting, abdominal pressing, violent coughing or sneezing, even after improvement. This almost always leads to complete recovery (Singleton 1986). If conservative therapy fails and disturbing vestibular symptoms persist, then exploratory tympanoscopy is indicated to examine the oval and round windows.

Surgical therapy

Surgical therapy with operative closure of the fistula is successful in only up to 50 to 70% of patients with vestibular vertigo. The preexisting hearing loss generally does not improve at all. The operative procedure involves the removal of the mucous membrane in the region of the fistula and its substitution with autologous material, such as perichondral tissue of the tragus or fascia by means of gel foam. Fistulas in the oval window adjacent to the stapes footplate require a stapedectomy and prosthesis. Even if the operation is successful, the postoperative sensitivity of the patients to extreme physical strain, such as abdominal pressing and barotrauma, is less than that of healthy subjects.

It is possible that a part of the fistulas presumed to be in the middle ear was actually a dehiscence of the superior semicircular canal because these can indirectly also lead to a pathological motility of the middle ear window. This probably explains in part the low rate of improvement after the aforementioned operations. The dehiscence of the superior semicircular canal can be treated neurosurgically by covering the bony defect or by occlusion, the so-called plugging, of the canal (Brandt et al. 2005; Minor et al. 2001). However, prospective studies to determine which procedure is more effective have not yet been performed.

Vestibular paroxysmia

Neurovascular cross-compression of the VIIIth cranial nerve

Definition and epidemiology

The cardinal symptoms of vestibular paroxysmia are brief attacks of rotatory or postural vertigo lasting seconds or rarely a few minutes, with or without ear symptoms such as tinnitus and hypoacusis (Brandt et al. 2005). These symptoms frequently depend on certain head positions and can occasionally be induced by hyperventilation. Hearing loss and tinnitus can also be present during the attack-free intervals.

Vestibular paroxysmia is a rare condition, accounting for about 2% of the cases in dizziness units. It is probably often underdiagnosed. Men are affected twice as often as women. There seem to be two peaks of frequency, one that begins early in cases of vertebrobasilar vascular anomalies and a second between the fifth and seventh decades with vascular elongation during old age. The course is generally chronic.

Diagnosis

Vestibular paroxysmia is suspected if brief and frequent attacks of vertigo are accompanied by the following features (Brandt and Dieterich 1994a):

- Short attacks of rotational or to-and-fro vertigo lasting for seconds to minutes with instability of posture and gait,
- Triggered in some patients by particular head positions, hyperventilation or influenced by changing the head position,
- Unilateral hypoacusis or tinnitus occasionally or permanently,
- In the course of the disease measurable vestibular and/or cochlear deficits that increase during the attack and are less pronounced during the attack-free interval. Neurophysiological function tests include audiogram, acoustic evoked potentials, caloric testing, subjective visual vertical,
- Attacks improved or lessened by carbamazepine, even low dosage effective, without the presence of central vestibular/oculomotor disorders or brainstem signs.

Conclusions can be drawn from the type of complaints whether vestibular, originating from the canals or otolith organs, or cochlear symptoms, about the portion of the nerve affected. If there is a combination of symptoms of various nerves, even the lesion site can be deduced. Thus, for example, simultaneously occurring symptoms of the VII and VIIIth cranial nerves with contraction of the frontal muscle, vertigo and double vision (Brandt 1999) indicate an irritation of both nerves in the internal acoustic meatus where both lie in close proximity.

Differential diagnosis

Important differential diagnoses are benign paroxysmal positioning vertigo, paroxysmal brainstem attacks, vestibular migraine, somatoform phobic postural vertigo, an occlusion syndrome of the vertebral artery (dependent on head position) and central positional/positioning nystagmus.

The differential diagnosis is generally not very problematic because of the characteristic brevity (seconds up to a few minutes) of the frequently recurring attacks of vertigo. Only paroxysmal brain stem attacks with vertigo and, for example, ataxia, can be difficult to distinguish because they too respond to low dosages of carbamazepine. It is assumed that they are caused by a brain stem lesion, for example, multiple sclerosis or infarction, which also leads to errors in the transmission of ephaptic activation to neighboring fibers of the brainstem paths. In such cases, the use of MRI of thin brain stem slices is expedient for establishing the diagnosis.

Benign paroxysmal positioning vertigo due to canalolithiasis can be diagnosed by the typical crescendo-decrescendo nystagmus caused by the positioning maneuver. This sign does not typically occur with vestibular paroxysmia and is triggered as regularly by positioning.

Pathophysiology

It is assumed that a neurovascular cross-compression of the VIIIth cranial nerve is the cause of the short episodes of vertigo that occur in trigeminal neuralgia, hemifacial spasm, glossopharyngeal neuralgia or oblique-superior myokymia (Brandt and Dieterich 1994a; Møller et al. 1986). Aberrant, in part arteriosclerotically elongated and dilated, and consequently more pulsating arteries in the cerebellopontine angle are thought to be the pathophysiological cause of a segmental pressure-induced lesion with demyelination of the central myelin. A loop of the AICA seems to be most often involved. The symptoms are trig-

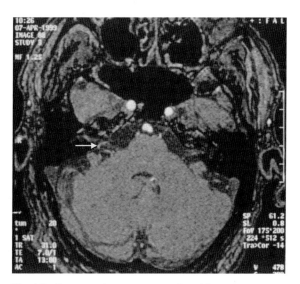

Fig. 6.3. Neurovascular cross-compression of the vestibulo-cochlear nerve by a loop of the anterior inferior cerebellar artery (arrow) in an MRI with 3D-CISS sequences (three-dimensional constructive interference in steady-state sequences) with a resolution of 0.5 mm and a slice thickness of 0.7 mm.

gered by direct pulsatile compression and/or ephaptic discharges, such as pathologically paroxysmal interaxonal transmission between neighboring and in part demyelinized axons. Another cause under discussion is central hyperactivity in the nucleus, which is induced and maintained by the compression. Finally, in addition to elongation and increased looping, a vascular malformation or arterial ectasia of the posterior fossa can also cause the nerve compression.

Despite signs of an arterial compression of the VIIIth cranial nerve, the definite consequences of which are visible on MRI (CISS; Fig. 6.3), prospective clinical studies are still lacking as to how frequent such neurovascular contacts can be imaged. These studies are necessary because neurovascular contacts are also seen in healthy persons, thus raising the question of which region of the myelin sheath of the vestibulo-cochlear nerve is the most vulnerable (distance measured precisely in millimeters from the nerve exit zone out of the brain stem). For patients with oblique superior myokymia of the trochlear nerve, a neurovascular contact was determined 0 to 1 mm from the nerve exit zone, whereas a neurovascular contact was proven in 14% of healthy subjects at a mean distance of 3.4 mm (Yousry et al. 2002).

In addition to neurovascular contact, vertigo attacks lasting seconds and occasionally caused by head movements point to an arachnoid cyst that stretches across the vestibulocochlear nerve (Brandt et al. 2005). This pathogenesis can result in a combination of longer-lasting lesion symptoms in one direction (hours to days) and paroxysmal symptoms of excitation (for seconds) in the opposite direction.

Therapy

Therapy with a low dosage of carbamazepine or oxcarbamazepine (200–600 mg/day) is expedient and useful for establishing the diagnosis (Brandt and Dieterich 1994a). In cases of intolerance gabapentine, valproic acid or phenytoin are possible alternatives. Despite the report of partial successes (Møller et al. 1986), operative microvascular decompression should be avoided for two reasons: On the one hand, there is the danger of intra- or postoperative vasospasms that could lead to a brainstem infarction (around 3–5%), and on the other, the affected side cannot be determined with sufficient accuracy. However, if there are additional causes, such as the aforementioned arachnoid cyst in the cerebellar pontine angle, the operation is recommended because drug therapy only rarely leads to a complete absence of symptoms.

Central vestibular forms of vertigo

To differentiate central vestibular forms of vertigo from other forms, it is helpful to refer to the duration of the symptoms:

- Short: Rotatory or postural vertigo attacks lasting seconds to minutes or for a few hours are caused by transient ischemic attacks within the vertebrobasilar territory, basilar migraine/vestibular migraine, paroxysmal brainstem attacks with ataxia/dysarthria in multiple sclerosis and the rare vestibular epilepsy.
- Hours to several days long: Persisting rotatory and postural vertigo attacks, generally with additional brainstem deficits, can be caused by an infarction, hemorrhage, or multiple sclerosis plaque in the brain stem, seldom by a long-lasting basilar migraine attack.
- Several days to weeks: Permanent postural vertigo which is seldom permanent rotatory vertigo, are combined with a tendency to fall and usually caused by persisting damage to the brain stem or the cerebellum bilaterally, for example, downbeat

nystagmus syndrome due to Arnold-Chiari malformation or upbeat nystagmus syndrome due to paramedian pontomedullary or pontomesencephalic damage, which suggests infarction, hemorrhage, multiple sclerosis plaques or tumor.

Vestibular migraine

Definition and epidemiology

The main symptoms of basilar type of migraine are recurring attacks of various combinations of vertigo, ataxia of stance and gait, visual disorders and other brain stem symptoms accompanied or followed by occipitally located head pressure or pain, nausea and vomiting which last for seconds, minutes or hours. As any movement increases the complaints, patients often have a need for rest. If the attacks of vertigo are associated with other brain stem symptoms, more rarely also disturbances of consciousness, psychomotor deficits or changes of mood, one speaks of basilar type of migraine. However, the attacks can also be monosymptomatic, manifesting with only vertigo and perhaps also with a hearing disorder; then they are called vestibular migraine. Monosymptomatic audiovestibular attacks predominate in about 75% of such cases if vertigo or dizziness is the cardinal symptom (Dieterich and Brandt 1999). They are more difficult to recognize if the headache is missing, which is the case about 30% of the time (Dieterich and Brandt 1999).

The frequency of vestibular migraine amounts to 7% to 9% in special outpatient clinics for dizziness (Dieterich and Brandt 1999; Neuhauser et al. 2001). The prevalence of vestibular migraine is not known. Naturally, the prevalence of migraine without aura is clearly higher and has a one-year rate of 12% to 14% for females after puberty and 7% to 8% for males after puberty. Women are affected two to three times more often than men. The duration of attacks of vertigo varies greatly and lasts either seconds to minutes or several hours to days (Cutrer and Baloh 1992; Dieterich and Brandt 1999; Neuhauser et al. 2001).

Originally, basilar type of migraine was described by Bickerstaff (1961) as a typical illness of adolescence, which clearly predominated in females. However, retrospective studies have shown that basilar type of migraine with dizziness and vestibular migraine can develop throughout the patient's entire life, most often between the third and sixth decades (Dieterich and Brandt 1999; Neuhauser et al. 2001). The mean age of women at its first occurrence was approximately 38, and that of men around 42. The ratio of women and men affected is 1.5:1.

Diagnosis

If the attacks are usually or always followed by occipital pressure in the head or a headache and if there is a positive family or personal history of other types of migraine (about 50%), the diagnosis is easy. It is easier to establish the diagnosis if the following symptoms occur: light and sound hypersensitivity, need for rest, tiredness after the attack and urine urge. A number of authors have called for the introduction of a new category into the classification of migraine named "vestibular migraine" or "migraine with vestibular aura" for auras with clearly rotatory vertigo or positional vertigo, excluding nonspecific vertigo sensations, analogous to hemiplegic or ophthalmoplegic migraine (Brandt and Strupp 2006; Neuhauser and Lempert 2004; Olesen 2005). The "vertigo experts" have therefore agreed to the *diagnostic criteria* proposed by Neuhauser and coworkers (2001), which are based on a combination of migraine symptoms and associated vertigo attacks:

1. Recurrent attacks with vestibular vertigo
2. Migraine without aura according to the IHS classification
3. Migraine symptoms during at least two vertigo attacks (migraine headache, phonophobia, photophobia, aura symptoms)
4. Exclusion of other causes of vertigo

When all of the above criteria are fulfilled, the term "certain vestibular migraine" is applied, whereas the term "probable vestibular migraine" is used if three of these criteria are met. Contrary to other forms of migraine, more than 60% of persons with vestibular migraine also show slight central ocular motor disorders during attack-free intervals, which manifest by a gaze-evoked nystagmus, smooth-pursuit saccades beyond those normal for the patient's age, a horizontal or vertical spontaneous nystagmus or central positional nystagmus (Dieterich and Brandt 1999; Neuhauser et al. 2001). The patients are generally hypersensitive to movements and motion sickness, particularly during the migraine attack (Cutrer and Baloh 1992). This is similar to phonophobia and pho-

tophobia during migraine attacks, which is induced by a neuronal sensory overexcitability, for example, of the inner-ear receptors.

Differential diagnosis

Differentiating vestibular migraine from transient ischemic attacks, Menière's disease or vestibular paroxysmia can occasionally be difficult. In some cases, the diagnosis can only be established on the basis of the patient's response to a "specific" therapy. Transitional and mixed forms or pathophysiological combinations are now being recognized especially for Menière's disease and vestibular migraine. Currently, there are no reliable data, in part because patients with primarily vestibular symptoms are more frequently misdiagnosed as having Menière's disease.

Since BPPV occurs three times more frequently in migraine patients than in trauma patients, according to a recent retrospective study (Ishiyama et al. 2000), it has been speculated that a relapsing functional deficit in the inner ear could be the underlying cause of the migraine attacks, for example, in the form of a vasospasm. The therapy for benign paroxysmal positioning vertigo in migraine patients corresponds to the liberatory maneuvers used to treat idiopathic benign paroxysmal positioning vertigo.

The rare episodic ataxia type 2 is also characterized by episodic attacks of dizziness with central ocular motor deficits, even during the attack-free interval. In this situation a trial of acetazolamide can be successful.

Transient ischemic attacks (TIA) in the vertebrobasilar system, basilar artery thrombosis, and brain stem/cerebellum hemorrhage can also accompany headache centered primarily in the nuchal region. These important symptoms should be rapidly clarified in a differential diagnosis. Basilar artery thrombosis and brain stem hemorrhage usually develop quite rapidly along with vigilance disorders and can worsen to coma, increasing deficits of the cranial nerves and paresis, or sensory deficits in the extremities. A vertebral artery dissection can occur after head trauma or chiropractic maneuvers. It is associated with occipital head and neck pain, neck pressure, dizziness and other brain stem symptoms. Because brain stem ischemia, which is induced in the context of various mechanisms, is part of the differential diagnoses that have acute life-threatening significance, it is especially important to consider the possibility of this dangerous brain stem ischemia during the appearance of the first or first three migraine attacks to quickly obtain adequate diagnostic testing.

Pathophysiology

As regards the pathogenesis of vestibular migraine, it is interesting that the rare episodic ataxia type 2, which is due to a mutation of a gene on chromosome 19p in the calcium channel, occurs in several families in combination with hemiplegic migraine, which is due to a mutation which is also located on chromosome 19 (Ophoff et al. 1996). Moreover, the central findings in the ocular motor system during the symptom-free interval, as in episodic ataxia, also indicate that patients with vestibular migraine may have a hereditary neuronal disorder in the brain stem or cerebellar nuclei, perhaps a channelopathy. Neuronal deficits in the brainstem are also discussed as factors in the pathophysiology of migraine without aura. The serotonergic dorsal raphe nucleus in the midbrain seems to play an important role. PET studies have shown that this region and that of the dorsal pons including the nucleus coeruleus are also activated in patients during migraine attacks without aura (Weiller et al. 1995).

Therapy

The same principles of therapy that have proven effective in migraine without aura are used to treat the attacks as well as for migraine prophylaxis, although the symptoms of dizziness and the accompanying headache can respond differently. To stop attacks lasting 45 minutes and longer, it is advisable to administer an antiemetic, such as metoclopramide or domperidone, early and in combination with a non-steroidal antiphlogistics, such as ibuprofen or diclofenac, and an analgesia such as acetylsalicylic acid as soluble tablet or paracetamol as a suppository, or an ergotamine such as ergotamine tartrate. The triptans, which are very effective against migraine attacks without aura and act at the 5-HT$_{1B/1D}$ receptors of the vessels, are contraindicated for the treatment of migraine with aura because of the danger of a cerebral or cardiac infarction due to the drug-induced vasoconstriction of the arteries. However, in individual cases they have been reported to have also positive effects on attacks of vertigo.

The treatment of first choice for migraine prophylaxis is the administration of the beta-receptor blocker metoprolol retard (100 mg/day) for about six months or topiramate (100 mg/day), valproic acid (600–1200 mg/day), lamotrigine (50–100 mg/day) and the calcium antagonist flunarizine (1–2 capsules, 10 mg per capsule, in the evening). Sometimes a combination of two medications is necessary for a few months, for example, metoprolol plus topiramate. In a retrospective study a significant benefit of the migraine prophylaxis was proven (Baier et al. 2009).

Vertebrobasilar ischemia

Another differential diagnostic possibility for central vestibular paroxysmal vertigo attacks is the transient ischemic attack within the vertebro-basilar system, a disease of the elderly. However, isolated vertigo attacks or isolated vertigo attacks with hearing loss are not typical. Single or a very few (up to five) attacks may take place, but over time additional brainstem symptoms, such as dysarthria, double vision, numbness or drop attacks, regularly occur in varying combinations and to different extents. This syndrome is due to the steep pressure gradient from the aorta to the long circumferential terminal pontine arteries, which provide a highly vulnerable blood supply to the vestibular nuclei in the pontomedullary brainstem. A central vestibular vertigo syndrome – for example, in the yaw or roll plane – results. In addition to arteriosclerosis of the small arteries, there is rarely found a functional compression of the vertebral artery secondary to atheromas or cervical spondylosis or osteophytes, which narrow the transverse foramina. In such cases, vertigo, postural imbalance and nystagmus are induced when the head is maximally rotated or extended while standing. Because the blood supply to the inner ear, the labyrinthine artery, originates from the anterior inferior cerebellar artery, it is also possible that transient ischemia of a labyrinth can cause these transient attacks of vertigo. A rare mechanism is that of the "rotatory vertebral artery occlusion syndrome," that is, when the one vertebral artery is occluded by head rotation while the other is significantly hypoplastic. This leads to recurrent transient ischemic attacks of the medullary brainstem.

Antiplatelet agents and anticoagulants or dilatation of the stenotic artery may be effective for therapy.

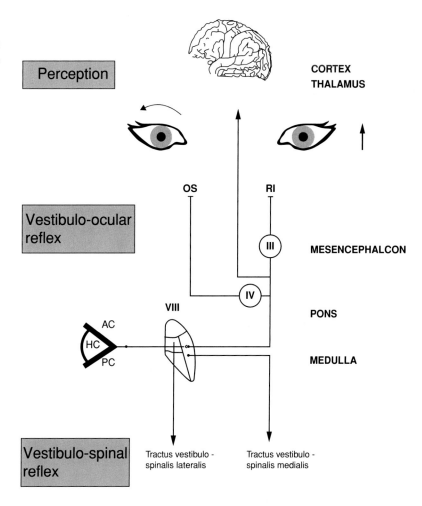

Fig. 6.4. Schematic drawing representing the vestibulo-ocular reflex (VOR) with its three-neuron reflex arc and its mediation of ocular motor, perceptual, and postural functions (reproduced with permission from Brandt et al. 2005).

Perception

Vestibulo-ocular reflex

Vestibulo-spinal reflex

CORTEX
THALAMUS

MESENCEPHALCON

PONS

MEDULLA

OS RI

III

IV

VIII

AC
HC
PC

Tractus vestibulo -
spinalis lateralis

Tractus vestibulo -
spinalis medialis

Central vestibular syndromes in the three planes of action of the vestibulo-ocular reflex

Central vestibular forms of vertigo are caused by lesions along the vestibular pathways, which extend from the vestibular nuclei in the medulla oblongata to the ocular motor nuclei and integration centers in the rostral midbrain, and to the vestibulocerebellum, the thalamus and multisensory vestibular cortex areas in the temporoparietal cortex (Brandt et al. 2005; Brandt and Dieterich 1995; Fig. 6.4). These forms of vertigo are often clearly defined clinical syndromes of various etiologies, with typical ocular motor, perceptual and postural manifestations that permit a topographic brain stem diagnosis. The analysis of nystagmus can also be helpful for localizing the lesion site (Büttner

et al. 1995). This section discusses such typical findings in detail. Depending on the size and site of the lesion, central vestibular syndromes can occur in isolation or as part of a complex infratentorial syndrome. Additional symptoms of supranuclear or nuclear ocular motor disorders and/or other neurological brainstem deficits can also occur, for example, Wallenberg's syndrome with ocular tilt reaction as well as Horner's syndrome, sensory deficits, ataxia, dysarthria and dysphagia.

The most important structures for central vestibular forms of vertigo are the neuronal pathways for mediating the vestibulo-ocular reflex (VOR; Fig. 6.4). They travel from the peripheral labyrinth over the vestibular nuclei in the medullar brain stem to the ocular motor nuclei (III, IV, VI) and the supranuclear integration centers in the pons and midbrain, which include the interstitial nucleus of Cajal (INC) and rostral interstitial nuclei of the medial longitudinal fasciculus (riMLF; Brandt and Dieterich 1994b, 1995). This three-neuronal reflex arc makes compensatory eye movements possible during rapid head and body movements. It is thus crucially responsible for regulating the ocular motor system. Another branch of the VOR system runs over the posterolateral thalamus up to the vestibular areas in the parietotemporal cortex, such as the parietoinsular vestibular cortex (PIVC), area 7, the inferior parietal lobule, and areas in the superior temporal gyrus, which are primarily responsible for perception of self-motion and orientation. Descending pathways lead from the vestibular nuclei along the medial and lateral vestibulospinal tract into the spinal cord to mediate postural control. In addition, there are also pathways to the vestibulocerebellum and to the hippocampus. Thus, disorders of the VOR are not only characterized by ocular motor deficits but also by disorders of perception due to impaired vestibulocortical projections of the VOR and by disorders of postural control due to impaired vestibulospinal projections of the VOR.

Central vestibular syndromes are the result of lesions of these pathways caused by infarction, hemorrhage or tumor, by multiple sclerosis plaques or, more seldom, by pathological irritations such as paroxysmal brain stem attacks (with ataxia and dysarthria) as occur in multiple sclerosis or in vestibular epilepsy. Table 6.2 provides an overview of ischemic lesions (Fig. 6.5) caused by lacunar or territorial infarctions in

Table 6.2 Overview of symptoms and lesion sites

Syndrome of the VOR	Clinical symptoms and lesion site
Horizontal plane (yaw)	"Vestibular pseudoneuritis," spontaneous horizontal nystagmus, horizontal past-pointing to the right/left (subjective straight-ahead), postural instability, falling tendency to one side, turning in the Unterberger-step test Unilateral lesions affecting the vestibular nucleus
Sagittal plane (pitch)	Downbeat nystagmus (DBN), upbeat nystagmus (UBN), deviation of the subjective horizontal upward or downward, postural instability with falling tendency forward or backward UBN: bilateral lesions of the medullary or ponto-mesencephalic brainstem at midline, midpontine lesion DBN: medullary lesions at midline and between the vestibular nuclei, bilateral flocculus lesions
Frontal plane (roll)	Ocular tilt reaction, skew deviation, ocular torsion, head tilt, deviation of the subjective visual vertical (SVV) clockwise or counterclockwise, postural instability withfalling tendency to one side Ipsilateral signs in unilateral pontomedullary lesions (vestibular nucleus), contralateral signs in ponto-mesencephalic lesions (MLF, INC)

the region of the central vestibular system along with the typical clinical syndromes and the arteries responsible.

Vestibular syndromes in the horizontal (yaw) plane are rare, for example, horizontal benign paroxysmal positioning vertigo due to a canalolithiasis in the horizontal canal of the labyrinth. As far as we know, central syndromes in yaw are caused only by lesions in the area of the entry zone of the vestibular nerve in the medulla oblongata, the medial and/or superior vestibular nuclei and the neighboring integration centers for horizontal eye movements, the nucleus prepositus hypoglossi and paramedian pontine reticular formation (Fig. 6.5). Other clinical signs are ipsilateral caloric hypo-responsiveness, horizontal gaze deviation, falling tendency to the affected side and a past-pointing corresponding to a deviation of the "subjective straight-ahead." The clinical symptoms are similar to those of an acute peripheral vestibular lesion as occurs in vestibular neuritis, and thus is also called "vestibular pseudoneuritis" (Fig. 6.6).

The most common causes include multiple sclerosis plaques or ischemic infarctions within the

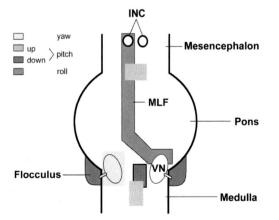

Fig. 6.5. Schematic drawing of the brain stem and cerebellum with the typical sites of lesions that induce vestibular syndromes in the three planes of the VOR yaw, pitch and roll (III, IV, VI, VII cranial nerve nuclei; MLF = medial longitudinal fasciculus; riMLF = rostral interstitial nucleus of the medial longitudinal fasciculus; INC = interstitial nucleus of Cajal).

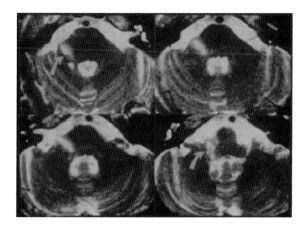

Fig. 6.6. MRI of a patient with "vestibular pseudoneuritis," a disorder of the VOR in the yaw plane. The T2-weighted and T1-weighted sequences show a pontomedullary brain stem infarction, which extends into the cerebellar peduncle and impairs the fascicle of the VIIIth cranial nerve as well as the region of the medial vestibular subnucleus.

vestibular nuclei or fascicles. If the lesion extends beyond the vestibular nuclei, other accompanying brain stem symptoms can be detected. Because a unilateral medullary ischemic or an inflammatory brain stem lesion are generally present, the prognosis is favorable because central compensation takes place over the opposite side. The symptoms can be expected to resolve slowly within days to weeks. Thus, central compensation together with simultaneous treatment of the underlying illness can be promoted by early balance training.

Vestibular syndromes in the sagittal (pitch) plane have so far been attributed to lesions in the following three sites: in the medullary and pontomedullary brain stem, paramedian bilaterally; the pontomesencephalic brainstem with the adjacent cerebellar peduncle; and the cerebellar flocculus bilaterally (Fig. 6.5).

The downbeat nystagmus syndrome (DBN) is characterized by a fixational nystagmus that is frequently acquired. It beats downward in primary gaze position, is exacerbated on lateral gaze and in head-hanging position, may have a rotatory component, and is accompanied by a combination of visual and vestibulocerebellar ataxia with a tendency to fall backward and past-pointing upward. The syndrome is frequently persistent. DBN is often the result of a bilateral lesion of the flocculus or the paraflocculus, for example, intoxication due to anticonvulsant drugs or caused by lesions at the bottom of the fourth ventricle or the cerebellum. Fifty percent are of unknown etiology; 25% of patients have craniocervical junction anomalies such as the Arnold-Chiari malformation, 20% have cerebellar degeneration and, more seldom but in decline, lesions secondary to multiple sclerosis (Wagner et al. 2008). It can more rarely be caused by a paramedian lesion of the medulla oblongata, by conditions like multiple sclerosis, hemorrhage, infarction or tumor.

Upbeat nystagmus (UBN) is rarer than downbeat nystagmus. It is also a fixation-induced nystagmus that beats upward in primary gaze position, and is combined with a disorder of the vertical smooth pursuit eye movements, a visual and vestibulospinal ataxia with a tendency to fall backward, and past-pointing downward. The anatomic location of most acute lesions is either near the median plane in the medulla oblongata in neurons of the paramedian tract (PMT), close to the caudal part of the perihypoglossal nucleus, or near the median plane in the tegmentum of the pontomesencephalic junction, the brachium conjunctivum, the pontine brain stem and probably in the anterior vermis. The symptoms persist for several weeks but are not permanent.

The course and prognosis depend on the underlying illness. It is therapeutically expedient to treat the symptoms of persisting downbeat or upbeat nystagmus syndrome by administering gabapentin (3 × 200 mg/day p.o.), baclofen (3 × 5–15 mg/day p.o.), clonazepam (3 × 0.5 mg/day p.o.), or 4-aminopyridine (up to 3 × 20 mg/day p.o.; Brandt et al. 2005).

Vestibular syndromes in the vertical (roll) plane indicate an acute unilateral deficit of the "graviceptive" vestibular pathways, which run from the vertical canals and otoliths over the ipsilateral medial and superior vestibular nuclei and the contralateral medial longitudinal fasciculus (MLF) to the ocular motor nuclei and integration centers for vertical and torsional eye movements (INC and riMLF) in the rostral midbrain (Brandt and Dieterich 1994b, 1995; Fig. 6.7). More rostral to the midbrain, only the vestibular projection of the VOR for perception in the roll plane (determination of the subjective visual vertical, SVV) runs over the vestibular subnuclei in the posterolateral thalamus to the PIVC in the posterior insula. The crossing of these pathways at the pontine level is especially important for topographic diagnosis of the brain stem. All signs of lesions in the roll plane whether a single or a complete ocular tilt reaction, that is, head tilt, vertical divergence of the eyes, ocular torsion, SVV deviation, show an ipsiversive tilt (ipsilateral eye is lowermost) in both the very rare, unilateral peripheral

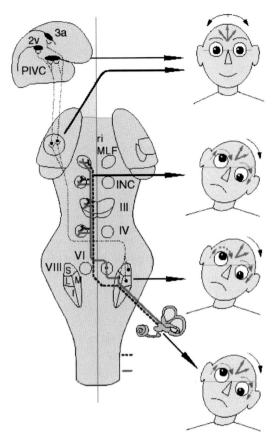

Fig. 6.7. Pathway of the roll plane.

tions of the paramedian thalamus (in 50% of cases) is caused by a simultaneous lesion in the paramedian rostral midbrain (INC and riMLF). Unilateral lesions of the posterolateral thalamus can cause thalamic astasia with moderate ipsiversive or contraversive SVV tilts, which indicate involvement of the vestibular thalamic subnuclei. This generally resolves within a matter of days or a few weeks. Unilateral lesions of vestibular cortex areas (e.g. the PIVC) cause moderate, mostly contraversive SVV tilts lasting several days. Perceptual deficits in the sense of pathological deviations of the SVV occur during unilateral deficits along the entire VOR projection and are one of the most sensitive signs of acute brain stem lesions, occurring in 90% of cases of acute unilateral infarctions. If instead of a functional deficit due to a lesion there is an excitation of the VOR projection on one side, the same effects will be triggered but in the opposite direction. If a torsional nystagmus occurs in the acute phase, the rapid nystagmus phase will be in the opposite direction of the tonic skew deviation and the ocular torsion.

The etiology of these unilateral lesions is frequently an infarction of the brainstem or the paramedian thalamus, which extends into the rostral midbrain. The course and prognosis depend also here on the etiology of the underlying illness. Often, one can count on a significant, generally complete recovery from the symptoms in the roll plane within days to weeks due to the central compensation over the opposite side.

References

American Academy of Ophthalmology and Otolaryngology. Committee on Hearing and Equilibrium guidelines for diagnosis and evaluation of therapy in Meniere's disease. *Otolaryngol, Head and Neck Surgery* 1995, **113**:181–185.

Baier B, Winkenwerder E, Dieterich M. "Vestibular migraine": Effects of prophylactic therapy with various drugs. A retrospective study. *J Neurol* 2009, **256**:436–442.

Baloh RW, Jacobson K, Honrubia V. Horizontal semicircular canal variant of benign positional vertigo. *Neurology* 1993, **43**:2542–2549.

Bickerstaff ER. Basilar artery migraine. *Lancet* 1961, I:15–17.

Blakley BW. Update on intratympanic gentamicin for Menière's disease. *Laryngoscope* 2000, **110**:236–240.

Brandt T. *Vertigo: its multisensory syndromes.* 2nd edn. London: Springer, 1999.

vestibular lesion or the more frequent pontomedullary lesion (medial and superior vestibular nuclei). The pathology is below the crossing in the brainstem. All signs in the roll plane (ocular motor, perceptual and postural) exhibit contraversive deviations (contralateral eye is lowermost) for unilateral pontomesencephalic lesions of the brain stem above the crossing and indicate a deficit of the MLF or of the supranuclear nucleus of the INC. In some cases an isolated perceptual deficit with an ipsilateral tilt of SVV was also seen in unilateral lesions of the anteromedial pontomesencephalic brain stem affecting a novel ipsilateral graviceptive pathway that runs from the vestibular nuclei close to and within the medial lemniscus to the posterolateral thalamus (ipsilateral vestibulothalamic tract, IVTT)(Zwergal et al. 2008). Unilateral lesions of vestibular structures located rostral from the INC manifest with only perceptual deficits (deviation of the SVV) without accompanying ocular motor deficits or head tilt. Ocular tilt reaction in unilateral infarc-

Brandt TH, Daroff RB. Physical therapy for benign paroxysmal positional vertigo. *Arch Otolaryngol* 1980, **106**:484–485.

Brandt T, Dieterich M. Vestibular paroxysmia: vascular compression of the 8th nerve? *Lancet* 1994a, **343**:798–799.

Brandt T, Dieterich M. Vestibular syndromes in the roll plane: topographic diagnosis from brainstem to cortex. *Ann Neurol* 1994b, **36**:337–347.

Brandt T, Dieterich M. Central vestibular syndromes in roll, pitch, and yaw planes. Topographic diagnosis of brainstem disorders. *Neuro-ophthalmology* 1995, **15**:291–303.

Brandt TH, Dieterich M, Strupp M. Vertigo and dizziness. *Common complaints*. London: Springer, 2005.

Brandt T, Steddin S, Daroff RB. Therapy for benign paroxysmal positioning vertigo, revisited. *Neurology* 1994, **44**:896–900.

Brandt T, Strupp M. Migraine and vertigo: classification, clinical features, and special treatment considerations. Clinical review. *Headache Currents* 2006, **3**: 12–19.

Büttner U, Helmchen C, Büttner-Ennever JA. The localizing value of nystagmus in brainstem disorders. *Neuro-ophthalmology* 1995, **15**:283–290.

Claes J, van de Heyning PH. Medical Treatment of Menière's disease: a review of literature. *Acta Otolaryngol (Stockh) Suppl* 1997, **526**:37–42.

Cutrer FM, Baloh RW. Migraine-associated dizziness. *Headache* 1992, **32**:300–304.

Dieterich M, Brandt TH. Episodic vertigo related to migraine (90 cases): vestibular migraine? *J Neurol* 1999, **246**:883–892.

Fife TD, Iverson DJ, Lempert T, et al. Practice parameter: therapies for benign paroxysmal positional vertigo (an evidence-based report): Report of the Quality Standards Subcommittee of the American Academy of Neurology. *Neurology* 2008, **70**:2067–2074.

Herdman SJ, Tusa RJ, Zee DS, Proctor LR, Mattox BE. Single treatment approaches to benign paroxysmal vertigo. *Arch Otolaryngol Head Neck Surg* 1993, **119**:450–454.

Ishiyama A, Jacobson KM, Baloh RW. Migraine and benign positional vertigo. *Ann Otol Rhinol Laryngol* 2000, **109**:377–380.

James A, Thorp M. Menière's disease. *Clinical Evidence* 2001, **5**:348–355.

Lempert TH, Tiel-Wilck K. A positional maneuver for treatment of horizontal-canal benign positional vertigo. *Laryngoscope* 1996, **106**:476–478.

Levat E, van Melle G, Monnier P, Maire R. Efficacy of the Semont maneuver in benign paroxysmal positional vertigo. *Arch Otolaryngol Head Neck Surg* 2003, **129**:629–633.

Magnusson M, Padoan S, Karlberg M, Johansson R. Delayed onset of ototoxic effects of gentamicin in treatment of Menière's disease. *Acta Otolaryngol (Stockh)* Suppl 1991, **481**:610–612.

Minor LB, Solomon D, Zinreich JS, Zee DS. Sound- and/or pressure-induced vertigo due to bone dehiscence of the superior semicircular canal. *Arch Otolaryngol Head Neck Surg* 1998, **124**:249–258.

Minor LB, Cremer PD, Carey JP, Della-Santina CC, Streubel SO, Weg N. Symptoms and signs in superior canal dehiscence syndrome. *Ann NY Acad Sci* 2001, **942**:259–273.

Møller MB, Møller AR, Jannetta PJ, Sekhar L. Diagnosis and surgical treatment of disabling positional vertigo. *J Neurosurg* 1986, **64**:21–28.

Neuhauser H, Lempert T. Vertigo and dizziness related to migraine: a diagnostic challenge. Review. *Cephalgia* 2004, **24**:83–91.

Neuhauser H, Leopold M, von Brevern M, Arnold G, Lempert T. The interrelations of migraine, vertigo and migrainous vertigo. *Neurology* 2001, **56**:436–441.

Olesen J. Vertigo and dizziness related to migraine: a diagnostic challenge. Letter to the editor. *Cephalgia* 2005, **25**:761–763.

Ophoff RA, Terwindt GM, Vergouwe MN, et al. Familial hemiplegic migraine and episodic ataxia type-2 are caused by mutations in the Ca2+ channel gene CACNL1A4. *Cell* 1996, **87**:543–552.

Parnes ES, McClure JA. Posterior semicircular canal occlusion in normal hearing ear. *Otolaryngol Head Neck Surg* 1991, **104**:52–57.

Schuknecht HF. Cupulolithiasis. *Arch Otolaryngol* 1969, **90**:765–778.

Singleton GT. Diagnosis and treatment of perilymph fistulas without hearing loss. *Otolaryngol Head Neck Surg* 1986, **94**:426–429.

Strupp M, Huppert D, Frenzel C, et al. Long-term prophylactic treatment of attacks of vertigo in Menière's disease – comparison of a high with a low dosage of betahistine in an open trial. *Acta Otolaryngol* 2008, **128**:620–624.

Van Cauwenberge PB, De Moor SEG. Physiopathology of H3-Receptors and pharmacology of betahistine. *Acta Otolaryngol (Stockh)* 1997, **526**:43–46.

Vanucchi P, Giannoni B, Pagnini P. Treatment of horizontal semicircular canal benign paroxysmal positional vertigo. *J Vestib Res* 1997, 7:1–6.

Wagner JN, Glaser M, Brandt T, Strupp M. Downbeat nystagmus: aetiology and comorbidity in 117 patients. *J Neurol Neurosurg Psychiatry* 2008, **79**:672–677.

Weiller C, May A, Limmroth V, Jüpter M, Kaube H, van Schayck R, Coenen HH, Diener HC. Brain stem activation in spontaneous human migraine attacks. *Nat Med* 1995, **1**:658–660.

Yabe T, de Waele C, Serafin M, Vibert N, Arrang JM, Mühlethaler M, Vidal PP. Medial vestibular nucleus in guinea-pig: histaminergic receptors. *Exp Brain Res* 1993, **93**:249–258.

Yousry I, Dieterich M, Naidich TP, Schmid UD, Yousry TA. Superior oblique myokymia: Magnetic resonance imaging support for the neurovascular compression hypothesis. *Ann Neurol* 2002, **51**:361–368

Zwergal A, Büttner-Ennever J, Brandt T, Strupp M. An ipsilateral vestibulo thalamic tract adjacent to the medial lemniscus in humans. *Brain* 2008, **131**:2928–2935.

Further Reading

Baloh RW, Halmagyi GM (eds.). *Disorders of the vestibular system*. New York, Oxford: Oxford University Press, 1996.

Baloh RW, Honrubia V (eds.). *Clinical neurophysiology of the vestibular system*. Philadelphia: FA Davis, 1990

Paroxysmal visual disturbances

Hans Wolfgang Kölmel and Christina Kölmel

Visual function is continuous during wakefulness. The system constantly analyzes information and is an essential component of maintaining alertness. Any change or apparent disruption of the input signal is immediately detected upon its initiation. Visual disturbances appear when the activity's constancy, an indispensable precondition of perception and our confidence in this perception, is no longer maintained due to functional or structural lesions in the brain.

Such impairments are manifest in various forms. Most have a structural etiology with different degrees of expression. They can be of a "negative" character, in the case of scotoma, or they can be of a "positive" one, where suddenly perceptions appear, which exceed what is natural, normal or expected. The latter will be described in this chapter.

Vision in the blind field

It has often been described that despite the loss of vision, patients still have maintained rudimentary visual perception (Matthews and Kennard 1993). They are able to perceive light stimuli that reach the anopic field, to detect and to locate them. A possible explanation for this phenomenon is the presence of a secondary, archaic visual field, which lies beyond the primary visual field, through connections from the lateral geniculate body or from the pulvinar of the thalamus. These forms of perception are not classified under the "paroxysmal" category.

Homonymous scotoma result as a consequence of a central lesion. Vision in a scotoma can be manifest in many ways, for example, as "paroxysmal," confusing both the patient who is affected as well as the examining doctors. This phenomenon of paroxysmal vision in scotoma becomes apparent as the patient can suddenly perceive and recognize objects in their anopic field. This can be either in the center or in the periphery of the field. Often the image is present only for a fraction of a second. Immediately following this, the ability "to see" is again lost, and the previous blindness in this area returns. The patient may suddenly see, for example, a few letters or a word or two in a newspaper and can consequently read them, but then reports immediately afterward that they can no longer see anything in the same position. Such paroxysmal "positive" visual ability suggests that there is still partial or residual function in the damaged structures that have resulted in the anopia, but this function is transient. However, this can be a good prognostic sign with respect to the improvement of an anopia.

Delusions

Delusions are subjective perceptions and do not correspond to that generally accepted as reality. They are individual misperceptions and can be mistaken for "false" realities. Visual delusions usually appear paroxysmally. Since Esquirol's description (1838), we separate delusions into illusions and hallucinations. Illusions deal with the conversion from perception of outer stimuli, which many times are determined individually and not necessarily categorized as pathological phenomena. In contrast, hallucinations are a pure endogenous product and occur more likely as a pathological discharge pattern. Usually, they do not show any relation between an outer stimulus and the corresponding sense organs. If we agree to adhere to the original definition of illusion – (fre.) *delusion, imagination* – and hallucination – (lat.) *to babble, to talk nonsense* – it appears that these definitions are more or less arbitrary. Actually, if both terms are evaluated for their practicality, one repeatedly encounters difficulties in the clinical field. This applies especially for vestibular delusions. It also applies to some forms of visual delusions, for example, visual perseverations, which can usually be counted among illusions but are also able to be categorized as hallucinations in many ways.

However, a phenomenological differentiation of delusions into illusions and hallucinations is generally useful. Both forms of visual delusions have typical clinical characteristics, which presumably account for different pathophysiological correlates. Thus, we differentiate between the true illusions or hallucinations and pseudo-illusions or hallucinations. The affected person cannot distance themselves from the true illusions. They are convinced that these correspond to reality and are "objective" perceptions. Conversely, the affected person recognizes pseudo-illusions/hallucinations as not corresponding to reality but rather phenomena, which arise from "within themselves," and then deals with them accordingly. People are more conspicuous if they have true illusions or hallucinations. These are often distressing, and the patient so states. If the patient regards their sudden delusions as the unreal truth, then they rarely complain and are almost never identified or are so only after being requested.

Differentiations can be made between:

Visual delusions, especially hallucinations, which appear in the physiological visual field,

In-field hallucinations (campine), and

Out-of-field hallucinations (extra-campine), which appear outside the visual field, perhaps beyond the affected person.

Usually, hallucinations appear within the physiological visual field. Out-of-field hallucinations are the exception. The hallucinations are reported by people in great affliction or in fear of death, for example, by those in distress at sea, who have recounted a protective hand or a guardian angel behind an endangered seaman. They can also occur as an epileptic aura alone or an aura preceding a seizure. They should be especially obvious and characteristic in Lewy body dementia (Harding, Broe and Halliday 2002). Sometimes suddenly, and sometimes slowly, the patient sees off to the side or behind him people who are of normal height and without relation to him. He lives with them and stays relatively unaffected by the delusions. These are usually true hallucinations.

Anyone studying visual delusion cases for the first time may think that it has less to do with neuroscience and more to do with meaningless phenomena. That is the reason why seldom will a patient volunteer

Table 7.1 Visual delusions in neurological diseases

– Migraine

– Vision loss due to ophthalmological disease

– Vision impairment due to lesions of the central visual pathway, mostly as a result of a posterior cerebral artery stroke

– Lesions in the thalamus or upper brainstem (peduncular hallucinations)

– Epilepsy

– Hypnagogic or hypnopompic states, for example, in narcolepsy

– Parkinson's disease

– Dementia

to report their misperceptions spontaneously. Many simply choose to ignore them or are understandably overcome by other discomforts or symptoms, which dominate this disease pattern, such as headaches, partial or total vision loss, that they have no sense of such secondary phenomena. Others live in fear of being labeled insane because they are unable to control their seemingly bizarre actions in response to the delusions they are experiencing. They try at all costs to avoid mentioning their delusions to others. Listening carefully to patients and not being distracted by other symptoms will easily show that delusions in general, and particularly visual delusions, play no small role in brain pathology. The acknowledgement of what is possible in visual delusions vis-à-vis plausible central vision impairment enriches diagnostic statements, and ultimately leads not only to a better understanding of what literally takes place before the patient but also of what may frighten them and what must be overcome.

Most visual delusions occur within a short timeframe, usually when visual impairment first develops or ultimately resolves. Most only last for seconds or fractions of seconds, and on rare occasions for days or weeks. Some tend to appear at night, others in mornings or evenings. Some develop slowly; others suddenly or are just suddenly noticed. Their nosological classification requires accurate semiology. Usually, there are other complaints or neurological findings to be dealt with to be able to correctly classify the disease pattern. Table 7.1 summarizes neurological (and neuro-ophthalmological) diseases, which are typical for visual delusions.

Visual illusions

A broad spectrum of visual illusions can occur in association with lesions of the visual pathway. These

Table 7.2 Objects' characteristics and corresponding illusionary alterations

Axis	– Images are tilted or inverted
Distance	– Pelopsia or teleopsia
Size	– Macropsia or micropsia
Form	– Metamorphopsia
Color	– Dyschromatopsia or achromatopsia
Brightness	– Pallor or blending
Movement	– Slow motion or fast motion
Number	– Diplopia or polyopia (multiple vision)
Extinction	– Perseveration
Memory	– Déjà vu or jamais vu

delusions tend initially to scare the patients considerably, although they are usually less dramatic than those unrelated to lesions of the visual pathway, namely those due to intoxication, either during or immediately after drug consumption, or conversely after withdrawal, and those delusions of delirium or psychosis. Depending on the dominant disturbance of the object, different forms of visual illusions can be distinguished (Table 7.2).

Thus, disorders with changed axial perception lead to tilted or inverted pictures. They are often the result of cerebellopontine lesions. Changed perception of size, macropsia or micropsia, allude to occipitotemporal lesions, changed perception of color allude to occipital lesions and changed brightness allude to occipital or thalamic lesions, whereas déjà vu or jamais vu indicate mesial-temporal lesions.

Visual perseveration

Visual perseveration occurs when the complex neuronal system for image extinction or suppression, which performs tasks in the retina, the lateral geniculate body and in the occipital and temporal lobes, is damaged. Visual perseveration is persistence of an image in the absence of its original external stimulus. Immediately after the external stimulus disappears, or after a certain latency period, the patient develops the impression that all or part of the stimulus persists. Even though it may appear different, the external stimulus is still recognizable as the source of the perception.

Visual perseveration of a perception in the absence of its stimulus may occur as a physiological or a pathological phenomenon. For example, retinal afterimages indicate physiological perseveration, whose detailed analysis dates from Purkinje (Grüsser 1984). Another

example of physiological visual perseveration include the so-called "images in memory" (Müller 1846), also the eidetic phenomena (Jaensch 1930) and déjà vu. Déjà vu gives the affected person the impression that they have already seen a particular visual scene. However, because this impression is not accompanied by a visual experience or perception it does not constitute genuine perseveration.

All forms of visual perseveration occur paroxysmally, and if they are the result of a brain lesion are usually unilateral and then contralateral to the lesion. Thus, many patients see the image lateralized but still almost directly in front of themselves, not in the periphery of the anopic field but instead in the transitional zone between the anopic and the intact field. Feldmann and Bender (1970) were of the opinion that visual perseveration only occurs during the development or the remission of homonymous anopia, as is the case with photopsias. They never occur in complete anopia because the capacity for visual perception is lost in this situation.

These illusions are subdivided depending on how much time elapses between the perception of reality and its revised illusionary appearance. They are categorized into immediate perseveration, palinopsia and hallucinatory palinopsia (Bekeny and Peter 1961; Kölmel 1982). Visual perseveration with its different facets has been described with numerous neurological diseases, as in the context of epilepsy (Swash 1979), intracranial tumor (Critchley 1951), cerebral infarction (Kömpf et al. 1983), migraine (Klee and Willanger 1966) or traumatic brain injury (Kinsbourne and Warrington 1963). The brain lesion is more often in the right hemisphere and predominately occipitally localized, but visual perseveration is certainly not generated by any one specific region of the brain.

Immediate perseveration

Le Beau and Wolinetz (1958) accurately described immediate perseveration as the true form of visual perseveration. The object disappears out of the visual field as a result of its own motion or displacement of the patient's gaze but the image is sustained, giving the impression of continuity between the perception of reality and illusion. The persistent image is so clear and distinct that it obscures real objects, and it is easy to understand why the patient initially mistakes the image for reality. The contours and colors of the illusion closely resemble those of the original. The persistent image maintains a constant relation to the coordinates of the retina or acts like a retinal after-image and moves with the gaze. The persistent image tilts with head movement. In most cases it is motionless, although there are reports of illusions moving like the original images (Cleland, Saunders and Rosser 1981). The illusion usually disappears suddenly, often within seconds or up to a maximum of several minutes, generally after its colors pale or its contours have become distinct. There is an obvious relationship between these perceptions and physiological afterimages, especially to those experienced in dazzling light. It is conceivable that prolonged afterimages might be the result of incomplete or delayed inhibition and could contribute to visual perseveration. However, studies of these images in affected people failed to produce consistent results. Some investigators have described conspicuously prolonged afterimages (Blythe et al. 1986), whereas others found none at all (Bender et al. 1968).

Whether or not prolonged afterimages could lead to immediate perseveration, there are characteristic differences between the two. Afterimages appear in front of a bright background in complementary colors, whereas illusions are independent of their background and appear in their original colors. Persistent images may demonstrate some degree of stereotyped motion, whereas afterimages are always stationary. There is a direct relationship between the intensity and duration of the original image and those of afterimages, but there is no evidence for such a relationship in the case of immediate perseveration.

Palinopsia

Palinopsia means "seeing again," meaning there is a latency period from several seconds to somewhat more than one hour, rarely some days, between perception of an object and a second illusionary experience. The time between can last from seconds to hours and sometimes for days. Just as with immediate visual perseveration, the objects seen in palinopsia correspond so greatly with the formerly seen true object that the patient initially cannot distinguish between the reality and palinopsia. Eye movement does not extinguish these illusions. On the contrary, they move synchronously with the view or appear repeatedly wherever the eye is focused.

Each episode can last several minutes and even occasionally extend over an entire day. The images are usually incomplete, representing single details such as a head, an eye, an arm or a sign. The assortment of

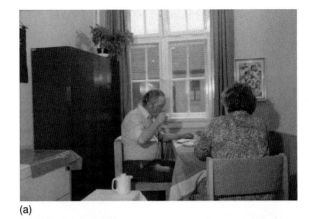

(a)

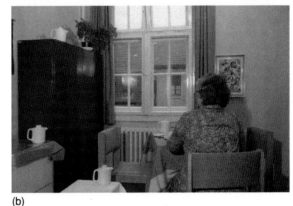

(b)

Fig. 7.1. Domestic situation of a patient. (a) Situation before the search for the coffeepot. (b) The husband lets the guest in. The patient searches for the coffeepot to pour the guest some coffee. Anywhere she looks, the pot appears.

details seen is not random. They are always meaningful for the patient or the current situation. Contrary to physiological afterimages, these perceptions do not change in size dependent on the projection's distance. They are more likely to adapt to the current environment. There are often symbolic relationships between the perceptions and the patient's surroundings, which can irritate the affected person and hinder the chance to distinguish the perceptions as illusions (Kölmel 1982; Kömpf 1983).

Case report

A 68-year-old patient (Fig. 7.1) had sustained right homonymous hemianopia as result of a left occipital brain infarction. She recovered fairly well. Partial vision was possible again in the right visual field. In the first six months of her disease, she repeatedly experienced palinopsia. She reported, for example, "As I searched for the coffee pot in order to pour some coffee for a guest who had just arrived, it was impossible for me to find the actual pot. Anywhere I looked, on the chair, the cupboard, the table… the coffee pot appeared, but without actually being there. I experienced similar perceptions sometimes multiple times per day."

Pötzl (1954) has termed this characteristic of palinopsia *"kategoriale Einordnung,"* which is consistently semantic or category specific. It could be possible that this displays a distinct visual logic. One searches for the coffee pot only in those places where it might be, and for taxi-stand signs only where they should be attached. Although no corresponding observation for this exists, it could be assumed that palinopic images keep their coordinates constant and retain their categorical arrangement even when the head is tilted. In any case, these characteristics suggest that cerebral processes independent of the retina may generate palinopsia.

Various casuistic data reveals how different the pathogenesis of visual palinopsia can be: epilepsy, intracranial tumor, cerebral infarction, migraine, traumatic brain injury and so on. The brain lesion is always contralateral to the side of perseveration. When the lesion is lateralized, it more often is on the right hemisphere. Critchley named the place of the lesion the occipital lobe, whereas Le Beau and Wolinetz (1958) pinpointed the lesion occipital and in adjacent brain regions. Results from computed tomography show always occipital, next to occipitoparietal and particularly occipitotemporal brain lesions (Cleland, Saunders and Rosser 1981; Kölmel 1982). It is assumed that the pathomechanisms for the different forms of visual perseverations are not identical, not connected and accordingly also not connected to certain lesion patterns.

Hallucinatory palinopsia

Rarely, the interval between the actual perception and illusionary recurrence can be up to days or weeks. In such a case, it is difficult to classify these phenomena as illusion. Pötzl therefore formed the concept of hallucinatory palinopsia (Pötzl 1954). Such palinopsia is extinguished by head or eye movement, which is less typical for perseveration images but more typical for complex hallucinations.

Visual perseveration and epilepsy

Just as with trying to distinguish between photopsias and complex hallucinations, it is difficult to differentiate between visual perseveration related to epilepsy and to non-epileptic causes. Swash (1979) described two patients who experienced visual perseveration during a partial epileptic seizure. There was no defect of their visual fields. From the descriptions, it was not possible to determine whether the perseveration was restricted to one visual hemifield, but it is unlikely. The same applies for the two patients, in whom Critchley (1951) described visual perseveration as the aura of a partial epileptic seizure without lateralization or homonymous visual field defect. The stated examples indicate that when visual perseveration is not lateralized and does not occur in connection with a homonymous visual field defect, it is most likely to represent an epileptic aura.

Visual perseveration which is lateralized to the side of the visual field defect is more likely a non-epileptic phenomenon. It is then generally an isolated phenomenon, independent from other positive motor or sensory symptoms and not mediated by cortical impulse propagation. This is the result of either the activation or the failure of inhibition of a specific neuronal pathway (Kinsbourne and Warrington 1963).

Polyopia

Polyopia presents a special type of visual perseveration. The patient suddenly sees a fovea-fixed object multiple times, not distributed randomly but rather like a string of pearls (Kömpf et al. 1983). The phenomenon is possible when the fixed object or the patient moves. In our experience, eye movement alone is rarely sufficient to cause this phenomenon. The appearance of double or multiple images is dependent on the velocity of the head movement and the severity of the brain lesion, and consequently the visual field defect. The distances of the outer images of this sequence correspond to the distance, which the patient or the object have created, but also to the angle of the saccade. One of the peripheral images corresponds to the original, whereas the second corresponds to the new point of fixation. Therefore, the outermost images are more distinct while the intermediate ones are identical in size and shape but have weaker outlines.

Either the object moved just before in front of the patient or the patient moved their eyes. The number of perseverated images and the frequency of their position are dependent on the velocity of the simultaneous movement. There is no clear explanation for the pathology of polyopia. Saccadic eye movement usually extinguishes the previous retinal image and allows perception of a new object of fixation. This effect appears to be disturbed in polyopia, which is explained partially by the function of the retina but also by other mechanisms (i.e., the awakening reaction or as the result of ocular movement). Excessively strong and prolonged afterimages may contribute to the development of polyopia.

Polyopia is a poor localizing sign. Often it appears in early stages of central vision failure, or when a vision failure recedes, for example, after hypoxia or during the recession of brain edema.

Monocular diplopia

Diplopia is a common sequela of eye muscle paresis. When one eye is closed, one image disappears and only the remaining image perceived by the eye, which is still open, is received; therefore, no diplopia occurs. Monocular diplopia is present even when one eye is closed. In the absence of pathological findings in the eye, patients with monocular double vision should be investigated for disease of the central visual pathway before a psychiatric diagnosis – for example, conversion syndrome – is considered.

There are few reports in the medical literature to date regarding monocular diplopia, although the phenomenon is not rare. The double image appears directly next to the real one. It always appears laterally in the direction of the relative or absolute visual field defect. It is not always found in a horizontal plane but may be slightly above or below the level of the true image. The visual field defect is not necessarily large, and monocular diplopia has even been reported adjacent to paracentral scotoma (Safran 1981).

The pathophysiology has yet to be elucidated. It is conceivable that conduction in the central visual pathway loses normal inhibition or that alteration in neuronal transmission results in a second pathway parallel to the original. It is also possible that diplopia is a manifestation of the fact that retinal neurones project to multiple different points on the visual cortex (Hubel and Wiesel 1965, 1968, 1972).

Visual hallucinations

Visual hallucinations can be simple or complex in nature. The simple hallucinations, often termed phosphenes (or photopsias), include colored or colorless perceptions, points, stars, lines, curves, circles, sparks or flames, singular or multiple, identical or contrasting, grouped or diffused, spread throughout

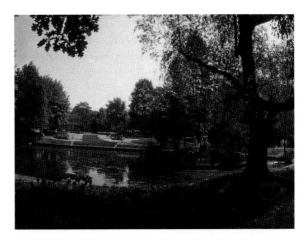

Fig. 7.2. Fortification lines in the right visual field approximately 8 minutes after the beginning of a visual aura of a migraine.

or in a part of the visual field. Complex hallucinations include the perception of single images, people or objects, motionless or in moving sequences or whole scenes. Visual hallucinations as the result of neuro-ophthalmological diseases are usually considered unreal by the patient, and are then termed pseudo-hallucinations. However, altered consciousness or inadequate visual matching of the objects seen within their environment, for instance by ocular, retinal, or central amblyopia or anopia, can limit the patient's ability to discriminate between reality and delusion. In the last case, the patient may be tempted to act as though complex hallucinations represent reality.

Photopsias

Photopsias, also called phosphenes or photomes, appear in different diseases. Before a neurological disorder is taken into consideration, diseases of the eye or intoxication and side-effects of medicine should be excluded. A systematic phenomenological description of the phenomenon of photopsias can be found by Gloning and collaboration (1967) and Kölmel (1984).

Photopsias in migraine

From the different visual symptoms which can accompany migraines (photopsias, complex hallucinations, dysmorphopsia, perseveration) special observations can be deduced from the so-called "fortification pattern" (Charcot 1886). This pattern ranges from colorless, very bright and lightly oscillating lines to a brilliant starburst (Fig. 7.2). It begins small and concentric, in direct juxtaposition to the fovea, and then extensively disturbs the vision, creating the impression that one has something in their eye but something not recognizable in a definite form. It is not until the pattern moves out of the central visual field, slowly initially then growing and speeding up, advancing toward the periphery of the visual field, that one can actually see the jagged pattern.

Photopsias are most often blinding, glare, white, consequently colorless, thus patients are usually only left with a memory of these characteristics. Exact observations also reveal colored parts of photopsias. After 15 to 20 minutes, they disappear. A narrow scotoma immediately follows them. During the photopsias or shortly thereafter, contralateral temporal headaches occur. Many of these auras also continue without the associated headaches. The regular angular pattern of the "fortification lines" correspond to the structures of the visual cortex, here particularly to the Area V_1 (Corwey and Rolls 1974; Richards 1971). This disturbance in the form of a continuous discharge begins immediately in the area of foveal representation, collecting in adjacent regions and spreading with continual and constant speed over the primary visual cortex. Accelerated extension with simultaneous enlargement of the photopsias is related to changes in the retinocortical magnification factor. The images are smallest near the fovea and increase in area to the periphery of the visual field. This is the result of an anatomical specialty whereby the neurons are layered in a homogenous concentration in the visual cortex, but cortical representation of the fovea is much larger than that of the peripheral retina.

Migraines' visual aura is thought to be triggered by ischemia. However, its expression is that of a pure neuronal phenomenon, namely in the initial discharge activity and the subsequent prostration depolarization or the spreading depression (Leao 1944). This is how a partly narrow, partly much wider, lightly flickering zone trails after a spreading starburst fortification pattern into an area of the visual field where it can no longer be seen. This scotoma, which originated subjectively as a blending effect, is then also frequently coupled with light sensitivity and expanding sometimes into a homonymous hemianopsia.

Case report

Silva B. has suffered since childhood with typical migraines. At the age of 15, she primarily experienced occipitally localized encephalitis of unclear etiology. She recovered from the severe disease. Fatiga-

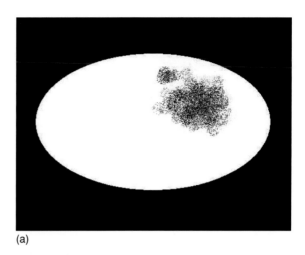

(a)

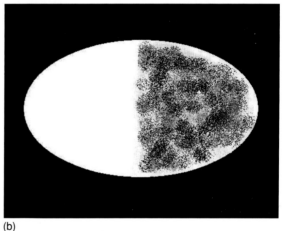

(b)

Fig. 7.3. Photopsias (a) in right visual field as partial epileptic seizure, and (b) filling almost the entire right visual field; a grand mal seizure is imminent (see color plate section).

bility in her central vision remained with correlation to a coarse shape of the occipital gyration. Since this episode of encephalitis, Silva experiences daily photopsias in her left visual field. She has sketched this (Fig. 7.3a, b) and writes, "The flicker can be in all areas of my visual field, but predominantly occurs on the left side. Sometimes in larger, sometimes in smaller areas, and occasionally also involving the entire half (of the visual field). It is composed of many small, colored dots, which flash variably. This is how this ungodly mess takes place. I can no longer see in this area. The remaining part of my vision is sharp, but I must discontinue my work and wait, until everything is gone, because I get distracted from these kinds of flickers. This can sometimes take a couple of seconds to 15 minutes. When the flickering occurs on the right side I

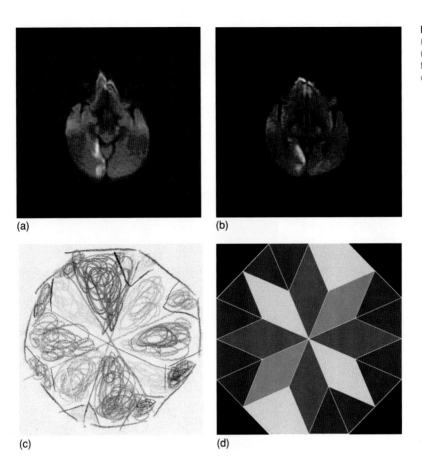

Fig. 7.4. Occipito-mesial brain infarction (right). (a, b) MRI of a head with DWI. (c) Photopsias of a patient in his left visual field, sketch of the patient. (d) Translation of the sketch (see color plate section).

have to be especially careful and concentrate intensely. Now there is the danger that I may lose consciousness and suffer a grand mal. This has happened four times in the four years since my disease began."

The interpretation of the symptoms is not so simple. It would have been even more difficult without the knowledge that the patient suffered from occipital encephalitis. Then one can assume, for example, that it is a case of idiopathic occipital epilepsy of adolescence. It seems possible that in this patient the photopsias occurring on the left side of the visual field is the symptom of a migraine, and if occurring of the right side of the visual field is the symptom of partial epilepsy.

Photopsias in the hemianopic field

A large portion of patients with occipital brain infarction are able to report photopsias in the hemianopic field. Occasionally, photopsias also precede the visual field defect. Photopsias are usually formed geometrically, sometimes monochrome, sometimes colored, or others in light white or in gray. They can appear for hours singularly, in groups or temporarily as "fireworks."

In the diversity of photopsias, one group stands out as repeatedly described by patients. Here it deals with very light squares or hexagons almost blending together, whose planes are the base colors of blue, yellow, red and green, and they are characteristically assembled in a design (Fig. 7.4a–d). They obviously reflect, again, a functional matrix of the visual cortex with at least stimulation of the orientation- and color-coding neurons. Their appearance indicates the functional ability of the substrate, and they may actually also be considered a beneficial prognostic sign (Kölmel 1984). How they should be nosologically categorized is unclear. It could be an ictal phenomenon (i.e., partial epileptic seizures) and, moreover, a matter of the status of focal seizures. On the other hand, it has never been reported that a generalized seizure had ever developed from such ictal phenomena.

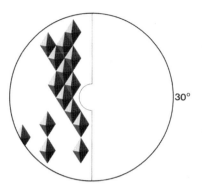

Fig. 7.5. Sharp, brightly colored pattern in left visual field immediately before the development of a homonymous hemianopsia left after infarction in the supply area of the right posterior cerebral artery (see color plate section).

Ultimately, such photopsias do not apply as evidence that epilepsy could later develop. Photopsias are probably more likely interpreted, as with migraines, as the expression of a locally terminated, self-limiting excitation.

Case report

Suddenly one night, a 72-year-old retired teacher experienced extremely colorful photopsias in his left visual field (Fig. 7.5). The photopsias appeared spatial in a pattern of pyramids lying adjacent to each other, where every side is either red, green, blue or yellow. The photopsias appear in a flash, and for fractions of a second very bright in different areas of the visual field, most often near the foveal area. Never having experienced this and very frightened, the man goes to the hospital emergency room. All findings are normal. The next morning a homonymous hemianopsia occurs on the left side. The photopsias now appear only sporadically. The imaging of the brain reveals a right-sided, relatively small infarction in the calcarine gyrus.

If the hemianopsia is completely evolved and persistent for weeks, then no spontaneous episodes of photopsias will occur. If this is still the case, then a partial epileptic seizure should be considered.

Complex hallucinations

Complex hallucinations and epilepsy

Such hallucinations can be quite varied, although an individual patient during seizures tends to repeatedly perceive the exact same hallucinations. If the character of the hallucinations changes, then a change in brain morphology should be assumed, for example, an increase of a brain tumor. Sometimes the hallucinations begin as photopsias, only in one half of the visual field, and then change over the course of the seizures into complex hallucinations involving the entire visual field. This is commonly a sign of occipital to temporal lobe excitation spread. Often the photopsias appearing hemispherically are followed by a tonic homolateral versive eye or head movement. Sometimes the patients report they wanted "to watch the photopsias." However, the tonic movement is involuntary, providing a clue for the spreading of the cortical discharge, and therefore a sign that a generalization is imminent. If the hallucinations in an epileptic seizure appear primarily as complex, then often no lateralization is recognizable. The patients, who primarily experience complex visual hallucinations, also lose consciousness more quickly than those whose aura initially began with photopsias.

The pathogenesis of such hallucinations is diverse; the visual hallucinations in epilepsy are most frequently the result of a traumatic brain injury, cerebral hemorrhage or, occasionally, cerebral ischemia or tumor.

Case report

Seventeen-year-old Oliver K. is on his way home in an unfamiliar city. Other adolescents, whom he asked for directions to the train station, pursue him. He tries to find protection in a telephone booth. For no reason, they pull him out and hit him multiple times with a baseball bat. The next day, his mother brings her somnolent son to the hospital. A subdural hematoma has developed under a compression fracture and must be operatively evacuated (Fig. 7.6).

About three months later, he experiences his first epileptic seizure: a round, colored disk appears in the right visual field. It grows concentrically into larger disks, which respectively turn and overlap one another. Suddenly, the outermost disk takes on a starburst shape and, almost at the same time, an object in the center of the circles appears which he had seen shortly before the seizure, often also a telephone booth. At this moment, he loses consciousness. The seizure initially begins purely partially, with photopsias in one half of the visual field. The photopsias are generated in different, contralaterally situated regions of the visual cortex. The discharges widen, then suddenly move to the outward temporal lobe (identifiable as palinopsia) and become a complex partial seizure.

The context of the experiences, which have played decisive roles directly or in connection with the trauma, are seen revised in the visual aura and have

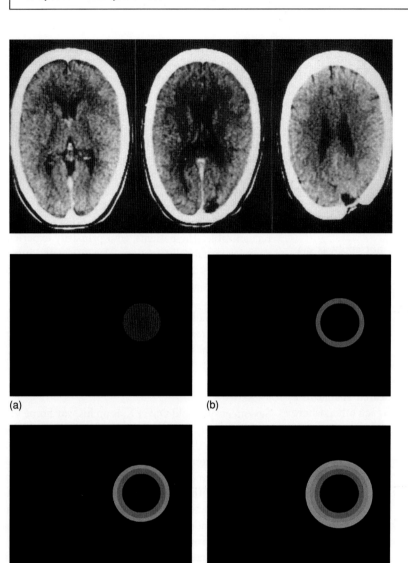

Fig. 7.6. Left occipital brain contusion after violent trauma.

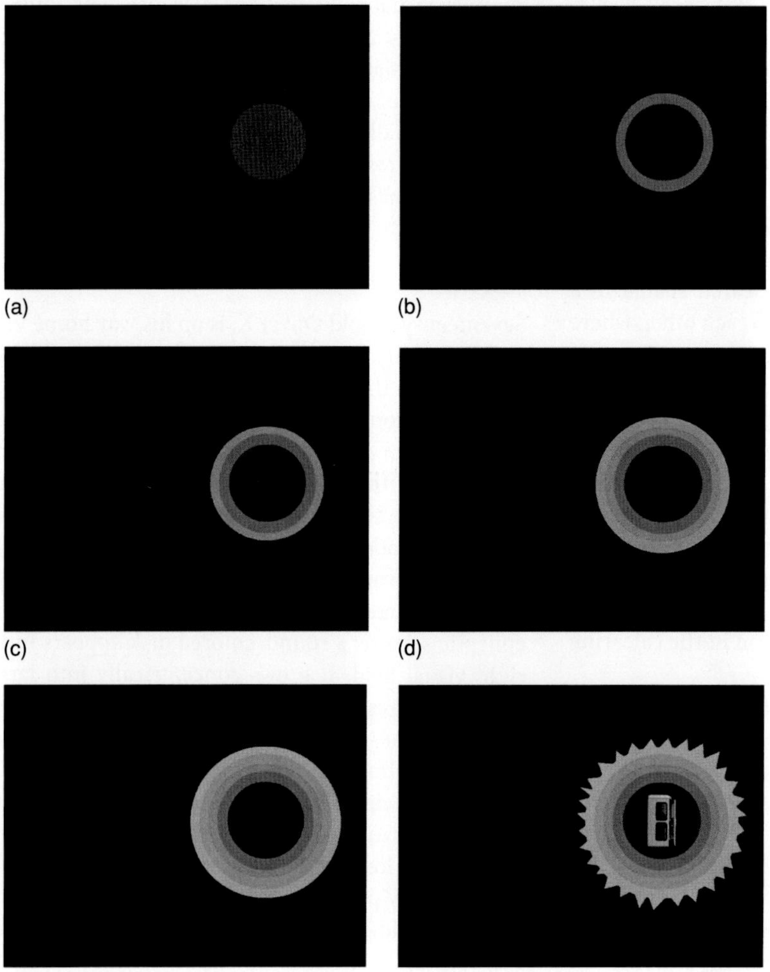

(a)

(b)

Fig. 7.7. Photopsias in right visual field with visual perseveration ("*Erregungsfang*") as partial epileptic seizure. Result of a brain contusion occipital on the left (see color plate section).

(c)

(d)

(e)

(f)

been identified by Pötzl (1954) as "*Erregungsfang*" (flashback) (Fig. 7.7a–f). A specific scene has been "branded" onto the brain and will always be recalled more quickly than others.

However, visual hallucinations in epilepsy also occur without morphological correlate to the brain. With idiopathic photosensitive epilepsy of the occipital lobe, the seizures are often triggered by strobe

Table 7.3 Characteristics of Charles Bonnet hallucinations

- Only visual in nature
- Over the entire visual field
- Often moving and multicolored
- With great variety, never stereotypical
- What is seen is often smaller than in actuality
- Eye movement extinguishes the hallucinations (temporarily)
- Episodes last several seconds to several minutes
- No connection with a specific time of day
- Can recur over a period of weeks to months
- Initially true, later increasingly pseudo-hallucinations

lights or other similar quickly changing light intensities. The seizures begin with seeing sharp, bright, small or large dots, usually in the periphery of the visual field, and often initially in small groups. Then they broaden quickly and it amounts to further symptoms, gaze deviation, symptoms of the temporal lobe and often also headaches.

Charles Bonnet syndrome

Eye diseases which lead to severe bilateral reduction of vision diminish the physiological flow of visual stimuli or can cause its complete disruption. The relatively prevalent hallucinations are then combined under the term "Charles Bonnet syndrome" (Table 7.3).

In the middle of the eighteenth century, Bonnet described the hallucinations of his grandfather, who suffered from an ophthalmological disease. As fate would have it, at a later age Bonnet himself experienced the same kind of hallucinations in the context of vision impairment (Berrios and Brock 1982). One should only be dealing with visual hallucinations under the term Charles Bonnet syndrome, which should occur in people as a result of their pronounced, acquired visual impairment. Due to the conspicuous connection of hallucinations with an eye disease, the term *"hallucinations des ophthalmopathes"* has been coined in French literature. It is in no way a rare phenomenon or mainly limited to the elderly. Why the hallucinations of elderly people do attract attention is due to the fact that older people have difficulties in identifying the hallucinations as unreal. Olbrich (1987) believed that reductions in the attention span observed in the elderly are responsible for these hallucinations. This is questionable, like the concept that the hallucinations allude to the onset of dementia. Likewise, the hallucinations appear also in younger people who later become blind, with whom one can have no reason to assume an age-related brain disease, for example, due to arteriosclerosis.

A psychodynamic interpretation of the origin and content of these hallucinations may be more plausible. Most apply to creative people for whom sight has been an essential way of communication and who suffer greatly at the loss. Hallucinations are more common when impairment of vision occurs rapidly and unexpectedly. They occur most often with acute-onset blindness, for example, as a result of retinal hemorrhage, retinal infarction or traumatic damage of the eyeball.

The hallucinations usually disappear within several months after the visual disorder develops. However, they may reappear in situations of physical or emotional stress. The therapy should be individually tailored. This always begins with assuring the patient that the perceptions are not real. In addition, psychotherapy may be useful to help the patient understand the association between the loss of sight and the appearance of the hallucinations.

Medication (e.g., neuroleptic drugs) is seldom successful and should only be tried in exceptional cases.

Peduncular hallucinations

In 1922, Jean Lhermitte described a patient who suffered from vivid visual hallucinations. His symptoms alluded to lesions in the midbrain and pons, and Lhermitte assumed that the mesencephalic lesion was particularly the cause of the hallucinations. Sometime later, van Bogaert (1927) described similar hallucinations with a patient. Because the autopsy of the deceased revealed lesions in the pedunculi cerebri, van Bogaert created the term "peduncular hallucinations". However, this term reveals nothing about the cause of the hallucinations and was not very precise, as Lhermitte and van Bogaert as well as others later found lesions, which were located in the mesencephalon and thalamus (Caplan 1980). The thalamus and especially the reticular formation in the thalamus and mesencephalon are more likely the crucial structures – as they are "portals for awareness" – for the pathogenesis of such hallucinations. Mostly these lesions are the result of a cerebral infarction, especially as a "top of the basilar" syndrome.

Such complex hallucinations are rare; often they are misjudged as psychiatric phenomena. The characteristics shown in Table 7.4 are always to be continually monitored. Usually, further neurological

Table 7.4 Characteristics of peduncular hallucinations

– Hallucinations are visual but can also be additionally auditory or somatosensory in nature

– Cover the entire visual field

– Versatile, motile, but more likely lacking in color

– Episodes last seconds to minutes

– Occur over a period of days to weeks

– Appear predominantly in evenings, by twilight or in the night

– Pertain to true hallucinations

– Effect of eye movement is not known

Table 7.5 Characteristics of hallucinations in the hemianopic field

– Exclusively visual

– Only in the hemianopic field

– Vivid but stereotyped, rarely animated, usually lacking in color

– Objects are usually smaller than in reality

– Eye movement extinguishes the hallucinations

– Length of individual episodes is seconds to minutes

– No limitation with regard to the time of day

– Total length of time is days to weeks

– Pseudo-hallucinations

symptoms are observed, such as ophthalmoplegia, ataxia and disturbance of circadian rhythm and of the consciousness.

Complex hallucinations in the hemianopic field

Complex hallucinations observed in the hemianopic field are a relatively common phenomenon (Fig. 7.2). As in other forms of sensory deprivation, here the physiological flow from the "outer world" to the "inner world" is discontinued. The anopic field becomes a projection screen for already saved visual engrams. Because the "outer world" can be registered relatively unaltered by means of the intact contralateral visual pathway, the hallucination's correct categorization is quickly perceived by affected persons. That means that the patients can associate their misperception with their visual impairment and can recognize it as unreal. Therefore, they have critical advantages over those patients with Charles Bonnet syndrome or with peduncular hallucinations, where a correction is not possible offhand, once through the severe binocular vision impairment, once through the disturbance of consciousness.

The hallucinations in the hemianopic field (Table 7.5) are to be understood as deprivation or release-phenomena and not as ictal phenomenon. Complex hallucinations which are symptoms of a partial or initially partial epileptic seizure appear in the entire visual field and are only lateralized as an exception. Generally, the entire visual field is maintained or exhibits only marginal, usually hidden, functional losses. However, the epileptic visual aura can be followed with a homonymous quadrant- or hemianopsia equivalent to the Todd phenomenon.

Visual hallucinations never occur simultaneously with the onset of the visual field defect; several hours to several days elapse before the anopic field is used as a projection screen. The hallucinations always disappear when function in the visual field returns. If the visual field defect persists, hallucinations occur less frequently over the succeeding days, weeks or months and ultimately cease altogether.

The perceptions never correspond with complete reality. They are colorless, usually infused with different grey or brown tones. Often the patients have the impression that the persons or objects they see are smaller than in reality. Many hallucinations are static and fixed, others demonstrate proper motion. They consistently awaken memories of a specific object not seen for quite a while, or of certain scenes, which were actually experienced. Sometimes they give the impression that one has just seen their own image. Such a reduplicative hallucination (heautoscopy) occasionally appears with febrile illness. It has also been described as a visual aura preceding epileptic seizures (Lhermitte 1951; Janz 1969). If the self-image appears younger, which is not rare, the patients may not recognize what they are seeing until the image appears multiple times, or after being questioned with an analytical technique.

A connection between hemianopic complex hallucinations and the person's pool of experiences cannot be denied, and it is to be expected that similar principles govern the development of visual hallucinations and dreams. Visual hallucinations appear initially as unrecognizably disguised, occurring seemingly senselessly and unrelated, but then reveal after exact analysis the connection between the patients' entire personal collection of experiences, to their wishes, fears and perceptions of the world.

All patients have the experience that the hallucinations disappear then, just when they want to examine them more closely. Many patients then use these

Table 7.6 Characteristics of complex visual hallucinations as an epileptic aura

- Predominantly in the entire visual field
- No loss of visual field
- Episodes last for seconds
- Identical or similar images from seizure to seizure
- True hallucinations
- No extinguishing effect by saccades
- Related to tonic head turning
- Connected with vegetative symptoms

Table 7.7 Conditions and findings, which occur concurrently with hypnagogic hallucinations (Mavromatis 1987)

- Psychophysical relaxation
- Reduced perception of outer and inner stimuli
- Reduction in ability to be awakened from sleep
- Tendency toward passiveness
- Reduction of conscious thought process
- Psychological withdrawal/recession
- Introversion
- Quicker thought alternation
- Deceleration of EEG waves

mechanisms to rid themselves of the hallucinations. Complex hallucinations in the hemianopic field are thus extinguished by saccadic eye movement. During the visual aura of an epileptic seizure, this only appears exceptionally (Table 7.6).

No definite ideas exist about the localization of brain lesions which generate the hallucinations as well as the hemianopsia. Two morphological findings stand out as essential for complex hallucinations: the first is the occipital lesion, which has created the hemianopsia and has interrupted the physiological stimulus transmission to the parietal and especially temporal lobes, and the other is the further rostral, primarily mesiotemporal lesion (also in the form of an edema), which is responsible for the occurrence of visual engrams (Kölmel 1985). It is still debatable whether the hallucinations have a tendency toward being generated from lesions in the left or right brain hemispheres. Lance (1976) believed that the lesion is predominantly seen in the right hemisphere under the notion that the more rational section is represented by the left and the more emotional and non-verbal by the right hemisphere. However, in larger samples no preferences to brain hemispheres have been found (Kölmel 1985).

Hypnagogic and respectively hypnopompic hallucinations

Such hallucinations appear in the transitional phase from wakefulness to sleep and vice versa, and are therefore considered physiological. In EEGs, occipital, predominantly alpha waves are still observed. Generally, complex hallucinations develop slowly from simple hallucinations and to some extent from entopic phenomena, which occur even more in sleep phase 1. They are often found pleasant and sleep-supporting. Hypnagogic hallucinations with narcolepsy occur in a

sleep phase, where inability of movement exists and rapid-eye movements are observed. These hallucinations are less pleasant, often developing into nightmares. Table 7.7 summarizes the conditions and findings, which accompany the occurrence of hypnagogic hallucinations.

Literature

(See original edition in German.)

References

Bekeny G, Peter A. Über Polyopie und Palinopsie. *Psychiatria Neurologia* 1961, **142**:154–175.

Bender MB, Feldman M, Sobin AJ. Palinopsia. *Brain* 1968, **91**:321–338.

Berrios GE, Brook P. The Charles Bonnet syndrome and the problem of visual perceptual disorders in the elderly. *Age Ageing* 1982, **11**:17–23.

Blythe IM, Bromley JM, Ruddock KH, Kennard C, Traub M. A study of systematic visual perception involving central mechanisms. *Brain* 1986, **109**:661–675.

Caplan LR. "Top of the basilar" syndrome. *Neurology* 1980, **30**:72–79.

Charcot JM. Über Migraine ophthalamique in der Initialperiode der progressiven Paralyse. *In:* Freud S. (ed.) *Neue Vorlesungen über die Krankheiten des Nervensystems insbesondere über Hysterie*. Leipzig: Toeplitz & Deuticke, 1886, pp. 60–61.

Cleland PG, Saunders M, Rosser R. An unusual case of visual preservation. *Journal of Neurology, Neurosurgery and Psychiatry* 1981, **44**:262–263.

Corwey A, Rolls ET. Human cortical magnification-factor and its relation to the visual acuity. *Exp Brain Res* 1974, **21**:447–454.

Critchley M. Types of visual perseveration "palinopsia" and "illusory visual spread." *Brain* 1951, **74**:267–299.

Esquirol JED. *Die Geisteskrankheiten in Beziehung zur Medizin und Staatsarzneikunde.* Berlin: Ross'sche Buchhandlung, 1838.

Feldmann M, Bender MB. Visual illusions and hallucinations in parieto-occipital lesions of the brain. In: Kemp W. (ed.) Origin and mechanism of hallucinations. *Proceed 14 Ann Meetings at the Eastern Psychiat Res.* New York: Plenum Press, 1970, pp. 23–25.

Gloning I, Gloning K, Hoff H. Über optische Halluzinationen. *Wien z Nervenheilkd* 1967, **25**: 1–19.

Grüsser OJ. J.E. Purkyně's contributions to the physiology of the visual, the vestibular and the oculomotor systems. *Hum Neurobiol* 1984, 3:129–144.

Harding AJ, Broe GA, Halliday GM. Visual hallucinations in Lewy body disease relate to Lewy bodies in the temporal lobe. *Brain* 2002, **125**:391–403.

Hubel DH, Wiesel TN. Binocular interaction in striate cortex of kittens reared with artificial squint. *J Neurophysiol* 1965, **28**:1041–1059.

Hubel DH, Wiesel TN. Receptive fields and functional architecture of monkey striate cortex. *J Physiol* 1968, **195**:215–243.

Hubel DH, Wiesel TN. Laminar and columnar distribution of geniculo-cortical fibers in the macaque monkey. *J Comp Neurol* 1972; **146**:421–450.

Jaensch ER. *Eidetic imagery and typological method of investigation.* London: Paul Kegan, 1930.

Janz D. *Die Epilepsien. Spezielle Pathologie und Therapie.* Stuttgart: Thieme, 1969.

Kinsbourne M, Warrington EK. A study of visual preservation. *JNNP* 1963, **26**:468–475.

Klee A, Willanger R. Disturbance of visual preservation. *Acta Neurol Scand* 1966, **42**:400–414.

Kölmel HW. Visuelle Perseveration. *Nervenarzt* 1982, **53**:560–571.

Kölmel HW. *Visuelle Halluzationen im hemianopen Feld.* Berlin: Springer, 1984.

Kölmel HW. Coloured pattern in hemaniopic fields. *Brain* 1984, **107**:155–167.

Kölmel HW. Complex hallucations in the hemianopic field. *JNNP* 1985, **48**:29–38.

Kömpf D, Piper HV, Neundörfer B, Dietrich H. Palinopsie (visuelle Perseveration) und zerebrale Polyopie – klinische Analyse und computertomographische Befunde. *Fortschr Neurol Psychiatr* 1983, **51**:270–281.

Lance JW. Simple formed hallucinations confined to the area of a specific visual field defect. *Brain* 1976, **99**:719–734.

Leao AAP. Spreading depression of activity in cerebral cortex. *J. Neurophysiol* 1944, 7:359–390.

Le Beau J, Wolinetz E. Le phenomène de persévération visuelle. *Rev Neurol* 1958, **99**:524–534.

Lhermitte J. Sydrome de la calotte du pédoncle cérébral. Les troubles psychosensorielles dans les lesions du mésencephale. *Rev Neurol* 1922, **38**:1359–1365.

Lhermitte J. Visual hallucination of the self. *Br Med J* 1951, 1:431–434.

Matthews TD, Kennard, C. Residual vision following geniculostriate lesions. In: Kennard C. (ed.) *Visual perceptual defects, Baillière's clinical neurology.* London: Baillière Tindall, 1993.

Mavromatis A. *Hypnagogia – the unique state of consciousness between wakefulness and sleep.* London: Routledge, 1987.

Müller J. *Über phantastische Gesichtserscheinungen.* Coblenz: Jacob Hölscher, 1846.

Olbrich HM. Optische Halluzinationen bei älteren Menschen mit Erkrankungen des Auges (Charles-Bonnet-Syndrom). In: Olbrich HM (ed.). *Halluzinationen und Wahn.* Berlin: Springer, 1987, pp. 33–41.

Pötzl O. Über Palinopsie. *Wien Z Nervenheilkd* 1954, **8**:161–186.

Richards W. The fortification illusion of migraine. *Scient Am* 1971, **224**:89–96.

Safran AB, Kline LB, Glaser JS, Daroff RB. Television-induced formed hallucinations and cerebral diplopia. *Br J Ophthamol* 1981, **65**:707–711.

Swash M. Visual perseveration in temporal lobe epilepsy. *JNNP* 1979, **42**:569–571.

Van Bogaert L. L'Hallucinose pedunculaire. *Rev Neurol* 1927, **43**:608–617.

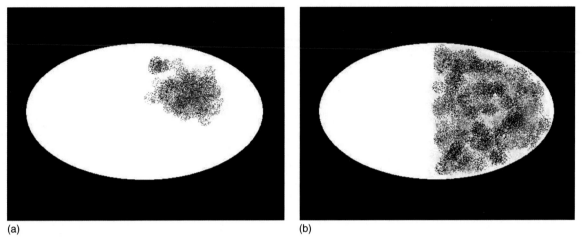

Fig. 7.3. Photopsias (a) in right visual field as partial epileptic seizure, and (b) filling almost the entire right visual field; a grand mal seizure is imminent.

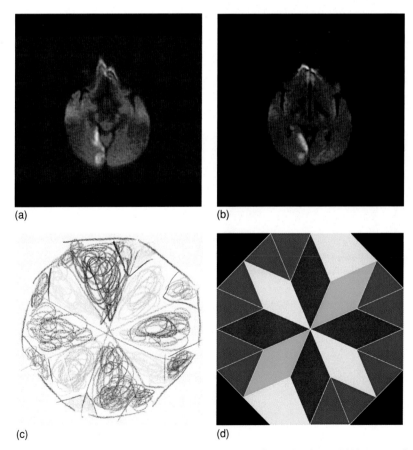

Fig. 7.4. Occipito-mesial brain infarction (right). (a, b) MRI of a head with DWI. (c) Photopsias of a patient in his left visual field, sketch of the patient. (d) Translation of the sketch.

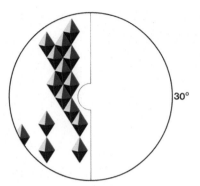

Fig. 7.5. Sharp, brightly colored pattern in left visual field immediately before the development of a homonymous hemianopsia left after infarction in the supply area of the right posterior cerebral artery.

30°

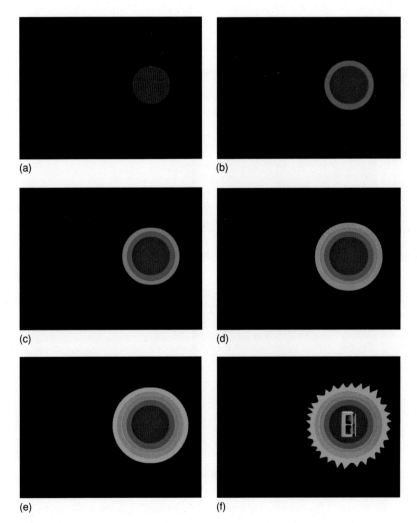

(a)

(b)

(c)

(d)

(e)

(f)

Fig. 7.7. Photopsias in right visual field with visual perseveration ("*Erregungsfang*") as partial epileptic seizure. Result of a left occipital brain contusion.

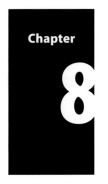

Paroxysmal paresis

Barbara Tettenborn

In general, paroxysmal focal weakness or paresis can be differentiated from paroxysmal generalized weakness or paresis. Focal paresis includes hemiparesis, paraparesis, tetraparesis or monoparesis. The anatomical distribution as well as the occurrence of associated symptoms can give a hint toward the most likely localization of a lesion, but it does not differentiate between etiological causes. The patient's history can be one of a paresis of one arm or a weakness of one side of the face, and only a careful neurological examination reveals additional paresis of one leg. The weakness does not usually affect all parts of an extremity equally. The distribution pattern of the weakness can give important topodiagnostic information. The evaluation of a patient with a paroxysmal paresis is made difficult by the fact that in most patients, the clinical neurological examination will be normal at the time when the patient presents to the doctor, and the doctor is dependent on history only.

If a traumatic cause can be excluded, a sudden onset paresis is most likely due either to a vascular event, for example, ischemia or bleeding, or due to certain toxic or metabolic causes. In contrast, paresis due to neoplastic, infectious or autoimmune diseases of the central or peripheral nervous system are rather subacute or slowly progressive, and only in exclusive cases paroxysmal. Pareses due to hereditary or degenerative diseases are usually slowly progressive.

In the following, the different causes of focal and generalized paroxysmal pareses are discussed.

Localized paroxysmal paresis

Localized or focal pareses can occur as a weakness of one side of the body as a hemiparesis or, in the case of complete paresis, a hemiplegia, as paraparesis of the arms or legs, or as monoparesis of one extremity (Table 8.1).

The topodiagnostic localization can help to limit the number of differential diagnoses. It has to be kept in mind that the usual neurological symptoms of central or peripheral nervous diseases are not present in paroxysmal disturbances such as spasticity due to central nervous diseases or atrophy in peripheral nervous disease. Other signs, like a positive Babinski sign in patients with pyramidal tract lesion, can already be present in the acute phase (Table 8.2).

Hemiparesis or hemiplegia

The distribution of pareses and the associated clinical symptoms depend on the exact anatomical localization. The localization of a lesion causing hemiparesis can be in the cerebral cortex, the subcortical white substance, in the basal ganglia, the brain stem or in the spine. The clinical neurological signs and symptoms are more important in the localization of a lesion than the etiology.

Topodiagnosis
Cortical and subcortical lesions

The topographical organization of the cerebral cortex is well known, and the representation of the singular parts of the body in the precentral gyrus is called homuncule. The leg is represented in the interhemispheric fissure, arm and face lateral in the hemisphere. Small cortical lesions can lead to marked paresis of an extremity, but hemiplegia is unlikely to occur if there is not extensive damage of the cortical region. Cortical lesions are often associated with non-motor symptoms of cortical dysfunction, such as aphasia in cases of cortical lesions of the dominant hemisphere. Motor symptoms are almost always associated with sensory symptoms because the motor and sensory cortical areas lie closely together. Hemianopia occurs in patients with cerebral lesions when the optic radiation is involved.

The Paroxysmal Disorders, ed. Bettina Schmitz, Barbara Tettenborn and Donald L. Schomer. Published by Cambridge University Press. © Cambridge University Press 2010.

Table 8.1 Evaluation of a focal motor deficit

distribution of the focal motor deficit

   hemiparesis/ hemiplegia

      relative affectedness of face/arm/leg

      associated motor signs

         muscle tone

         impairment of coordination

         pathological spontaneous movements

paraparesis/paraplegia

   level of motor signs

tetraparesis/ tetraplegia

   with/without cranial nerve involvement

monoparesis/monoplegia

   centrally caused monoparesis

   peripheral nerve lesion

      radicular nerve lesion

      lesion of the plexus

      lesion of a singular peripheral nerve

Table 8.2 Localization by associated neurological symptoms and signs

hemiparesis/hemiplegia

   speech disturbance

   neglect

   visual field defect

   apraxia

   orientation in space

paraparesis/paraplegia

   sensory disturbances

   bladder/bowel dysfunction

   sexual dysfunction

tetraparesis/tetraplegia

   sensory disturbances

   course of onset of pareses

   cranial nerve involvement

monoparesis/monoplegia

   distribution of sensory disturbances, e.g., congruence with distribution of motor symptoms

   disturbance of sweating for differentiation of radicular lesions

If a patient has an isolated cortical lesion, the occipital cortex must be involved to cause a hemianopia.

A small lesion of the cerebral cortex or the respective projections can lead to a localized paresis, for example, of the contralateral hand. Lesions within the territory of the anterior cerebral artery typically cause a paresis of the contralateral leg; lesions within the territory of the middle cerebral artery cause a paresis of the contralateral side of the face and the contralateral arm. More extended cortical or subcortical lesions lead to a more-or-less marked paresis of the contralateral side of the body, including the face, and can be associated with multiple other symptoms like aphasia, visual field defect or sensory symptoms.

Lesions in the internal capsule

A lesion in the internal capsule usually results in a marked paresis of the contralateral side of the body, including the face, because the descending fibers from the cortex are located closely together.

Brain stem lesion

Depending on the localization, a lesion in the brain stem can lead to uni- or bilateral pareses. Often these are accompanied by cranial nerve lesions depending on the level of the brain stem lesion. Owing to the closed anatomical relationship between cranial nerve nuclei and the pyramidal tract running through, typi-cal crossed syndromes of brain stem lesions can occur, mainly cranial nerve lesion on one side and hemipare-sis of extremities on the other side of the body.

Spinal lesion

A unilateral lesion of the spinal gray matter above the fifth cervical segment but below the brain stem leads to an ipsilateral hemiparesis sparing the face and the cranial nerves. Differential diagnoses of paroxysmal hemiparesis are listed in Table 8.3.

Ischemia

Clinical findings

The most common cause of paroxysmal paresis of one side of the body with or without other associated symptoms is transient cerebral ischemia (Fig. 8.1). The duration of the neurological symptoms is divided into transient ischemic attacks (TIA) if the neurological symptoms subside completely within 24 hours. Most TIAs are of very short duration, usually from seconds to 30 minutes. One has always to keep in mind that a TIA is a clinical description. MRI findings in recent years have demonstrated that even in cases of transient clinical findings, a morphological lesion can be seen. It depends on the cerebral region involved in transient ischemia which neurological

Fig. 8.1. Acute neurological deficit (modified from Berlit 2006).

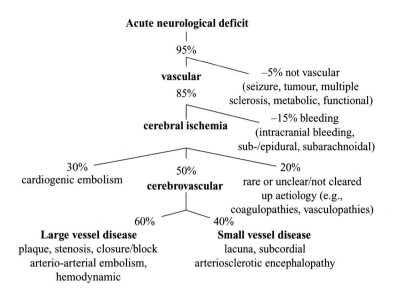

Table 8.3 Causes of acute-onset hemiparesis/hemiplegia

cerebral ischemia
intracerebral bleeding
subarachnoid bleeding
sinus/venous thrombosis
spinal lesion above the fifth cervical segment (face not affected)
multiple sclerosis
ADEM
sporadic hemiplegic migraine
familiar hemiplegic migraine
Todd's paresis after epileptic seizure
ictal paresis
tumor with acute bleeding
acute encephalitis, especially herpes encephalitis
acute encephalopathy
metabolic disturbance (hyponatremia, hypoglycemia)
hypertensive encephalopathy
psychogenic hemiparesis

symptoms are occurring. Most TIAs are associated with transient hemiparesis, which in the common case of middle cerebral artery ischemia is brachiofacially pronounced. Pure motor hemipareses are the most common clinical presentation of lacunar strokes, most commonly in the region of the internal capsule of the pons.

TIAs are warning symptoms of an impending stroke, and have therefore to be handled like an emergency. Up to 10% of TIA patients will suffer a stroke within the next 48 hours, the stroke risk naturally depending on the etiology of the ischemia (European Stroke Organisation [ESO] 2008). Patients at risk for a stroke are predominantly those above the age of 60 years with TIA of more than 10 minutes' duration.

Diagnostic procedures

TIA as a differential diagnosis urges an emergency work-up of the pathophysiology of the ischemia to initiate effective secondary prevention as soon as possible. The majority of patients with a paroxysmal paresis will need a cerebral imaging. In the emergency setting, cranial computed tomography excluding cerebral bleeding is usually sufficient. MRI, including diffusion-weighted images, can often show an ischemic area even in the very acute phase or in patients with transient neurological symptoms and signs, even if there are not signs of a morphological lesion in follow-up examinations.

If there is suspicion of a paroxysmal hemiparesis due to a tumor, a vascular malformation or an encephalitis, a MRI has to be performed and possibly also a lumbar puncture. If acute imaging has not shown bleeding or a intracerebral space-occupying lesion, a cerebral ischemia as cause of the clinical symptoms has to be suspected, and the immediate work-up of pathogenesis and treatment of risk factors for stroke is necessary.

The following pathogenetic mechanisms have to be considered:

Large vessel disease. Due to arteriosclerotic disease of the large brain-feeding vessels, an intra-arterial embolism can lead to occlusion of an intracerebral vessel, or a local thrombus can cause a hemodynamical ischemia in the dependant region of the brain.

Small vessel disease. Hyalinosis of the small penetrating arteries and arterioles can lead to small lacunar infarctions. Just these small lacunar infarcts in the internal capsule or in the brain stem at the pontine level can lead to isolated motor symptoms or pure motor stroke.

Cardiac embolism. The most common cause of embolic stroke is non-rheumatic atrial fibrillation with absolute arrhythmia. Besides cardiac valve disease, stenosis as well as insufficiency can lead to embolization as well as endocarditis or post-myocardial infarction. The risk of embolization in cases of patent foramen ovale (PFO) is not well defined yet. The combination of PFO with atrial septal aneurysm is accompanied by an increased embolic rate.

Coagulation disturbances. Possible causes for cerebral ischemia due to coagulation defects are genetic AT III-deficiency, protein S and protein C-deficiency, APC-resistance (factor V mutation) and factor II mutation, increased coagulation due to polyglobulinemia or exsiccosis.

Rare causes

Dissections of the brain-feeding vessels, vasculitis, cocaine consumption and so on belong in this group. For differentiation of the underlying pathogenetic mechanisms, brain imaging, laboratory examinations, ultrasonography of the brain feeding vessels, electrocardiography as well as echocardiography are necessary as well as the clinical neurological examination.

The decision if further examinations are necessary including transoesophageal echocardiography, Holter (long-term) ECG, transcranial duplex sonography as well as determination of cerebral reserve capacity depends on the results of the preceding examinations and the general clinical impression.

Therapy
Treatment of the risk factors

Some vascular risk factors are not treatable, for example, age and genetic predisposition. But arterial hypertension, atrial fibrillation, other cardiac embolic sources, smoking, hyperlipidemia, diabetes mellitus, obesity and inactivity can be influenced. Optimal management of these vascular risk factors includes regular checking of blood pressure and blood glucose (PROGRESS 2001; Schrader et al. 2005). Statin therapy is recommended in patients with non-cardioembolic stroke (Amarenco et al. 2006). Cigarette smoking and

heavy use of alcohol are discouraged. Regular physical activity is recommended. A diet low in salt and saturated fat, high in fruits and vegetables, and rich in fiber is recommended (ESO 2008). Regarding PFO, drug abuse, migraines, hyperhomocysteinemia, hypercoagulability as well as antiphospholipid antibody syndrome, no congruent data from larger studies are available. Therefore, no precise therapeutic recommendations can be given in patients with these conditions. When the PFO is combined with an atrial septal aneurysm or in patients with cryptogenic stroke, PFO and recurrent ischemic events endovascular closure of PFO is feasible (Mas et al. 2001).

Thrombocytic aggregation inhibitors

Thrombocyte aggregation inhibitors have a substantial impact on the avoidance of stroke following TIA (Antithrombotic Trialists' Collaboration 2002). Meta-analyses demonstrate thrombocyte aggregation inhibitors can reduce the risk of stroke following TIA by 11% to 15% and the combined vascular risk (stroke, myocardial infarction, vascular death) by 15% to 22%. It is not clear which drug and what dose should be given. Between the Food and Drug Administration (FDA) and the ESO, every dose of acetylsalicylic acid between 50 and 325 mg per day has been recommended (Department of Health and Human Services and FDA 1998; European Stroke Initiative 2004; ESO 2008). In most countries, therapy with 100 mg acetylsalicylic acid per day is given.

Another thrombocyte antiaggregant is clopidogrel. In a dosage of 75 mg per day, it reduced stroke risk in a randomized, double-blind study that compared 325 mg ASS per day in patients following cerebral ischemia, myocardial infarction or peripheral vascular disease by 8.7%, absolute by 0.5% with the endpoint being stroke, myocardial infarction or vascular death (CAPRIE Steering Committee 1996). The safety regarding side-effects of clopidogrel as compared to ASS is very good, as there are only 0.1% severe neuropenia reported so far, but there are also cases of thrombotic-thrombopenic purpura described (Bennett et al. 2000).

The third clinically relevant thrombocyte antiaggregant substance is dipyridamole. The combination of 400 mg dipyridamole with 50 mg acetylsalicylic acid per day led in a randomized, placebo-controlled study to a relative risk reduction of 37% compared to placebo, whereas ASS or dipyridamole alone reduced the stroke risk by 18% and 16%, respectively (Diener et al. 1997; Halkes et al. 2006). A multicenter study including almost 7600 high-risk patients with TIA or ischemic stroke (MATCH study) showed that the combined application of ASS and clopidogrel is not superior to clopidogrel alone in the secondary prevention of cerebral ischemia (Diener et al. 2004). Similarly, in the CHARISMA study the combination of aspirin and clopidogrel did not reduce the risk of myocardial infarction, stroke or death from vascular causes compared with aspirin alone (Bhatt et al. 2006).

Outside of randomized studies, the combination of ASS with clopidogrel is used in singular patients with recurrent ischemias under monotherapy or with rapidly progressive areteriosclerotic disease. The newer GP-IIb/IIIa antagonists, which have shown to be very effective in patients with acute coronary syndrome, did not show effectiveness in oral application in cardiovascular secondary prevention, so that clinical studies in the secondary prevention of ischemic stroke had to be stopped prematurely (Diener and Hamann 2003).

Anticoagulation

In patients with a cardiac embolic source, especially with atrial fibrillation, oral anticoagulation with an intended INR of 2 to 3 is recommended. In the European Atrial Fibrillation Trial, oral anticoagulation led to a risk reduction of 70% for recurrent cerebral ischemia as compared to only 15% risk reduction under ASS alone (EAFT 1993). In patients with cardiac valve replacement, oral anticoagulation is necessary as well. For PFO, no evidence-based data are available yet. In a European multicenter study, the recurrence rate under ASS 325 mg per day was very low, with 0.6% per year in patients with pure PFO (Mas et al. 2001). Only patients with PFO combined with intraseptal aneurysm had an increased stroke risk. Therefore, in these patients oral anticoagulation is recommended at the moment, either up to the time point of interventional closure or if intervention is not feasible.

Carotid endarterectomy

Patients with a more than 70% symptomatic stenosis of the internal carotid artery and symptoms within the preceding six months profit from carotid endarterectomy as long as the perioperative complication rate in the specific center is not above 6% (ECST 1991; NASCET 1991). The relative risk reduction of the oper-

ation as compared to drug treatment alone was 60% to 80% for patients with greater than 70% symptomatic carotid stenosis. Patients with less than 50% stenosis do not profit from the operation. Only in patients with 50% to 69% stenosis is the advantage of the operation very low (Rothwell et al. 2003).

Several trials have compared carotid artery angioplasty and stenting with carotid endarterectomy in the secondary prevention of stroke. In CAVATAS (Carotid and Vertebral Artery Transluminal Angioplasty Study, 2001), the majority of the patients in the endovascular group underwent angioplasty but only 26% were treated with a stent. The two most recent studies revealed slightly different results (SPACE and EVA3S). SPACE (stent-protected angioplasty versus carotid endarterectomy in symptomatic patients) marginally failed to prove the non-inferiority of carotid artery stenting (CAS) compared to carotid endarterectomy (CEA); for the endpoint of ipsilateral stroke or death up to day 30, the event rates after 1200 patients were 6.8% for CAS and 6.3% for CEA patients (Ringleb et al. 2006). The French EVA3S (endarterectomy versus stenting in patients with symptomatic severe carotid stenosis) trial was stopped prematurely after the inclusion of 527 patients because of safety concerns and lack of efficacy (Mas et al. 2006).

Vascular malformations and space-occupying lesions

In rare cases, small intracerebral bleeding, a vascular malformation or an intracerebral space-occupying lesion can mimic the clinical symptoms of a TIA with paroxysmal paresis. A subdural hematoma can also lead to fluctuating hemiparesis of varying degrees. In these cases, brain imaging is necessary for the differential diagnosis.

Sinus- and cerebral-vein thrombosis

In singular cases, a sinus thrombosis or thrombosis of cerebral veins can become symptomatic with transient or fluctuating hemiparesis of varying degrees.

Encephalitis

In the intial phase of encephalitis, transient focal neurological symptoms can occur including paresis which poses like a TIA. If the clinical picture is consistent with meningoencephalitis, further investigations in this direction are necessary. In questionable cases, lumbar puncture has to be performed following brain imaging.

Metabolic disturbances

Metabolic disturbances like low potassium and low sodium cause most commonly a diffuse encephalopathy, but singular patients can also present with focal symptoms like hemiparesis, which improve parallel to improvement of the metabolic disturbance.

In recurrent attacks, the motoric deficit can occur on the same side on different occasions. Commonly, these patients have a preexisting intracerebral lesion like a cerebral ischemia or a multiple sclerosis plaque. In other patients, brain imaging demonstrates no structural lesion, and the precise pathogenesis for the transient focal symptoms remains unclear. Similarly, an acute encephalopathy due to a hypertensive crisis can cause a rapidly occurring transient hemiparesis, often associated with headache and disorientation.

Migraine

Patients with migraines can develop focal neurological symptoms, including hemiparesis, as part of the initial phase of the neuronal depression in the sense of migraine with aura. Most of these patients have a history of migraines but not necessarily a history of hemiplegic migraines. The name hemiplegic migraine is used if a patient develops hemiplegia in the context of an otherwise typical migraine attack. (Migraines are covered in more detail in Chapter 5).

Regarding therapy, it has to be considered that triptans are ineffective and also contraindicated in the aura phase of the migraine attack. A migraine attack with prolonged aura can clinically look like a stroke, which can necessitate further diagnostic procedures like CT or MRI. Lately, the possibility of migraine-associated stroke is discussed more commonly.

Postictal paresis

After an epileptic seizure, a transient postictal paresis can occur (Todd's paresis), most commonly in the form of hemiparesis, which can have a localizing singnificance regarding the origin of the seizure. The history is important for differentiation if disturbance of consciousness or motor symptoms occurred before the paresis.

Ictal paresis

On the other hand, with frontal lobe or parietal lobe seizures ictal paresis can occur like ictal hemiparesis (Sareen 2001), which has to be differentiated from TIAs. For differential diagnosis ictal EEG is helpful, as EEG in the interval between seizures can be normal.

Therapeutically, these ictal pareses react well on treatment with anticonvulsants.

Multiple sclerosis

An acute relapse of multiple sclerosis can in rare cases develop and remit so suddenly that it appears as paroxysmal paresis. In most cases, the history is crucial. In newly diagnosed patients, a diagnosis is made based on the results of cranial and cervical MRI, spinal fluid examination and neurophysiological testing.

Alternating hemiplegia of childhood

This is possibly a special form of basilar migraine. It usually starts in the first decade of life and goes along with progressive psychomotor retardation. Attacks of hemiplegia occur at alternating sides and have a duration between 15 minutes and several days. They are accompanied by dystonic attacks, choreoathetotic movements, tonic crisis, nystagmus and irritability. Naloxan as well as the calcium antagonist flunarizine are therapeutically effective.

Paraparesis or paraplegia

Acute paraparesis or paraplegia consists in most cases in incomplete (paresis) or complete (plegia) paresis of the legs. The rare paresis of both arms is called diplegia brachialis.

Topodiagnosis

Spinal lesion

In cases of an acute paraparesis or paraplegia, a spinal lesion has to be suspected primarily. Depending on the level and extent of the lesion in cross-section, accompanying sensory symptoms and dysfunction of bladder and/or bowel function can be present (Table 8.4). Lesions of the cervical spinal cord predispose for tetraparesis, and lesions of the thoracic spinal cord for paraparesis of the legs. A special situation is the conus syndrome with an acute bladder paresis as the leading symptom. It always has to be kept in mind, especially when requesting imaging, that the morphological lesion may lie above the clinical level of lesion.

Parasagittal lesion

An intracranial parasagittal lesion in the cortical representative area of the legs in the precentral region on both sides leads typically to a paresis of both legs. Differential diagnoses of paroxysmal paraparesis are listed in Table 8.5. As acute, non-traumatic causes of

Table 8.4 Paraplegia and tetraplegia in dependance of lesion level

Level	Motor symptoms	DTR (*)	Sensibility	Bladder/Bowel
Upper cervical spinal cord	Tetraparesis/-plegia, breathing insufficiency	All increased, Bab.pos.	Disturbed below	Loss of control
Thoracic and lumbar spinal cord (until L3)	Paraparesis/-plegia of the legs	Arms normal, legs increased, Bab.pos.	Disturbed below	Loss of control
Conus-cauda	Paraparesis/-plegia of the legs (most marked distally, initially often of mild extent)	Arms normal, legs diminished, Bab.neg.	Disturbed below L4/5 (typically saddle anesthesia)	Bladder and bowel incontinence (flaccid paresis)

Notes: (*) in spinal shock before increase of DTR areflexia possible; Bab. = Babinski-sign (pos. = positive, neg. = negative); DTR = Deep tendon reflexes

Table 8.5 Causes of acute-onset paraparesis/paraplegia

Spinal lesions

    acute segmental ischemia

    acute peridural process (e.g., abscess)

    intramedullary bleeding

    autoimmune: transverse parainfectious myelitis, multiple sclerosis, lupus erythematodes

    germ associated viral transverse myelitis, poliomyelitis, coxsackie viral infection, space occupying : tumor, disc prolapse, abscess

Mantelkanten syndrome

Psychogenic paraparesis

intermittent compression of the spinal cord in a previously healthy person, inflammation in the sense of transverse myelitis or spinal ischemia have to be considered primarily. Spinal space-occupying lesions including metastatic carcinoma, epidural hematoma or abscess show a rather subacute, slowly progressing course.

Spinal ischemia

The anterior spinal artery syndrome causes a functional disturbance in the spinal areas, which are perfused by the anterior spinal artery leading to an affection of the pyramidal tracts with paresis below the lesion level. A lesion of the lateral spinothalamic tract leading to loss of pain and temperature sensation is usually present. At the same time, posterior tract function with superficial sensation and proprioceptive sense remains intact.

A patient with an anterior spinal artery syndrome therefore presents with a complete paresis (plegia) of both legs and disturbance of pain and temperature sensation below the lesion level with preserved superficial sensation. Due to the intact sensation for light touch, the wrong diagnosis of a psychogenic paresis is sometimes made. An intermittent anterior spinal artery syndrome with recurrent pareses of the legs can occur in cases of TIA in the territory of the anterior spinal artery, that is, vascular spinal claudication, as well as with arteriovenous fistulas. In singular cases, ischemia in the lower cervical region of the territory of the anterior spinal artery can lead to isolated paraparesis of the arms. An MRI is necessary if an ischemic spinal lesion is suspected. Pathogenesis of the ischemia as well as the therapy are similar to the cerebral ischemias.

Spinal bleeding

In rare cases, an epidural, subdural or intraspinal bleed can cause a sudden paraparesis. This is one of the main differential diagnoses in patients with sudden paraparesis on oral anticoagulation.

Bilateral ischemia in the territories of the anterior cerebral arteries can lead to an acute paraparesis of the legs or to a tetraparesis. Due to transient ischemia, paroxysmal pareses can occur. In the differential diagnoses, bilateral ischemia in the territory of the anterior chorioidal arteries, or in exceptional cases in the territory of the basilar artery, have to be included.

Myelitis

Rarely, paroxysmal pareses can occur in transverse myelitis. In most patients, progressive paraparesis of the legs including sensory loss and disturbance of the sphincter function, often associated with local pain, is prominent.

Spinal space-occupying lesion

Spinal space-occupying lesions, especially an epidural tumor, can sometimes clinically lead to paroxysmal

95

paresis depending on the local pressure on the myelin. The clinical symptoms depend on the location of the space-occupying lesion (Table 8.4). The most common cause of a spinal space-occupying lesion is a disc prolapse.

Epidural abscess

In the same way, an epidural abscess can lead to intermittent pareses if the extent of compression of the myelin varies. An abscess is in most cases accompanied by high fever, often disorientation and in all cases back pain and radicular pain. The epidural abscess can be the sequel of infectious foci on other locations like skin infection, sepsis, vertebral osteomyelitis and intravenous drug abuse. The most common infective agents are staphylococcus and gram-negative bacteria. Predisposing factors are HIV infection and iatrogenic immunosuppression.

Disc prolapse

A disc prolapse can lead to intermittent pressure on the myelin or the rami, depending on the localization, and therefore leading to varying degrees of paresis. It can be paraparesis or monoparesis. In cases of median disc prolapse, pain is less prominent and paresis is the leading symptom; in cases of lateral disc prolapse, radicular pain is the most prominent sign due to compression of the nerve root. In some cases, the neurological symptoms are dependent on movement and can lead to paroxysmal paresis.

Cervical myelopathy

Degenerative bony changes of the cervical spine can also lead to intermittent pressure on the myelin or the nerve roots and therefore lead to paresis at varying degree. This can be paraparesis or monoparesis. As a further pathogenetic mechanism, compression of the spinal vessels by bony degenerative changes has to be considered which causes, depending on movement, varying degrees of compression and therefore varying degrees of paroxysmal paresis.

Tetraparesis or tetraplegia

Topodiagnosis

Spinal lesions

In patients with acute teraparesis or tetraplegia (Table 8.6), the first differential diagnosis is a spinal lesion in the upper part of the cervical spine. Associ-

Table 8.6 Causes of acute-onset tetraparesis/tetraplegia

Brain stem lesion
Ischemia, bleeding, space-occupying lesion, inflammation
Drop attacks
Lesion in the upper cervical spine
Spinal ischemia
Space-occupying lesion: tumor, disc prolapse, abscess, bleeding
Myelitis
Polyradiculitis
Toxic acute polyneuropathies
Psychogenic tetraparesis

ated are commonly sensory symptoms and bladder or bowel function disturbance.

Brain stem lesion

A brain stem lesion can cause a tetraparesis. Depending on the localization, accompanying cranial nerve lesions can help to localize the lesion within the brain stem (Table 8.2).

Differential diagnosis of paroxysmal tetraparesis

As non-traumatic causes of acute tetraparesis, spinal lesions in the upper cervical spine of vascular, space-occupying or inflammatory etiology have to be considered primarily. Also, brain stem lesions of different etiologies can be the cause of an acute tetraparesis. In some cases, a rapidly progressive polyradiculitis (GBS) can be the cause of the clinical syndrome of acute tetraparesis.

Ischemia

Ischemic lesions in the brain stem can lead to tetraparesis in cases of bilateral localization. A thrombus in the basilar artery, which intermittently compresses the rami ad pontem, can lead to bilateral pontine ischemia. In some cases this can cause paroxysmal pareses, depending on the extent of the varying perfusion disturbance. Besides the tetraparesis cranial nerve lesions can occur, which can help in localization. A special form is probably the drop attack. The clinical picture, diagnostic procedures and therapy of the ischemic lesions in the brain stem are similar to the ischemic lesions mentioned previously. Tetraparesis can also occur in patients with ischemia in the upper part of the cervical spine in the territory of the anterior spinal artery.

Drop attacks

Drop attacks are non-epileptic falling attacks with the patient falling while walking or standing without any preceding warning symptoms and preserved consciousness. It is more a paroxysmal loss of muscular tone than a paroxysmal paresis, but from the history it cannot be differentiated. Immediately following the fall, the neurological examination is already normal again (Remler et al. 1996).

Drop attacks are most likely vascular in origin due to transient ischemia in the vertebrobasilar territory. Transient ischemia of the corticospinal tracts or the paramedian formatio reticularis are discussed as causes. Most of the time, the patients complain about other symptoms like dizziness, vertigo, double vision or ataxia. Other possible causes are a tumor in the third ventricle or the posterior fossa (Lee et al. 1994). The same clinical phenomenon can also occur in ischemia in the territory of the anterior cerebral arteries bilaterally. Drop attacks due to ischemia in the anterior vascular territory are the sequel of ischemic perfusion disturbances of the parasaggital premotor or motor cortex. Most of the time, drop attacks are an exclusion diagnoses. Most likely, the drop attacks of elderly women – often called *syndrome des genoux bleus* or "syndrome of the blue knees" – also belong in this group (drop attacks are covered in more detail in Chapter 3).

Disc prolapse

A disc prolapse in the upper cervical region can be the cause of a tetraparesis without facial involvement.

Polyneuroradiculitis

The acute polyneuroradiculitis (Guillain-Barré syndrome, or GBS) develops acute or subacute with typically distal to proximal ascending symmetrical flaccid pareses, which develop most often days to weeks after an infection, a vaccination, an operation or in autoimmune diseases, for example, lymphoma or systemic lupus erythematosis. The accompanying sensory disturbances, which have a sock- or glove-like distribution, ascend distally to proximally. The pareses are mostly rapidly progressive and often involve the trunk- and head-stabilizing muscles until tetraparesis exists. In this stage, there is the danger of breathing paralysis. In rare cases, the pareses can be so rapidly progressive that breathing insufficiency occurs within hours after the first extremity pareses. Cranial nerve involvement is common even in milder cases, especially the facial nerves and the ocular motor nerves. As signs of autonomic nervous system involvement, bladder dysfunction, blood pressure fluctuations, tachycardia and less commonly bradycardia can occur.

The exact pathophysiological mechanism of the occurrence of GBS is not known. It comes to an acute lesion of the nerve roots (polyradiculitis) and the peripheral nerves with histologically proven lymphocytic infiltration. Primarily, an autoimmune process with circulating immune complexes is suspected. Cellular reactions also seem to play a role. In most patients loss of myelin develops, in severe cases with secondary axonal degeneration.

In the clinical neurological examination, the actual extent of the paresis can be recorded. The suspected diagnosis is proven by spinal fluid examination with typically isolated increase of protein content without pleocytosis as well as by electrophysiological examination of the peripheral nerves. In severe cases with rapid progression and impending or already existing breathing insufficiency, intensive care unit treatment is necessary. Treatment is either with intravenous application of immunoglobulins (0.4 g/kg/day for five days) or plasmapheresis. The indication for a transient cardiac pacemaker should be made broadmindedly because of the often unpredictable occurrence of cardiac arrhythmias.

The main complication is often acute onset of breathing insufficiency, even if the pareses of the extremities do not show any further progression. The protein elevation in the spinal fluid can still be absent in the first couple of days of the disease. In questionable cases, a second lumbar puncture will be necessary.

The differential diagnosis is compression of the cervical spinal cord, which can also lead to acute ascending sensomotoric symptoms. The spinal fluid findings can be similar with isolated increased protein content. In these patients, the electrophysiological examinations with nerve conduction studies help to differentiate. In GBS, there is typically a marked slowing of the nerve conduction velocity.

Other polyneuropathies due to toxins, diphtheria or porphyria have to be discriminated as well as acute spinal cord disease or ventral brain stem lesions. Pure motor polyneuritis has to be delimited against poliomyelitis in people not vaccinated. The asymmetric distribution of the pareses and the spinal fluid findings usually help to differentiate poliomyelitis

Table 8.7 Causes of acute onset monoparesis/monoplegia

Brain stem lesions with consecutive isolated cranial nerve lesion

Very localized cerebral cortical lesion

Localized spinal lesion

Acute myogenic or neurogenic process

Nerve compression lesion

    Compression syndrome in anatomical narrowness

    Neuropathy with tendency to compression lesion

Psychogenic monoparesis

Table 8.8 Causes of acute onset monoparesis of one arm

Cerebral cortical lesion in the medial central gyrus

    Ischemia, bleeding, space-occupying lesion, inflammatory lesion

Migraine accompagnée

Epileptic seizure with ictal or postictal paresis

Spinal lesion in the cervical part

    Ischemia, bleeding, space-occupying lesion, inflammatory lesion

Lesion of the brachial plexus

    Neuralgic shoulder amyotrophy

    Compressive syndrome of the brachial plexus (e.g., backpacker paresis)

    Acute ischemia of the brachial plexus

    Hereditary brachial plexus neuropathy

Compressive nerve lesion

    Compressive syndrome in anatomical narrowness (thoracic outlet syndrome, carpal tunnel syndrome, sulcus ulnaris syndrome)

    Neuropathy with tendency to compressive lesions

    Long-term pressure on peripheral nerves

Acute anterior poliomyelitis

Subclavian steal syndrome

Acute localized myogenic process

Dissection of the vertebral artery (compression of the cervical roots by periarterial hematoma)

Weakness due to pain related to primary articular or spondylogenic problems (e.g., periarthropathia humeroscapularis)

Psychogenic monoparesis

Table 8.9 Causes of acute monoparesis of one leg

Cerebral cortical lesion in the region of the Mantelkante

    Ischemia, bleeding, space-occupying lesion, inflammatory lesion

Migraine accompagnée

Epileptic seizure with ictal or postictal paresis

Spinal lesion in the region of the lumbar spine

    Ischemia, bleeding, space-occupying lesion, inflammatory lesion

Lesion of the lumbosacral plexus

    Retroperitoneal hematoma around the psoas muscle

    Compression or distension syndrome of the lumbar plexus following long-term sitting or working in squatting position

    Acute ischemia of the lumbosacral plexus

Nerve compression lesion

    Neuropathy with tendency to compressive lesions

    Long-term pressure on peripheral nerves

Acute anterior poliomyelitis

Acute localized myogenic process

Weakness due to pain inhibition in primary articular or spondylogenic problems

Psychogenic monoparesis

Monoparesis/Monoplegia

In cases of an acute paresis of one extremity or even only singular muscle groups of one extremity, a monoparesis or monoplegia is present depending on the fact if the paresis is incomplete or complete. Paresis of singular cranial nerves can also be called monoparesis.

Topodiagnosis and differential diagnosis of paroxysmal monoparesis

The cause of sudden-onset, non-traumatic monoparesis or monoplegia can be a cortical cerebral lesion as well as a localized spinal, radicular nerve lesion or a peripheral nerve lesion (Table 8.7). Depending on the localization, it is a monoparesis of one arm (Table 8.8) or one leg (Table 8.9). In localized brain stem lesions, an isolated cranial nerve lesion can occur. In the following, some of the most important causes in neurological differential diagnosis are described in more detail.

Acute double vision

Primary muscular dysfunction due to myogenic or neurogenic disease can lead to double vision as well

from GBS. Critical illness polyneuropathy with distally pronounced motor and sensory symptoms develops only in polypathic or polytraumatized patients in the course of the intensive care unit treatment, often with sepsis and multiple organ failure.

as ophthalmological causes including the possiblity of monocular double vision.

Especially in myasthenia, intermittent double vision can occur very early in the disease manifestation at a variable extent with or without other symptoms. The double vision is usually worse in the evening as compared to the morning or only present in the evening or after long-term exertion like long car rides or prolonged reading.

Peripheral facial nerve palsy

Peripheral facial nerve palsy is an acute paresis of the facial muscles supplied by the facial nerve, most commonly on one side. The idiopathic facial nerve palsy is also called Bell's palsy. Often, the patient wakes up in the morning with a newly developed paresis of the mimic muscles of one side of the face, most commonly including vegetative (autonomic) fibers for tear and saliva secretion and afferent sensory fibers, which supply the frontal two thirds of the tongue. The mimic muscles are flaccid on the affected side, and the forehead is without wrinkles.

Often the paresis is first detected by relatives who notice that the patient cannot close the eye completely on the affected side, or that the lateral edge of the mouth shows no motion on laughing. The attempt to close the eye on the affected side leads to an uprolling of the eyeball (Bell phenomenon). Often patients complain of pain behind the ear and a subjective numbness at the cheek. Additionally, there is often a disturbance of hearing with hyperacusis due to the affected stapedius muscle.

Etiologically, the so-called idiopathic peripheral facial nerve palsy is possibly due to an inflammatory process at the bony facial canal at the base of the skull. In the acute phase, an MRI can often demonstrate signal intensities in the facial canal. Symptomatic facial nerve paresis can occur with, for example, zoster oticus or borreliosis.

If there is incomplete eyelid closure, a watch-glass bandage to avoid lesions of the cornea and/or eye cream is necessary. In cases of severe pain, oral corticosteroids (e.g., 60 mg/day prednisolone) for a few days duration can be favorable.

Frequently, patients with an acute facial nerve palsy are hospitalized with the proposed diagnosis of a suspected central lesion or a stroke. The most important differentiating sign is that patients with a central facial paresis can close the eye on the affected side due to the centrally bilateral supply of the forehead, whereas this is not possible in cases of a complete peripheral facial nerve palsy.

Subclavian steal syndrome

The subclavian steal syndrome is the consequence of a high-grade stenosis or occlusion of the left subclavian artery proximal from the origin of the vertebral artery or of the right brachiocephalic truncus. The subclavian artery does not receive enough blood supply and, therefore, the blood flow in the affected vertebral artery is retrograde on exercising the arm, which can lead to a steal effect from the cerebral circulus possibly leading to the clinical symptoms of a brain stem ischemia. More commonly, a patient with this vascular pathology develops a painful paresis of the arm on exercising the arm because the steal phenomenon from the basilar vascular territory is often not sufficient for the oxygen supply of the arm. There is always a measurable blood pressure difference between the two arms.

Compression syndromes in anatomical narrowings

Latent compartment syndrome

Compression of a peripheral nerve in an anatomically vulnerable region to variable extents can lead to intermittent paresis in these muscles which are fed by the affected nerve. Most common syndromes of this type are the carpal tunnel syndrome and the sulcus ulnaris syndrome.

Thoracic outlet syndrome

The anatomical conditions in the upper thoracic region predispose to pressure lesions of the brachial plexus. Often the exact pathogenesis cannot be found. Therefore, it is called syndrome of the upper thoracic aperture or thoracic outlet syndrome (TOS). The cervical rib syndrome and the scalenus syndrome also belong into this group. If the brachial plexus runs through the gap between anterior scalenal muscle and medial scalenal muscle together with the subclavian artery, pressure can occur on the brachial plexus and sometimes on the subclavian artery as well. But it has to be mentioned that most of the cervical ribs are without any clinical symptoms. In some people the space between clavicle and first rib is relativly narrow, which can cause pressure on the brachial plexus, or the costoclavicular syndrome.

Altogether, these local compression syndromes are rarer than generally expected. There must be objective signs of a mostly lower brachial plexus lesion or marked symptoms of compression of the subclavian artery. A variety of provocative tests like the Adson maneuver – where the head is tilted to the affected side with elevation of the chin and deep inspiration – have been described. However, great skepticism is necessary because a lot of healthy people will also have their pulse disappear doing the same provocative test of the radial artery.

The therapy of these compression syndromes in patients without motor or sensory disturbances usually consists of physiotherapy including strengthening of the shoulder girdle muscles and avoidance of certain precipitating external factors. Surgical cutting of the anterior scalenal muscle, with removal or partial resection of the first rib, is only indicated and necessary in rare cases where there are objective motor symptoms.

Neuralgic amyotrophy (brachial neuropathy)

This is an acute, most likely inflammatory lesion of the brachial plexus. The right arm is affected more commonly than the left, but sometimes the symptoms are bilateral. In most patients, the upper part of the plexus is more markedly affected than the lower part. The etiology is not uniform: In some patients, the lesion is thought to be due to circulating immune complexes. Before the onset of the pareses, most patients suffer from pain in the shoulder and the upper part of the arm for the duration of a few days. Disturbance of sensory function is comparatively low or can be completely absent. Long-term prognosis is relatively good but the improvement of pareses and the treatment of the commonly developing secondary shoulder freezing can last up to one year. In a few patients, recurrence is observed. Therapeutically, corticosteroids, pain-killers, resting the arm in abduction and, as soon as the pain allows it, passive and active movement are started.

Acute nerve root compression

Acute nerve root compression can lead to radicular pareses. An accompanying – often even preceding and leading – symptom in most patients is acute pain in the lumbar or, rarer, in the lower cervical region with often paravertebral or radicular, in one extremity radiating pain. Additionally, most patients also suffer from sensory disturbances, and in cases of compression of the cauda equina disturbance of bladder and bowel function can occur. About 80% of patients with acute lumbar nerve root compression do have pain on passive straight leg-raising – the positive Lasègue sign. In most cases, the radicular pain is restricted to one extremity; in rare cases, for example, medial disc prolapse, both arms or legs can be affected. In the so-called conus-cauda equina syndrome, pain and sensory changes are perianal in a saddle-like distribution, bladder and bowel function are disturbed and pareses can be completely missing, at least initially.

The most common etiology is the displacement of disc tissue with protrusion or prolapse of the nucleus pulposus with pressure on the spinal nerve root. Preferred localization are LWK 4/LWK 5 and LWK 5/SWK 1 in the lumbar region, with far less common higher lumbar nerve roots or the lower cervical segments. Rare differential diagnoses of acute nerve root compression are other space-occupying lesions, for example, local tumors, metastases, epidural abscesses or diseases of other organs nearby. They have to be considered, especially if atypical root lesions or thoracic root compression syndromes are present.

Diagnosis and therapy

Patients with acute onset radicular paresis or bladder/bowel dysfunction need emergency MRI, segmental CT or, if these methods are not available, conventional myelography. If a patient with acute onset radicular paresis proves to have a disc prolapse in the equivalent radicular segment, an emergency operation has to be discussed depending on the clinical findings. The reversibility of the neurological symptoms is dependent on their duration. Especially in patients with acute bladder/bowel dysfunction, an emergency operation is usually indicated. Pareses in the extremities can be reversible on conservative management. If conservative management is favored, the neurological status has to be controlled regularly because operation can become necessary if pareses are progressive or if new radicular symptoms occur. An absolute emergency indication for the operation is acute bladder/bowel dysfunction, which has to be observed very carefully as the damage is otherwise irreversible.

A disc prolapse in the lower conus-cauda region can cause symptoms solely in a saddle-like distribution in the perianal region and easily be overlooked, but it is an absolute emergency situation because of the accompanying bladder/bowel dysfunction. A radiculitis should always be included in the differential diagnosis.

Table 8.10 Causes of acute onset generalized weakness

Diseases of the neuromuscular junction

    Myasthenia gravis

    Lambert-Eaton syndrome

    Drugs and toxins

Cataplexy and sleep paralysis

Episodic paresis

Myopathies

    Metabolic, endocrine, toxic, inflammatory

Generalized weakness of non-organic origin

Functional pareses

Functional paresis includes a conversion reaction as well as simulation or malingering. Patients with a conversion reaction cannot realize consciously that their symptoms are of non-organic origin. In cases of simulation, the patient willingly produces a paresis. These pareses can occur in each degree of clinical intensity, including hemiparesis, tetraparesis or monoparesis. It can be of diagnostic help for differentiation between psychogenic versus organic paresis to observe the patient in supposed unobserved moments and to watch them undertaking certain activities, such as removing or putting on clothes. One can also try to divert the patient during the examination – for example, by calculating – to reduce the concentration on the paresis and possibly evoke unattended movements with a presumed paretic extremity. Attention should be paid to joint innervation of agonists and antagonists on examination of the muscular strength in detail. Neurophysiological examinations like electromyography and the motor evoked potentials can help in the differential diagnosis.

Generalized paroxysmal motor weakness (paresis)

Different diseases such as disorders of the neuromuscular junction as well as direct muscular disorders can lead to paroxysmal generalized pareses (Table 8.10). Fluctuation of symptoms within short periods of time with rapid generalized muscular fatigue on activity and rapid regain of muscular strength at rest is typical for a disease at the neuromuscular junction like myasthenia gravis or the very rare Lambert-Eaton syndrome. Of course, patients with psychosomatic diseases like the chronic fatigue syndrome can have similar symptoms that include abnormal fatigue, subjective

muscular weakness on exertion and return to normal strength at rest. But the recovery is in these patients often much slower than in patients with myasthenia gravis, and the subjective feeling of tiredness, malaise and fatigue is more prominent than in patients with myasthenia gravis.

Myopathic syndromes are the expression of a primary muscular disease including internal medicine diseases with leading muscular symptoms. Clinically, it is a pure motor weakness without sensory disturbances, mostly painless and accompanied by decreased tendon reflexes. The muscular weakness can occur acutely within hours – for example, paroxysmal hypokalemic paresis – or within a few days with changeable intensity and changing localization. In myasthenia, the weakness changes in intensity from one hour to the next, depending on the level of activity. Included in the differential diagnosis of these myopathic syndromes are anterior horn cell diseases, polyradiculitis, polyneuropathy or psychogenic weakness.

Myasthenia gravis

Myasthenia gravis is an autoimmune disease with the production of auto-antibodies against acetylcholine receptors located on the postsynaptic membrane of the muscular endplate, leading to exercise-induced muscular weakness. The leading clinical symptom of myasthenia is the weakness and abnormal fatigue of voluntary movements, which involve either only a group of muscles, for example, ocular form, or all muscles, generalized form. The exercise-induced weakness increases on repetitive or ongoing muscular activity during the day and improves at rest (sleep) or following the application of anticholinergic drugs. Light touch sensation and reflexes are not disturbed.

About half of patients have initial involvement of external ocular muscles; during the course of the disease this number increases to approximately 90%, leading to double vision and ptosis as the most common symptoms. On the extremities, the proximal muscles are more involved than the distal muscles. Commonly, the extent of the complaints and symptoms fluctuates from day to day as well as over longer periods of time. Involvement of breathing muscles as well as the complications of myasthenic or cholinergic crisis can lead to emergency situations and to the need for admission to an intensive care unit.

To confirm the diagnosis of myasthenia, electromyographic investigations including muscular end plate stimulation and even single-fiber electromyography are useful or necessary. Antibodies against muscular endplate can be positive in the blood serum. The sensitivity of this test is relatively low.

Emergency situations can occur as myasthenic or cholinergic crisis, the latter induced by drug therapy. The myasthenic and cholinergic crises have a very similar clinical picture, as both go along with rapidly progressive generalized pareses of the voluntary muscles with difficulties swallowing and talking as well as breathing difficulties. Myasthenic crises are most commonly diagnosed in patients previously not known to have myasthenia or just recently diagnosed to suffer from the disease but can also be seen in patients treated for infections or mistakes in drug therapy. In cholinergic crisis, which is an overdosage crisis, side-effects such as fasciculations, miosis, sweating, excessive saliva production, anxiety, abdominal cramps and diarrhea can be observed. A slight breathing insufficiency is usually preceded by tachycardia, sleeplessness and paresis on coughing in the case of infections. An increased sleepiness reaction or difficulties swallowing have to be judged as alarming symptoms.

Pathophysiology

The pathophysiological background is the change of the neuromuscular endplate due to antibodies against acetylcholine receptors. The myasthenic crisis is the sequel of a more-or-less rapidly developing deficiency of acetylcholine at the endplate either due to insufficient therapy with cholinesterase inhibitors that may occur from rapid discontinuation of drugs or increased need of acetylcholine because of a coexistent acute viral or bacterial infection. Certain drugs like local anaesthetics, muscle relaxants, neuroleptics and magnesium-containing antibiotics can cause a myasthenic crisis due to inhibition of the neuromuscular transmission. The cause of a cholinergic crisis is a (relative) overdose of cholinesterase inhibitors.

First aid pocedures

Myasthenic patients with marked muscular weakness, difficulties swallowing and beginning breathing insufficiency have to be intubated and ventilated and hospitalized after inspection of the pharnyx and possibly removal of food remnants. Any untargeted change of dose of cholinesterase inhibitors should be avoided because it can cause an acute crisis-like deteriora-

tion, especially if the differential diagnosis between cholinergic and myasthenic crisis is not obvious. In the case of a definite myasthenic crisis, an injection of 1 to 2 ampullas of neostigmine intravenously is recommended; in cases of a cholinergic crisis, the therapy of choice is 1 to 2 ampullas of atropine intravenously.

In patients with marked muscular weakness and breathing insufficiency, vital capacity has to be measured and arterial blood gas analysis may be necessary. If the clinical picture is not unequivocal, securing vital functions comes first and the differentiation between myasthenic and cholinergic crisis should be undertaken. For differentiation, 1 ml of the rapidly effective cholinesterase inhibitor edrophoniumchloride (Tensilon) can slowly be given intravenously under intensive care unit conditions. In cases of myasthenic crisis, a fast and short-lasting improvement of the clinical symptoms is observed. On the other hand, in cases of a cholinergic crisis respiratory arrest can be provoked.

In patients with a myasthenic crisis, plasmapheresis has to be discussed to reduce circulating antibodies and therefore improve the clinical picture. In patients with a cholinergic crisis, therapy consists of transient withdrawal of all cholinesterase inhibitors under ventilation and application of anticholinergics such as atropine.

Because respiratory arrest can occur in patients with cholinergic crisis, the often announced "trial" with a rapidly effective cholinesterase inhibitor edrophonium (Tensilon) in the acute emergency situation should only be done under intensive care unit conditions. Generally, 0.25 mg atropine sulfate has to be ready in a syringe in each test for immediate treatment of cholinergic symptoms.

If antibiotics have to be given in patients with a bacterial infection, which often leads to acute exacerbation of myasthenic symptoms, such drugs should be avoided which can lead to a deterioration of myasthenic symptoms themselves. Primarily, these are aminoglycosides and tetracyclines; alternatively, for example, cephalosporines can be given.

Lambert-Eaton syndrome

In Lambert-Eaton syndrome, the exercise-induced weakness is generalized and symmetric, whereas in myasthenia gravis the exercise-induced paresis is initially often restricted to certain muscle groups, especially eyelid elevators, swallowing and chewing muscles, and in generalized weakness the distribution is often asymmetrical.

The symmetrical exercise-induced pareses in Lambert-Eaton syndrome are often predominant in the hip and thigh region. Typical is their improvement under muscular work. In addition, a dry mouth and problems with accommodation can be found. A sudden deterioration can occur after ingestion of aminoglycosides, magnesium, calcium antagonists or iodine-containing contrast agents.

To establish a diagnosis of Lambert-Eaton-syndrom, an electromyographic examination including muscular endplate testing is necessary. On serial stimulation with 3 Hz, a decrement is seen only initially with a following increase of amplitude on repetitive nerve stimulation as opposed to myasthenia gravis. In addition, antibodies against voltage-dependant calcium channels can be positive. Often, the Lambert-Eaton syndrome is found as a paraneoplastic syndrome in patients with small-cell bronchial carcinoma.

Differential diagnoses to myasthenia and Lambert-Eaton syndrome are botulismus and alkylphosphate intoxication. The tensilon test is positive in patients with myasthenia gravis, although the effect is far less obvious in Lambert-Eaton syndrome and negative in other diseases of the neuromuscular junction including cholinergic crisis.

Muscular weakness due to toxic influence on the motoric endplate

There are several drugs, toxins and chemicals which can lead to weakness and paresis due to their effect on the motoric endplate. It can be a transient impairment of the normal function of the motoric endplate leading to a myasthenic-like syndrome, or a preexisting change of the motor endplate becomes symptomatic due to a toxic effect or the recovery after a neuromuscular blockade in anesthesia is delayed. Several drugs and toxins with effects on the motor endplate are listed in Table 8.11.

Botulism

Botulinum toxin is a metabolic product of the bacterium *Clostridium botulinum*, which augments in insufficiently sterilized and anerobically sealed food. The toxin presynaptically blocks the release of acetylcholine at the neuromuscular junction and in the autonomic nervous system and causes a progressive

Table 8.11 Drugs and toxins with effect on the motoric endplate

antibiotics
aminoglycosides, erythromycin, penicillin, sulphonamide, tetracycline fluorochinolone, polymyxin, colomycin
phenytoin
beta blockades and calcium antagonists
steroids
lithium
D-penicillamine
organophosphates
botulinum toxin
tick bites
snake poison

paresis which leads to death if not diagnosed and treated in time. The treatment of choice is specific botulinum antitoxin as early as possible. It can only neutralize free circulating toxin and not bind toxin on the neuromuscular synapse. Otherwise, symptomatic treatment is indicated in patients with generalized pareses, including respiratory insufficiency ventilation when necessary. Very rarely, botulism can also originate in wounds. In the therapeutic application of botulinum toxin, the nerve ends recover by formation of new presynaptic terminations, a process of 7 to 12 weeks duration.

Cataplexy and sleep paresis

Cataplexy describes a sudden paresis of the skeletal muscles caused by rapidly occurring emotions. Cataplectic seizures occur in 60% to 100% of patients with narcolepsy (Bassetti 2007), but only few patients have all four cardinal symptoms of sleep attacks, sleep paresis, hypnagogic hallucinations and cataplexy. Most commonly, cataplectic seizures are reported in association with sudden laughter but also with surprise, excitement or, more rarely, negative emotions like fear or anger. The weakness (paresis) can be restricted to the cranial muscles but can spread caudally and finally also involve leg muscles, leading to falls. The fall itself is recognized with full attention and can be associated with paroxysmal breathing difficulties and vegetative (autonomic) symptoms. The duration of the seizure is usually less than 60 seconds. In singular cases, prolonged cataplectic episodes of up to 20 minutes duration can occur (Guilleminault et al. 2007).

Pathophysiologically, the loss of muscular tone during cataplectic seizures is associated with a reduction of activity in the locus coeruleus within the brain stem. A disturbance of the hypothalamic hypocretin system seems to be associated with sleep attacks and occurrence of cataplectic symptoms in a dog model of narcolepsy as well as in men (Siegel et al. 2001).

Cataplectic seizures are within the differential diagnosis if typical emotional triggers for falls with preserved consciousness are obvious and if further symptoms of the narcoleptic triad are present.

In sleep paralysis, there is a short period of inability to move after awakening. This can be generalized or localized, for example, it can only involve the inability to open the eyelids. Further diagnostic evaluation necessitates a polysomnography in a sleep laboratory as well as the determination of specific human leucocyte antigene (HLA) markers and low cerebrospinal fluid levels of hypocretin-1. However, a negative result does not exclude the diagnosis of cataplexy or narcolepsy (Bassetti 2007).

Episodic pareses

Episodic pareses are characterized by paroxysmal, completely reversible attacks of pareses with symmetrical, proximally pronounced pareses up to tetraparesis, reduced muscle tone and decreased or lost tendon reflexes. The pareses develop within minutes or hours and usually start proximally. Consciousness, speech, breathing as well as bladder and bowl function are almost always preserved. The differentiation from tetraparesis or tetraplegia of other causes is possible due to preserved light touch sensation and proprioception. During the episodes, a progressive electrical inexcitability of the involved muscles develops together with an accompanying decrease of the evoked muscle action potentials. The duration of the episodic paresis varies between minutes and days. Discriminations are on the basis of changes of potassium serum levels into hyperkalemic and hypokalemic paresis, with both forms sometimes being triggered by rest after exertion. Recessive inherited myotonia and paramyotonia can go along with periodic paresis with normal potassium level. These are diseases of the sodium and calcium channels, which are described in more detail later.

Diseases of the sodium channel

There are eight phenotypically different diseases of the sodium channel, which are all inherited in an autosomal dominant way. The sodium conductivity of the channels is increased, depending on the temperature and the concentration of the local potassium concentration. An increase of the sodium conductivity leads to hyperexcitability of the membrane, leading to the clinical picture of myotonia, with further increases leading to inexcitability, the clinical paresis. Therefore, the leading symptoms of singular sodium-channel diseases are myotonia and paroxysmal paresis depending on muscle temperature and local potassium concentration, which can change during muscular exercise. The two most common sodium-channel diseases are the paramyotonia congenita and the hyperkalemic episodic paralysis.

Paramyotonia congenita

At room temperature, patients usually have no symptoms. These occur in cases of cooling, especially in the face and the hands. The involvement of the mimic muscles can lead to eye cramps of the orbicularis oculi muscle. First, there is a myotonic stiffness which rapidly changes into weakness, and arms and hands can be plegic. The diaphragm is not involved. The paresis continues for several hours even if the room temperature is returned to normal. It is important for diagnosis that creatine kinase is often elevated in paramyotonia, and in electromyography there are serial myotonic discharges even at room temperature. In cases of provocation of paramyotonic stiffness, electromyography shows dense fibrillation like spontaneous activity. The disease is often recognized in neonates, for example, if a cool washcloth is wiped over the face. The originally mutated gene lies on chromosome 17 and codes a subunit of a voltage-dependent sodium channel.

Hyperkalemic episodic paresis

In hyperkalemic paresis, the attacks predominantly occur at rest after exercise. Other triggers are starvation, stress and coldness as well as the ingestion of potassium. Symptoms are first seen in early childhood. The attacks can be mild, hardly notable, and last only a few minutes. But there are also severe generalized attacks which mostly occur in the morning before getting out of bed. Patients then lie in bed with pareses, where movement of head and voluntary facial muscles is possible but breathing is restricted. These episodes usually do not last longer than 2 to 3 hours. They have to be differentiated from usually shorter sleep pareses in the presence of narcolepsy.

During an attack of paresis in hyperkalemic episodic paresis, potassium is elevated and decreases during an attack to subnormal values. This can give rise to a dangerous misdiagnosis of a hypokalemic episodic paresis. Creatine kinase is hardly ever elevated in patients with hyperkalemic episodic paresis. Electromyography at intervals demonstrates myotonic series in some patients. In others, EMG at interval is normal. During the attack, myopathic changes can be seen which are congruent with the extent of the paresis up to electrical silence in case of plegia.

Therapy and Course

The symptoms of paramyotonia congenita and the hyperkalemic episodic paresis are of life-long presence, but many patients with hyperkalemic paresis improve after age 50. Most patients do not need continuous drug therapy. Slight physical exercise prevents or delays the occurrence of the hyperkalemic paresis, as well as food intake at the beginning of the paresis.

Patients with paramyotonia can be treated symptomatically for a short period of time, for example, before events when they definitely have to be symptom-free, with mexiletin or tocainid. For anesthesia, depolarizing drugs have to be avoided.

Patients with hyperkalemic episodic paresis should ingest frequent, small meals with a high carbohydrate content to avoid attacks. The drugs of choice are potassium-lowering diuretics, for example, hydrochlorothiazide or azetazolamide. In most cases, the attacks themselves do not urge any treatment. Most of the patients know that they can ameliorate a beginning attack with muscular exercise. Glucose-insuline infusions should not be given because of the subsequent hypokalemia. After several years of disease, permanent weakness as well as irreversible changes in the muscles can develop.

Diseases of the calcium channels

Out of four known pathogenic mutations of the gene for the voltage-dependant calcium channel of the voluntary muscles, three lead to the clinical picture of the hypokalemic episodic paresis. The inheritance is autosomal dominant. In hypokalemic episodic paresis, the serum potassium is decreased during the attack (more than 3 mmol/l); on the other hand, an attack can be provoked by a decrease of potassium, for example, by glucose-insulin infusion. The resting potential of muscular fibers is not really changed during an attack, but the electrical excitability is markedly reduced.

Hypokalemic episodic paresis

Leading clinical symptoms of this condition are paroxysmal attacks of paresis of variable degree. In severe cases, the first attacks occur in school-age children. In less severe cases, symptoms start in the second decade of life. In mild attacks, only slight pareses of single muscle groups occur. More severe attacks can produce tetraplegia, difficulty in talking and swallowing, as well as mimic expression. Breathing is sometimes affected to a life-threatening extent in severe attacks. The severe attacks especially occur predominantly in the second half of the night or in the morning. These attacks can be preceded by major physical exercise or a carbohydrate-rich meal during the prior evening. The duration of the attacks is between a few hours and 2 to 3 days. Between attacks, patients have a normal neurological examination. Only very severely affected patients have ongoing paresis between attacks. The paresis is least pronounced in the morning and worst in the evening. In mildly affected patients, only a few minor attacks occur during their whole life. They can be avoided or delayed by physical exercise. These attacks are sometimes misinterpreted as psychogenic.

Diagnosis

In cases of paresis, the voluntary muscles are at different extents paretic or plegic. Muscular tone is flaccid, and tendon reflexes are lost. Sometimes there is bladder and bowel atonia. Sensory functions are undisturbed. Serum creatine kinase can be slightly increased, and potassium is normal between attacks. Low potassium of 2 to 3 mmol/l during the attack is of diagnostic value. If it is possible to observe an attack, a serum potassium level should be taken several times. ECG shows signs of low potassium during the attack. Electromyography typically shows normal results between two attacks. During an attack, there is mainly electrical silence, even after electrical nerve stimulation. If there are myotonic series at EMG, the diagnosis has to be re-evaluated. In patients with long-standing severe disease, myopathic changes can be demonstrated by EMG. Muscular biopsies show characteristic vacuoles within the muscular fibers at different frequencies. In a long-standing disease, degenerative changes can occur.

Therapy and course of disease

An attack of paresis is treated by oral potassium administration as early as possible, for example, 2 to

3 potassium tablets. Parenteral potassium substitution should be avoided if at all possible and limited to exceptional cases because of possible cardiac complications.

For prophylaxis, carbohydrate-rich meals and physical exercise have to be avoided. If this is not sufficient, acetazolamide is the drug of choice. The dose should be as low as possible, for example, 125 mg every two days; an increase up to 250 mg twice daily is possible. If this is not sufficient, diclofenamide can be tried up to 25 mg three times per day. If the effect of these carbonic anhydrase inhibitors does not eliminate the symptoms, a strict low-sodium diet in combination with a potassium-saving diuretic, such as spironolactone 100 to 200 mg per day, can be tried. On this medication, the application of potassium during attacks of paresis is contraindicated.

The course of the disease cannot yet be influenced by drug therapy. In patients with a less severe disease, attacks decrease during the lifespan and can even stop completely. Aside from these attacks, some patients develop a progressive myopathy involving hip and leg muscles, the cause of this being unknown.

A symptomatic form of the low-potassium periodic paresis with Conn's syndrome has to be mentioned, the hyperaldosteronism with sodium retention and increased potassium excretion. The same clinical picture can symptomatically also occur in patients with thyreotoxicosis; therefore, thyroid hormones should be determined in patients with a family history of this condition. The episodic paresis in these patients is also accompanied by low serum potassium levels. Clinically, tachycardia and increased body temperature can be found in most patients. The symptoms disappear if the euthyroid status is reinstituted.

Normokalemic periodic paresis

Less common than the disease mentioned previously is normokalemic periodic paresis. The same gene defect and the same pathogenesis as in hyperkalemic paresis is suspected. The pareses occur especially during sleep and in early morning hours, at rest after physical exercise, following fasting or alcohol ingestion, in the cold and in the state of anxiety. In this type, the paresis involves the cranial muscles as well. Application of potassium provokes attacks.

Therapy during the attack is the application of sodium chloride. As prophylaxis, a low-carbohydrate diet and the intake of fluorohydrocortisone and acetazolamide is recommended.

Table 8.12 Muscular weakness due to electrolyte disturbances

Hypo- and hyperkalaemia
Hyponatraemia
Hypo- and hypercalcemia
Hypomagnesaemia
Hypophosphataemia

Table 8.13 Differential diagnosis of metabolic myopathies with exercise-induced weakness

Disturbance of glycogen metabolism
Enzyme defect: phosphorylase, phosphofructokinase, lactate dehydrogenase
Disturbance of fat metabolism
Enzyme defect: carnitine deficiency, carnitine palmitoyltransferase
Purine nucleotide cycle disturbance
Enzyme defect: myoadenylate deaminase
Mitochondrial myopathies

Muscular weakness due to electrolyte disturbance

In principle, with electrolyte disturbance like the one mentioned previously of any etiology, acute muscular weakness can occur and sometimes be the leading symptom (Table 8.12).

Metabolic myopathies

Metabolic myopathies are due to disturbances of the intermediate metabolism, and structural changes are secondary if present at all. Chronic progressive myopathies with permanent muscular weakness and the so-called exertion-induced myopathies have to be differentiated. The exertion-induced myopathies present with pareses, myalgias and cramps which occur on muscular exertion and are reversible at rest. Metabolic myopathies can be divided into defects of the glucose and glycogen metabolism, of fat metabolism and of oxidative phosphorylation (Table 8.13). In general, metabolic myopathies are rare.

Glycogenose type V (muscle phosphorylase deficiency, McArdle's disease)

The muscle enzyme phosphorylase splits glucose molecules from the outer glycogen chains. The result of a defect in this enzyme is the storage of glycogen within the muscle. Clinical characteristics of this metabolic disturbance are transient muscular weakness, muscular cramps, muscle pain, muscular stiffness and contractures provoked by exercise. The symptoms usually first present in childhood or adolescence. The extent of the symptoms differs individually. Some patients cannot walk more than a few paces, others tolerate more extensive exercise without a problem. The intolerance to exercise can vary intraindividually from day to day.

The classical examination is a load test with the forearm in which ischemia is induced by applying a cuff. A venous blood puncture from the exercised arm shows a reduced or missing increase of lactate. Relevant for the diagnosis is this only with an accompanying increase of ammonium. At the same time, the EMG shows electrical silence in the contracted muscle. Histologically, the biopsies with routine coloring show no, or only very slight, pathological changes. The presently known mutations enable diagnosis by DNA analysis from a simple blood probe in 90% of patients.

Glycogenose type VII (phosphofructokinase-deficiency, Tarui disease)

The phosphofructokinase is the limiting enzyme in the glycolysis. The deficiency is much rarer than the phophorylase deficiency, and was so far mainly diagnosed in the United States and Japan in patients of Jewish descent. In Europe, only a few cases have been described. The symptoms and signs of Tarui disease are very similar to the ones in McArdle's disease with exercise-induced symptoms.

In general, serum creatine kinase and uric acid are elevated. This so-called myogenic hyperuricemia is the consequence of an excessive exercise-induced degradation of purine nucleotides in muscles. The ischemia test does not display production of lactate. Biopsy shows an accumulation of glycogen of different degree.

Differential diagnosis

The differential diagnosis of metabolic myopathies includes the symptom of an exercise-induced transient muscular weakness and progressive persistent muscular weakness. Regarding the exercise-induced symptoms, functional (psychogenic) disorders like fibromyalgia or chronic fatigue syndrome have to be considered as well as myasthenia gravis and angiological or orthopedic diseases. If progressive pareses and atrophies are the leading signs, then limb girdle dystrophies, spinal muscular atrophy or myositis have to be differentiated.

Table 8.14 Muscular weakness due to endocrinopathies

Hyperthyroid disease/thyrotoxic crisis
Hypothyroid disease
Acute adrenocortical insufficiency
Anterior pituitary insufficiency
Hypercalcemic crisis
Acute Cushing syndrome/steroid myopathy
Hypoglycemia
Organic hyperinsulinism
Hypoparathyroidism
Hyperparathyroidism
Conn's syndrome
Acromegaly

Therapy

Myopathies and defects of the carbohydrate and lipid metabolism symptoms are commonly provoked by exercise or certain food intake when the muscular energy supply is especially dependent on the defected metabolic way. Even though the therapeutic options in metabolic myopathies are actually still very limited, dietetic measurements often lead to alleviation. Often a protein-rich therapy is recommended in glycogenoses.

In patients with McArdle's disease, the intake of glucose and fructose can ameliorate the symptoms but the same substances lead to an increase of symptoms in phosphofructokinase deficiency. The parenteral application of long-chain fatty acids or the oral intake of median-chain fatty acids is of advantage in both enzyme defects, but it is not feasible for long-term therapy.

Often patients with exercise-induced myopathies learn not to cross the symptom-free tolerable burden limits. In patients with cardiac and respiratory insufficiency, additional symptomatic measurements are helpful.

Endocrine myopathies

Myopathies can occur with different endocrine diseases and then lead to pareses of sudden onset (Table 8.14). Pathophysiological bases are changed electrolyte concentrations or metabolic disturbances due to the endocrinopathy.

Thyrotoxic episodic weakness (paresis)

This type of episodic paresis occurs primarily in Asian men. It is said to develop in up to 13% of all Asian men

Table 8.15 Toxic and drug induced myopathies

Acute alcohol myopathy (rhabdomyolysis)
Cocaine, heroine, amphetamines
Colchicine and vincristine
Chloroquine, doxorubicin, amiodarone
Low potassium myopathy due to diuretics, laxants, licorice or alcohol
Emetin
Petrol vapor, toluene
Lipid-lowering drugs
Inflammatory myopathies with penicillin and cimetidine
Steroid myopathy
Procainamide
Malnutrition, Vitamin E deficiency

Table 8.16 Inflammatory acute myopathies

polymyositis
dermatomyositis
polymyositis and dermatomyositis with malignant tumors
polymyositis with collagenoses
sarcoidosis
myositis with infections

with thyrotoxicosis. Clinically, the symptoms are similar to low potassium episodic weakness with paresis of singular muscles or groups of muscles or a generalized weakness. Facial muscles, speech muscles, muscles for swallowing as well as the diaphragm are always spared. The weakness usually lasts several minutes, but can last up to several days. The attacks of paresis are provoked by intense body exertion followed by rest, by coldness or by high-carbohydrate and sodium-content meals. During the period of paresis, the potassium level drops but not always below the reference value. If the hypothyroid status is treated adaequately, the periodic pareses stop. During the acute attack of paresis, application of potassium is of help. Propanolol can diminish the frequency of the attacks of episodic paresis.

Toxic and drug-induced myopathies

A number of toxic substances including drugs can cause myopathies (Table 8.15). Muscular damage due to drugs leads to a rapidly progressive proximal or proximally pronounced muscular weakness, often associated with pronounced muscular pain, and has to be differentiated from polymyositis. Sometimes the rapid destruction of muscle can lead to myoglobinuria.

Acute alcohol myopathy

Within hours to days, a rapidly progressive proximal, sometimes asymmetrical weakness develops with marked myalgias, rhabdomyolysis, myoglobinuria, creatine kinase increase and hypokalaemia (low potassium). Recommended therapy is alcohol abstinence.

Malignant hyperthermia

Malignant hyperthermia can be caused by different inhalation anesthetics and muscle relaxants used as narcotics. The liability is inherited autosomal dominantly on chromosome 17 and 19. Together with tachycardia, drop in blood pressure, acidosis and rise of temperature above 41°C, muscular tremor and muscle stiffness occur. As complication rhabdomyolysis, kidney insufficiency and disseminated intravascular coagulation can occur. The therapy of choice is dantrolene intravenously as well as external cooling.

Malignant neuroleptic syndrome

The malignant neuroleptic syndrome is clinically very similar to the malignant hyperthermic syndrome. The cardinal symptoms are extrapyramidal motor disturbances and hyperthermia, probably due to an acute relative dopamine deficiency in basal ganglia and hypothalamus. Very similar clinical symptoms can occur with acute L-dopa deprivation. Therapeutically, dantrolene or dopamine agonists can be given.

Inflammatory myopathies

The inflammatory myopathies are a heterogeneous group of diseases, some of which are associated with acute-onset muscular weakness, for example, polymyositis and dermatomyositis (Table 8.16), whereas other forms are more slowly progressive, such as inclusion body myositis. Myositis can occur in patients with systemic disease or in association with collagenoses as well as with infectious diseases. The exact differential diagnosis is important because, due to the different underlying pathologies of certain myositides, a differenciated therapy has to be implemented.

Generalized weakness of non-organic origin

Generalized motor weakness can be of psychogenic origin if all organic causes are excluded, which have to be considered in the differential diagnosis. Beside the aforementioned primarily neurological etiologies of a generalized paroxysmal muscular weakness, internal medicine diseases with generalized asthenia have to be kept in mind, which can be interpreted as muscular weakness by the patient. To be mentioned especially are diabetes mellitus, different endocrinopathies, consuming diseases, electrolyte disturbances and diseases with impaired immune resistance. If neither an underlying neurological nor an internal medicine organic disease can be found, a psychogenic cause is likely. Muscular weakness can often be seen as the somatic correlate of a depression with other signs of depression as leading symptoms. The "chronic fatigue syndrome" also has to be mentioned here.

Case history

Case 1: S.B., male, 22 years. Paroxysmal exercise-induced monoparesis right arm.

S.B. was referred for evaluation of paroxysmal weakness of the right arm. The patient reported that the symptoms started in mid-November 2003. During that time, he was given more responsibility in his work as roofer in the new position as foreman, and therefore had more stress than before. The first episode happened while swinging a 2-kg burner with the right arm. He was doing this pendicular movement for 3 to 4 hours per day, distributed over the whole day. During this movement, he first noticed a sudden weakness in the upper and lower part of the right arm, and the right arm was falling down following gravity. After a few seconds, he noticed a tremorous movement in the muscles of the right arm, especially in the lower part, of 10 to 30 seconds duration. Following that, the strength in the arm returned over the next three minutes and the patient could continue with his work. Initially, one to two episodes of this type of weakness occurred per day. At the end of December, the frequency of these paroxysmal attacks decreased to two episodes per week. The paresis comes on without warning each time when repetitive movements with the right arm for 10 to 30 minutes were performed. For example, the shovel of gravel or the frequent pouring from a two-liter bottle could provoke these attacks. Apart from some pain in the right elbow during the first attack, the patient never experienced pain, sensory disturbances or dizziness during or after an attack. From the personal history, a fall from 4-m height onto the back without loss of consciousness and without fractures in autumn 2002 has to be mentioned. No regular medication, and a family history negative for neurological dis-

eases. Social history revealed he worked for five years as a roofer.

Neurological examination: patient awake, fully conscious and orientated. Right-handed, head free and moveable. On hyperextension and flexion of the head, drawing pain in the nape of the neck, no paresis of the arm, Adson negative. No meningism, skull not painful on knocking; speech normal; cranial nerves normal. Deep tendon reflexes symmetrical, no pyramidal tract signs. No motor symptoms; coordination intact. Sensory system: discrete, distally pronounced diminution of pain, light touch and temperature sense on the right arm. Vibration sense 8/8 on both hands. Gait and standing normal. In conclusion, a slight diminution of light touch, pain and temperature sensation in the distal part of the right arm; otherwise normal examination.

Additional test results included laboratory examination with hematological blood tests: normal. Chemistry: slightly elevated creatine kinase of 180 U/l, otherwise normal. Coagulation tests normal; urine chemistry normal. Erythrocyte sedimentation rate of 22 mm/hr. Spinal fluid: total cell count 1/μl (less than 3), total protein content and glucose within normal limts.

Chest x-ray revealed minimal extraction of the cranial medial part of the first rib on the right side, and a slightly hypoplastic left first rib. Otherwise, age- and habitus-appropriate normal cardiac and pulmonary findings. The minimal bony extraction can be taken as an indirect hint toward a thoracic outlet syndrome.

Cranio-cerebral and vertebro-spinal (C0 – Th5) MRI showed a small AV-malformation in the cerebrum frontal left as well as in the left cerebellum; otherwise, a normal MRI. Normal cervical spine and normal cervical myelon. Normal MRI of the upper chest and brachial plexus, normal MR-angiography of the supraaortal branches with the normal variant of Truncus bicaroticus. With elevation of the arm, a slight impingement of the left subclavian artery between first rib and clavicle; normal right subclavian artery.

EEG and sonographic examination of the brain-feeding vessels revealed normal results. Electroneurographically normal results for right axillary, median and ulnar nerve. Electromyography at rest and after exercise revealed normal results in the deltoid muscle. Motor-evoked potentials at cortical magnetic stimulation and recording on arms and legs showed no signs of pyramidal tract lesion.

Somato-sensory evoked potentials of the median nerve with good reproducibility of the potentials on all leads (cortical, cervical, near plexus). There was a non-significant delay of the cortical N20 response with normal central conduction time and a significant side-to-side difference of the N9-response (near plexus) in disfavor of the right side. Therefore, the pathological absolute latency is most likely due to a peripheral lesion of the right median nerve. In conclusion, a pathological median nerve SEP on the right side with suspicion of a peripheral lesion.

The 22-year-old patient suffers from an exercise-induced, paroxysmal painless weakness of the right arm without accompanying sensory symptoms since mid-November 2003. The symptoms were always reversible within a few minutes. The clinical neurological examination was normal apart from a slight impairment of light touch, pain and temperature sensation on the distal part of the right arm, not consistent with a dermatome or the territory of a peripheral nerve distribution, especially where there were no pareses or reflex asymmetries. Differential diagnosis included compression of the myelon or affection of radicular structures, which could be excluded by vertebrospinal MRI. Electrophysiological examinations revealed no signs of a lesion of the axillary, median or ulnar nerve on the right side. There were also no signs of exercise-induced weakness of the deltoid muscle or the axillary nerve, respectively. With normal motor-evoked potentials in the interval, there were no signs of a permanent pyramidal tract lesion. Despite adaequate exercise, it was not possible to provoke the weakness the patient described. With respect to the patient's description, with only intermittently occurring weakness dependent on repetitive movement of the arm, a central etiology is highly unlikely to be compatible with the normal MRI results. Besides, small AV-malformations in the left frontal region of the cerebrum as well as in the cerebellum on the left side were seen without pathological meaning. The actual EEG showed neither focal slowing nor paroxysmal epileptic activity. Ultrasound sonography of the brain-feeding vessels was normal as well, especially with no sign of subclavian stenosis. Extensive laboratory work-up did not reveal any major abnormalities, especially normal electrolytes without signs of low potassium paresis. On lumbar puncture, no signs of acute CNS infection, tests for *B. burgdorferi* and Treponemen were negative. Oligoclonal bands as sign of autochthonous intrathecal IgG production in chronic inflammation was negative.

The only abnormal finding on additional tests were pathological somatosensory-evoked potentials of the right side with significantly delayed P9 response at Erb with reduced amplitude but normal central conduction time, consistent with a syndrome of the upper thoracic aperture. Conventional x-ray examination could not rule out a cervical rib but demonstrated a slight bony extension of the first rib on the right side as indirect sign of a possible thoracic outlet syndrome (TOS). MRI of the upper thoracic aperture and the brachial plexus as well as magnetic resonance angiography of the supraaortal branches did not unequivocally confirm the diagnosis of TOS. A functional etiology of the symptoms also has to be discussed but there are neither hints in the history nor on the impression from the personal examination and the time of the patient in the ward as an in-patient toward a funtional etiology. The paroxysmal exercise-induced weakness of the right arm was therefore diagnosed as the consequence of a compression syndrome near the brachial plexus in the sense of a TOS or a costoclavicular syndrome, respectively.

Therapeutically, physiotherapy for strengthening of the shoulder girdle- and body-bearing muscles was recommended. A decompressive operation was regarded as not indicated, especially as the postoperative results in the available studies are very variable. Follow-up examinations demonstrated stable clinical symptoms without deterioration.

References

Amarenco P, Bogousslavsky J, Callahan A, Goldstein L, Hennerici M, Rudolph A, Sillesen H, Simunovic L, Szarek M, Welch K, Zivin J. High-dose atorvastatin after stroke or transient ischemic attack. *N Engl J Med* 2006, **355**:549–559.

Antithrombotic Trialists' Collaboration. Collaborative meta-analysis of randomized trials of antiplatelet therapy for death, myocardial infarction, and stroke in high risk patients. *BMJ* 2002, **524**:71–86.

Bassetti C. Spectrum of narcolepsy. In: Bassetti CL, Billiard M, Mignot E (eds.) *Narcolepsy and hypersomnia.* New York, London: Informa Healthcare, 2007, pp. 97–108.

Bennett CL, Connors JM, Carwile JM, Moake JL, Bell WR, Tarantolo SR, MsCarthy LJ, Sarode R, Hatfield AJ, Feldman MD, Davidson CJ, Tsai HM. Thrombocytic thrombocytopenic purpura associated with clopidogrel. *N Engl J Med* 2000, **342**:1773–1777.

Berlit P. Schlaganfall – Differentialdiagnostische Übersicht. In: Berlit P (Hrsg.) *Klinische Neurologie*. Heidelberg, New York: Springer, Berlin, 2006, pp. 941–950.

Bhatt D, Fox K, Hacke W, Berger P, Black H, Boden W, Cacoub P, Cohen E, Creager M, Easton J, Flather M, Haffner S, Hamm C, Hankey G, Johnston S, Mak K, Mas J, Montalescot G, Pearson T, Steg P, Steinhubl S, Weber M, Brennan D, Fabry-Ribaudo I, Booth J, Topol E. Clopidogrel and aspirin versus aspirin alone fort he prevention of atherothrombotic events. *N Engl J Med* 2006, **354**:1706–1717.

CAPRIE Steering Committee. A randomised, blinded trial of clopidogrel versus aspirin in patients at risk of ischaemic events (CAPRIE). *Lancet* 1996, **348**:1329–1339.

CAVATAS. Endovascular versus surgical treatment in patients with carotid stenosis in the Carotid and Vertebral Artery Transluminal Angioplasty Study (CAVATAS): a randomized trial. *Lancet* 2001, **357**:1729–1737.

Department of Health and Human Services and FDA. Internal analgesic, antipyretic, and antirheumatic drug products for over-the counter human use. Final rule for professional labelling of aspirin, buffered aspirin and aspirin in combination with antacid drug. *Int J Clin Pract* 1998, **63**:56802–56819.

Diener HC, Forbes C, Riekkinen P, Sivenius J, Smets P, Lowenthal A, and the ESPS group. European Stroke Prevention Study 2: Efficacy and safety data. *J Neurol Sci* 1997, **151**:S1-S77.

Diener HC, Hamann GF. Primäre und sekundäre Prävention der zerebralen Ischämie. In: Brandt T, Dichgans J, Diener HC (Hrsg.) *Therapie und Verlauf neurologischer Erkrankungen.* 4. Aufl., Stuttgart: Kohlhammer, 2003, pp. 359–376.

Diener H, Bogousslavsky J, Brass I, Cimminiello C, Csiba I, Kaste M, Leys D, Matias-Guiu J, Rupprecht H. Aspirin and clopidogrel compared with clopidogrel alone after recent ischaemic stroke or transient ischemic attack in high-risk patients (MATCH): randomised, double-blind, placebo-controlled trial. *Lancet* 2004, **364**:331–337.

European Atrial Fibrillation Trial Study Group. Secondary prevention in non-rheumatic atrial fibrillation after transient ischemic attack or minor stroke. *Lancet* 1993, **342**:1255–1262.

European Carotid Surgery Trialists' Collaborative Group. MRC European Carotid Surgery Trial: interim results for symptomatic patients with severe (70–99%) or with mild (0–29%) carotid stenosis. *Lancet* 1991, **337**:1235–1243.

European Stroke Initiative. Recommendations for stroke management: update 2003. Prevention. *Cerebrovasc Dis* 2004, **17** (Suppl 2):15–29.

European Stroke Organisation (ESO) Executive Committee and the ESO Writing Committee. Guidelines for management of ischemic stroke and transient ischemic attack 2008. *Cerebrovasc Dis* 2008, **25**:457–507.

Guilleminault C, Lee JH, Arias V. Cataplexy. In: Bassetti CL, Billiard M, Mignot E (eds.) *Narcolepsy and hypersomnia.* New York, London: *Informa Healthcare* 2007, pp. 49–62.

Halkes P, van Gjin J, Kapelle I, Koudstaal P, Algra A. Aspirin plus dipyridamole versus aspirin alone after cerebral ischemia of arterial origin (ESPRIT): Randomized controlled trial. *Lancet* 2006, **367**:1665–1673.

Lee MS, Choi YC, Heo JH, Choi IS. "Drop attacks" with stiffening of the right leg associated with posterior fossa arachnoid cyst. *Movement Disorders* 1994, **9**:377–378.

Mas JL, Arquizan C, Lamy C, Zuber M, Cabanes L, Derumeaux G, Coste J, Patent Foramen Ovale and Atrial Septal Aneurysm Study Group. Recurrent cerebrovascular events associated with patent foramen ovale, atrial septal aneurysm, or both. *N Engl J Med* 2001, **345**:1740–1746.

Mas JL, Chatellier G, Beyssen B, Branchereau A, Moulin T, Becquemin JP, Larrue V, Lièvre M, Leys D, Bonneville JF, Watelet J, Pruvo JP, Albucher JF, Viguier A, Piquet P, Garnier P, Viader F, Touzé E, Giroud M, Hosseini H, Pillet JC, Favrole P, Neau JP, Ducrocq X, for the EVA-3S Investigators: endarterectomy versus stenting in patients with symptomatic severe carotid stenosis. *N Engl J Med* 2006, **355**:1660–1671.

North American Symptomatic Carotid Endarterectomy Trial Collaborators. Beneficial effect of carotid endarterectomy in symptomatic patients with high-grade carotid stenosis. *N Engl J Med* 1991, **325**:445–453.

PROGRESS Collaborative Group. Randomized trial of a perindopril-based blood-pressure-lowering regimen among 6,105 individuals with previous stroke or transient ischemic attack. *Lancet* 2001, **358**:1033–1041.

Remler BF, Daroff RB. Falls and drop attacks. In: Bradley WG, Daroff RB, Fenichel GM, Marsden CD. (eds.) *Neurology in Clinical Practice. Principles of Diagnosis and Management.* Volume I. 2nd edn. Boston: Butterworth-Heinemann, 1996, pp. 23–28.

Ringleb PA, Allenberg JR, Bereger J, Brückmann H, Eckstein HH, Fraedrich G, Hartmann M, Hennerici M, Jansen O, Klein G, Kunze A, Marx P, Niederkorn K, Schmiedt W, Solymosi I, Stingele R, Zeumer H, Hacke W. 30 day results from the SPACE trial of stent-protected angioplasty versus carotis endarterectomy in symptomatic patients: a randomised non-inferiority trial. *Lancet* 2006, **368**:1239–1247.

Rothwell PM, Eliasziv M, Gutnikov SA, Fox AJ, Taylor DW, Mayberg MR, Warlow CP, Barnett HJM. Analysis of pooled data from the randomized controlled trials of endarterectomy for symptomatic carotid stenosis. *Lancet* 2003, **361**:107–116.

Sareen D. Ictal hemiparesis: differentiation from stroke. *J Assoc Physicians India* 2001, **49**:838–840.

Schrader J, Luders S, Kulschewski A, Hammersen F, Plate K, Berger J, Zidek W, Dominiak P, Diener H. Morbidity and mortality after stroke. Eprosartan compared with nitrendipine for secondary prevention: principal results of a prospective randomized controlled study (MOSES). *Stroke* 2005, **36**: 1218–1226.

Siegel JM, Moore R, Thannickal T, Nienhuis R. A brief history of hypocretin/orexin and narcolepsy. *Neuropsychopharmacology* 2001, 25 (Suppl. 5):S14–20.

Further reading

Bassetti CL, Billiard M, Mignot E. (eds.). *Narcolepsy and Hypersomnia*. New York: Informa Healthcare, 2007.

Berlit P. (Hrsg.) *Klinische Neurologie*, 2. Auflage. Berlin, Heidelberg, New York: Springer, 2006.

Kaplan PW, Fisher RS. (eds.). *Imitators of epilepsy*, 2nd edn. New York: Demos, 2005.

Poeck K, Hacke W. (Hrsg.) Neurologie 12. *Auflage*. Berlin, Heidelberg, New York: Springer, 2006.

Paroxysmal dyskinesias

Ludwig D. Schelosky[*]

Introduction

Paroxysmal features occur in the majority of movement disorders (Table 9.1). Patients with Parkinson's disease fluctuate between states where they are "on" and "sudden off" ("yo-yoing"). Unexpected freezing leads to falls and serious injury. Facial or cervical dystonia changes according to accompanying environmental events. Action-specific dystonia only manifests itself during highly specialized movement sequences such as writing, playing musical instruments or practicing (professional) sports. Muscle spasms in the "stiff person" syndrome are paroxysmal. Choreatic, myoclonic, tic movements, startle reactions, restless-legs syndrome and periodic movements in sleep vary enormously in extent and may mimic paroxysms. Excitement or fear of social stigmatization increases the intensity of nearly all movement disorders. Yet they are not called "paroxysmal movement disorders." This term exclusively denotes a subgroup of movement disorders called "paroxysmal dyskinesias."

Definition

Paroxysmal dyskinesias are a heterogeneous group of disorders characterized by intermittent attacks of hyperkinetic involuntary movements without loss of consciousness. In 1892, Shuzo Kure was the first to give a detailed description of a young man with paroxysmal kinesigenic dyskinesia (PKD) but erroneously assigned the diagnosis "atypical case of Thomsen's disease." An early anecdotal report was found in the notes of Gowers in 1901. In 1965, Mount and Reback were

the first to describe a patient with paroxysmal non-kinesigenic dyskinesia (PNKD).

Initially, paroxysmal dyskinesias were differentiated by duration of symptoms (Lance 1977). Attacks of long duration were called non-kinesigenic and showed mainly dystonic and choreatic movements. All attacks of short duration were called kinesigenic and assumed to be choreatic. This classification was abandoned due to inaccurate differentiation of the subgroups of paroxysmal dyskinesias. The type of movement is insufficient to discriminate the disorders. In all paroxysmal dyskinesias, the movements are mainly dystonic (72% according to Demirkiran and Jankovic 1995), and chorea, ballism, unspecified or mixed types are rather rare.

Demirkiran and Jankovic (1995) suggested a new classification. Their proposal subdivided the paroxysmal disorders according to precipitating events that followed then by the duration of the attacks, and finally by possible underlying etiology. The precipitating event is predictive of a response to treatment and prognosis.

Paroxysmal dyskinesias comprise the following:

- Paroxysmal kinesigenic dyskinesia (PKD; DYT10)
- Paroxysmal non-kinesigenic dyskinesia (PNKD; DYT8)
- Paroxysmal exercise-induced dyskinesia (PED)
- Paroxysmal hypnogenic dyskinesia (PHD)

Each of these types may be of short (less than 5 minutes) or long (more than 5 minutes) duration. The etiology can be idiopathic, sporadic or secondary to known causes. The formerly used term paroxysmal kinesigenic choreoathetosis (PKC) is close to the currently used concept of short-duration PKD; the former paroxysmal dystonic choreoathetosis (PDC) resembles the long-duration PNKD of today (Bhatia 2001). The

---

[*] This chapter is dedicated to my esteemed teacher and mentor Prof. Dr. Werner H. Poewe, in deepest and sincerest gratitude.

Table 9.1 Paroxysmal dyskinesias – an overview (according to Jankovic and Demirkiran 2002)

	Paroxysmal kinesigenic dyskinesia (PKD)	Paroxysmal non-kinesigenic dyskinesia (PNKD)	Paroxysmal exercise-induced dyskinesia (PED)	Paroxysmal hypnogenic dyskinesia (PHD)
Trigger	Sudden movement	Alcohol, coffee, tea, spontaneous	Long duration exercise	Non-REM sleep stage II
Duration	Seconds to few minutes	Minutes to days	5–30 minutes	Mostly 30–45 seconds
Typical movement pattern	Dystonic, choreatic, ballistic	Dystonic	Dystonic	Dystonic, choreatic, ballistic
Frequency	Several per day	Few per day to some per year	1/day to 2/month	1–20/night to 5/year
Age at onset	7th–4th year of age	Earlier than PKD	9th–15th year of age	3rd–47th year of age, mean 21.8 years
Gender ratio	Male ≫ female	Male > female	Male > female	Male = female
Treatment	Antiepileptic drugs	Avoidance of triggers	Avoidance of long duration exercise	Antiepileptic drugs

classification by Demirkiran and Jankovic fits for most, but not all, of the patients. These paroxysmal dyskinesias are exceptionally rare and no information exists about their epidemiology.

Diagnosis

Paroxysmal kinesigenic dyskinesia (PKD; DYT10)

Trigger: Sudden movements, mainly of the whole body after a period of rest, rising after sitting, change of walking speed. Anxiety lowers the attack threshold in two thirds of patients. Rare precipitants are caffeine, starvation, cannabis, menstruation and cold weather.

Movement pattern: Mainly dystonic, infrequently choreatic, ballistic or unspecified (Fig. 9.1). Combination of different movement types is common. The paroxysmal movements may affect the arm or leg on one or both sides of the body, or all extremities. The head and trunk are less often involved, but falls and dysarthria have been described. The body parts involved and the side of the body may vary between the attacks. Consciousness is never lost, and the involuntary movements are very rarely painful. After a bout of dyskinesia, the person is refractory to the usual triggers for 5 to 20 minutes. The degree of dyskinesic movement is variable between the families and within the members of the individual families described. These movements range from slight movements allowing continued daily activity

to completely incapacitating storms of movements. The individual patient often gets familiar with a typical course of their attack, even though there may be some individual variability. Aura-like anticipation like a march of tingling, tight feeling or tremulousness of the affected extremities occurs in more than 80% of patients. Suspending or slowing down the intended movement during the premonitory feeling can avoid or mitigate the attack. Menstrual state can have an influence and can exacerbate this disorder.

There is an infantile-onset group where the disorder makes its clinical manifestation during the first year of life. Children have their attacks while playing or walking, sitting in a car seat, at times of excitement and during sleep. No loss of consciousness is observed. Movement, as the trigger, is less obligatory. The attacks are usually very short, sometimes only a few seconds.

Nearly 20% of the patients with PKC have a positive personal or family history of infantile convulsions. PKN may also be associated with migraine, writer's cramp and essential tremor.

Duration: Seconds to a few minutes. More than 95% of patients report attacks shorter than 1 minute.

Frequency: Several attacks per day, up to 30 or 40.

Age of onset: Disease starts at a mean age 6 to 15 years (range: 1–57), most often coinciding with puberty. Ninety percent have an onset before age 15, and it is unlikely to have the first attack of an idiopathic PKD after age 20. Males predominate anywhere from 4:1 to 8:1 (Fahn 1994a). There is an infantile group where the disorder manifests within

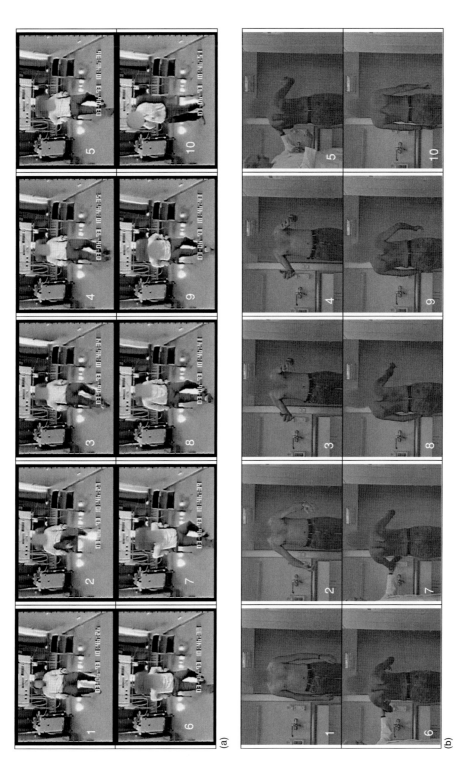

Fig. 9.1. (a) Paroxysmal kinesigenic dyskinesia. Patient is sitting in the chair (1) and voluntarily moves both legs in a cycling manner (2). Seven seconds later, the left leg extends dystonically, trunk is stretched and levers the patient out of the sitting position (3–7). The patient voluntarily pushes himself upward with his arms (8, 9). Seventeen seconds later the kinesigenic dyskinesia has stopped, the patient can stand upright (10) (Courtesy A. Nebe, MD). (b) Paroxysmal kinesigenic dyskinesias. The patient lifts both arms voluntarily (1–2). Muscles of the arms contract dystonically (3–4), and the shoulder girdle muscles are involved (5–6). Thirty-eight seconds later the left (7–8) and after a further 6 seconds the right arm release again (9–10).

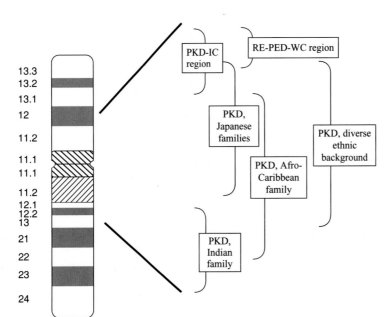

Fig. 9.2. Pericentromer of chromosome 16 containing the critical regions (grey bars) of the three paroxysmal dyskinesia loci. A: Szepetowski et al. 1997; B: Guerrini et al. 1999; D: Bruno et al. 2004; F: Bennett et al. 2000; Cuenca-Leon et al. 2002; H: Cuenca-Leon et al. 2002 (carrier); I: Cuenca-Leon et al. 2002 (non-carrier). RE-PED-WC denotes "Rolandic epilepsy, PED, graphospasm," PKD-IC is "PKD, Infantile convulsions," EKD2 stands for "Episodic Kinesigenic Dyskinesia 2." Centromere is indicated with an empty circle. Order and distances between markers are according to the Marshfield genetic map. The order of the markers concurs with that of the human genome sequence draft (genome.ucsc.edu). Figure reprinted with kind permission from Cuenca-Leon et al., Paroxysmal Kinesigenic Dyskinesia, *Neuropediatrics* (2002); **33**:288–293. Copyright 27.07.2007 Georg Thieme Verlag KG, Stuttgart.

the first year of life, called infantile-onset PKD. These statistics noted here are valid only for the idiopathic and familial types. Secondary cases appear to have more diversity and can present at different ages.

Therapy: Very good responses to low doses of anticonvulsant medication, particularly sodium-channel blockers, have been reported. There is up to a 90% response rate with carbamazepine and phenytoin. There are uncontrolled case reports of positive responses to phenobarbital, levetiracetam, oxcarbazepine and topiramate. Therapeutic success with acetazolamide, levodopa, tetrabenazine and flunarizine have also been reported. Overall, in the adult population 77% of patients lose their symptoms while an additional 14% experience attack reduction of more than 50% (Nagamitsu et al. 1999). Infantile cases are more variable in response to anti-epileptic drugs.

Etiology: Autosomal dominant inheritance pattern with variable, mostly high penetrance is noted. A positive family history is not mandatory for the diagnosis of idiopathic PKD but may ease significantly the need for a significant diagnostic workup. Sporadic forms are rare but must be suspected in patients with disease onset after age 20. Familial forms of the disease seem more frequent in Japan and China. The human earwax

phenotype (wet or dry) co-segregates with the PKC in several Japanese families and could be mapped within the PKC locus.

Initially, it was believed that PKD constituted a homogenous disease with one or at the most two closely related gene defects (Bhatia 2001). Spacey et al. identified the differences in triggering factors, clinical manifestation and concomitant neurological diseases between different families with the disorder and postulated genetic heterogeneity for PKD (Spacey et al. 2002). Gene loci for some of families are likely to lie in the pericentromeric region of chromosome 16 (Fig. 9.2), where candidate ion-channel genes are situated.

The ICCA syndrome (infantile convulsions, paroxysmal choreoathetosis) is mapped onto the same chromosomal region. PKD and ICCA are now believed to be essentially the same disorder, based on their clinical similarity and the overlap of the genetic loci (Bruno et al. 2004; Hattori et al. 2000). The genes of PKD have not been detected.

Course of disease: Attack frequency and intensity reach their peak level after several years and remain stable or decrease slowly over the years. The most common age of remission is the third decade. In one series, 27% of the patients became symptom-free, whereas another 25% showed marked improvement (Bruno et al. 2004). Females have a much higher rate of complete remissions and, during pregnancy, attacks are reduced. Infantile PKD may remit within the first or second decade of life.

In summary, the main diagnostic criteria for idiopathic PKD (Bruno et al. 2004) are:

1. Short (less than 1 minute) attacks following a kinesigenic trigger
2. No loss of consciousness
3. Respond to carbamazepine or phenytoin
4. Age of onset 1 to 20 years
5. Normal neurologic examination between attacks

Paroxysmal non-kinesigenic dyskinesia (PNKD; DYT8)

After identification of the *MR-1* gene, the proposal was made to divide typical (*MR-1* positive) and atypical (*MR-1* negative) forms. Patients with the typical clinical presentation, which is similar to PNKD as reported by Mount and Reback, are likely to harbor myofibrillogenesis regulator 1 (*MR-1*) gene mutations (see "Etiology," Bruno et al. 2007).

Trigger: Alcohol, coffee and tea frequently induce these movements 30 to 60 minutes after consumption. This sensitivity is one major clinical hint to the diagnosis of *MR-1* positive cases. Emotional stress may lower attack threshold. Menstruation (6%), heat (22%), exercise (12%), starvation (6%) and fatigue (12%) are less common precipitants. The movements may occur without a clear cause.

In *MR-1* negative patients, exercise is a trigger in 70%, followed by caffeine (38%), fatigue (32%), emotional stress (27%), heat (23%) and starvation (14%). Menstruation, alcohol and nicotine were not reported as triggers in any of these patients.

Movement pattern: *MR-1* positive patients experience a mixture of dystonia and chorea along with some ballistic elements. Dyskinesia can start in full intensity or may spread from one body part to the rest of the body. Dystonic muscle contraction is often painful. Consciousness is always preserved, but sometimes the patient is unresponsive because of dystonic contractions. Involuntary movements may eventually cause falling. Anticipatory symptoms in the affected extremities like tension, tightness, tenderness, numbness or tingling

dysesthesia were reported in nearly half of the *MR-1* patients. Epigastric aura can emerge (Lance 1977). Neurologic examination usually is unremarkable between attacks, but nearly half of the patients fulfill diagnostic criteria for migraine.

MR-1 negative patients mainly suffer from dystonic movements. Chorea and ballistic movements are rare, but combined movement sequences occur in about 30% of affected patients. Aura symptoms are common. The interictal neurologic examination is usually normal but one quarter of the patients have epilepsy or mild ataxia. The combination with other neurological signs or diseases has been reported such as myokymia, exercise-induced muscle cramps, focal dystonia and migraine (Hofele et al. 1997). Relatives of *MR-1* negative patients with no apparent movement disorder sometimes report short-lasting, painful exercise-induced tension or cramps in arms or legs. Some authors discussed a "forme fruste" of PNKD (Schloesser et al. 1996), whereas others assume this is a misclassification of PED-cases.

Duration: Symptoms may last 10 minutes to 1 hour in *MR-1* positive patients with some examples of cases lasting up to 12 hours. The *MR-1* negative patients usually have shorter attacks, several minutes to a few hours. Very long attacks up to 48 hours have been described.

Frequency: For *MR-1* positive patients, 1 to 3 attacks per day to 1 to 2 attacks per year is the range for the frequency, which varies over one's lifetime and seems to decline during pregnancy. *MR-1* negative patients have a lower frequency of attacks, with a range of several attacks per month to a few attacks per year.

Age of onset: *MK-1* positive cases usually start having symptoms at age 3 months to 12 years, with an average onset of four years. *MK-1* negative and sporadic cases have a more variable age of onset. The mean age at onset is 12 years with a range from the second month of age to age 40. The later onset is exceptionally rare. In typical familial cases there is no gender difference, and in *MK-1* negative cases male predominance is not as obvious as it is in PKN (1.4–2 : 1).

Therapy: Avoidance of trigger factors is of paramount importance. Some patients experience shortening of the attacks when they eat at onset. In about 70% of all typical patients, hyperkinetic movements resolve during sleep. Only one third of the *MR-1* negative cases report improvement with sleep. Diazepam, clonazepam or L-tryptophan (500–3000 mg/day) are the drugs of choice in typical patients, but these drugs are less beneficial in atypical ones. Anti-epileptic drugs are of no or poor benefit. Levodopa showed ambiguous results, with improvement in some and appeared to be associated with deterioration in others. Gabapentin helped one person, and a person with symptomatic disease they responded to oxcarbazepine. In summary, drug treatment of atypical PNKD is not very successful. Treatment with thalamic deep brain stimulation has been reported to be helpful. *Etiology*: The defective gene of the dominantly inherited PNKD is localized to the chromosome 2q and seems to be homogenous across the families described. The myofibrillogenesis regulator 1 gene (*MR-1*) on chromosome 2q33–35 is the gene associated with PNKD, with two known missense mutations at A7V and A9V. The function of *MR-1* is not known but it is homologous to HAGH (glyoxalase II), a member of the zinc metallohydrolase enzymes that hydrolyze methylglyoxal. This substance is contained in coffee and alcohol in high levels. These enzymes are expressed in the cerebellum, spinal cord and basal ganglia.

A second gene locus (*PNKD2*) was found on chromosome 2q31 and may be related to GABAergic metabolism. Although the phenotype is quite similar between the different genetic origins, the chromosome 2q31-family shows no provocation of attacks by alcohol and caffeine as was seen in the *MR-1* gene family. In a large German family, a slightly different syndrome, PNKD plus syndrome, was found where DYT9 has a location on chromosome 1p (Table 9.2).

Du et al. reported a large family with co-existing generalized epilepsy and PNKD. An autosomal dominantly inherited mutation of the chromosomal region 10q22 causes an $A \rightarrow G$ transition in exon 10 of the KCNMA1, encoding the pore forming α subunit of the Maxi-K channel. This region regulates the K^+ conductance of the channel, and this mutation resulted in an abnormal Ca^{++} affinity for the K^+ channel. In response to depolarization and Ca^{++} entry during action potentials, more mutant Maxi-K channels open. This causes a more rapid repolarization of the action potential, which enables a faster repriming of the channels and therefore greater firing frequency. The enhancement of the Maxi-K channel function is associated with brain hyperexcitability as expressed by epilepsy and PNKD.

Course of disease: Very variable across the families. Stable disease, improvement or worsening with age, all may occur.

In conclusion, together there are two main types of PNKD. The criteria for *MR-1* positive cases are defined by:

1. Hyperkinetic involuntary movement attacks with onset in infancy or early childhood, with dystonia, chorea, or a combination of both, typically lasting 10 minutes to one hour
2. Neurological examination normal between attacks
3. Precipitation of attacks by caffeine or alcohol consumption
4. Family history of the same movement disorder

The *MR-1* negative patients are more variable in their age at onset, precipitants, clinical features and response to medications.

Paroxysmal exercise-induced dyskinesia (PED)

Trigger: Long-duration exercise such as walking or chewing is often the trigger. Compared to PKD, the attacks start after 10 to 15 minutes of exercise, not immediately after movement onset. Rare precipitants are coldness, passive movement of extremities, vibration, alcohol and menstruation.
Movement pattern: Nearly always dystonic. Legs are involved most often. Very often spread from one extremity (the one with the long-standing exercise) to the whole body. Hemidystonic distribution with nearly no change of sides between attacks has been reported.
Duration: Five to 30 minutes, rarely up to 120 minutes. In most cases, dyskinesia stops a few minutes after the end of effort.
Frequency: The frequency varies from 1 per day to 2 per month.

Table 9.2 Genetics of paroxysmal dyskinesias (according to Bhatia 2001)

Author	Disease	Chromosomal location
Fouad et al. 1996	PNKD (DYT8)	2q33-q35, region has been narrowed to 4-cm interval (*FPD1*-Locus). The myofibrillogenesis regulator 1 gene (*MR-1/BRP17*) in this region is associated with PNKD
Spacey et al. 2006	PNKD (DYT8)	2q31 (between markers D2S335 and D2S152) (*PNKD2*-locus)
Du et al. 2005	PNKD (DYT8)	10q22, mutation in the α subunit of the Maxi-K channel
Auburger et al. 1996	PNKD and spasticity, perioral paraesthesia, headache, double vision, generalized myoclonia, epileptic seizures (DYT9)	Chromosome 1p13.3-p21 (Potassium-Channel, *CSE*-Locus)
Szepetowski et al. 1997	PKD/ICCA/Rolandic epilepsy, PED, graphospasm	16p12-q12, 16p11.2-q12.1, 16p12–11.2, 16q13–22.1 Two loci have been reported so far: Episodic Kinesigenic Dyskinesia 1 (*EKD1*) Episodic Kinesigenic Dyskinesia 2 (*EKD2*) At least one further locus must exist outside the chromosome 16
	PKD induced by passive limb movements, severe global retardation, thyroid hormone abnormalities	X-chromosomal mutation in the *MCT8* gene, encoding for a thyroid hormone transporter
Guerrini et al. 1999	PED, Rolandic epilepsy, writer's cramp	Chromosome 16p12–11.2 (overlapping with the region for ICCA and potentially allelic to the location of the PKD locus)
Münchau et al. 2000	PED and migraine without aura	Exclusion of a link to PNKD and ICCA-genes
Steinlein et al. 1995	ADNFLE (autosomal dominant nocturnal frontal lobe epilepsy)	Chromosome 20q13.2 (*CHRNA4*-Locus), acetylcholine-receptor Chromosome 15q24 (*?CHRNA3*-Locus), nicotinic acetylcholine-receptor ENFL3: Chromosome 1 (*CHRNB2*-Locus), β2 nicotinic acetylcholine-receptor subunit At least one further location

Age of onset: Onset of the disorder is usually the first or second decade (age 9–15). Men are affected three times as often as women (Münchau et al. 2000).

Therapy: Acetazolamide, trihexyphenidyl, diazepam, clonazepam and baclofen are used with variable benefit. Classic anticonvulsant drugs and levodopa have not proven useful. Avoidance of long-duration effort is the best therapeutic advice.

Etiology: PED is very rare. There exist only a few families with autosomal dominant heredity (Lance 1977; Münchau et al. 2000). Sporadic cases are even rarer. PED is not a forme fruste of PNKD because the gene locus on chromosome 2q was excluded. A PED-plus syndrome was localized on chromosome 16p12–11.2 (see Table 9.2). In this region, gene loci for families with ICCA and PKD were also found. There may be overlaps between these diseases.

Transcranial magnetic stimulation identified proprioceptive afferences from muscle spindles or tendons as crucial triggers of the attacks.

Course of disease: No reliable data exist in the literature to date. PED may continue unchanged (Münchau et al. 2000) or may taper off spontaneously and lasting (Spacey et al. 2002).

Paroxysmal hypnogenic dyskinesia (PHD)

Trigger: The trigger for these movements appears to be non-REM sleep, with stage II in most patients the most common stage (Lugaresi et al. 1986).

Movement pattern: Typically, the patient awakes with a cry and wide-staring eyes. EEG shows a preceding arousal reaction. Immediately or after a few seconds, the patient batters around with choreatic or ballistic movements. Dystonic postures of one extremity or the whole body can alternate with fast extending movements. Long-duration vocalization may accompany the spell. Tachycardia is common. Surface EEG displays no abnormality during the attack. At the end of the attack, the patient is awake and fully conscious, and can fall asleep again. The event is remembered the next morning. From attack to attack, the movements recur in a stereotyped manner. Some patients report focal sensible or motor seizures during daytime or generalized tonic-clonic seizures at night. PHD very rarely may even occur during daytime.

Duration: Thirty to 45 seconds. Longer attacks of 2 to 50 minutes duration have been described very rarely.

Frequency: One to 20 per night to 5 per year.

Age of onset: The onset is usually the first to third decade (mean age: 21.8 years). No gender preference is known.

Therapy: Low doses of carbamazepine or phenytoin reliably relieve the short attacks. Long-duration attacks may respond to haloperidol or acetazolamide but are often resistant to therapy.

Etiology: Nearly all or all patients with PHD suffer from frontal lobe epilepsy (Fish and Marsden 1994). The movements in PHD cannot be distinguished from the semiology of mesial frontal lobe seizures. Dystonic movements result from epileptogenic activity involving the basal ganglia, which are closely connected to the frontal lobes. Deep parenchymal electrodes verified the epileptic discharges in the mesial frontal lobes during PHD. In some families with typical PHD, the disorder was named autosomal dominant nocturnal frontal lobe epilepsy (ADNFLE). ADNFLE is a genetically heterogenous disorder with at least three known and several unknown mutations of the nicotinic acetylcholine-receptor gene (Table 9.2).

Course of disease: In the majority of cases, no change in frequency or intensity of seizures is identified during the lifetime. Usually, the disease responds very well to treatment.

Etiology

Idiopathic paroxysmal dyskinesias

Most sporadic and all familial (either autosomal-dominant or very rarely autosomal-recessive) paroxysmal dyskinesias are idiopathic. Genetics have been discussed previously (Table 9.2).

Secondary paroxysmal dyskinesias

An atypical presentation, for instance, an older age at onset, prolonged duration of attacks or inter-attack neurological symptoms, should raise the suspicion of secondary cases. Sometimes the movements are peculiar and cannot easily be separated from the underlying disease (Bressman et al. 1988). History often eludes the underlying cause.

Putaminal, pallidal, thalamic, brain stem or spinal lesions and very rarely even impairment of peripheral nerves have been reported in these patients. Paroxysmal kinesigenic activity may be released by reduced inhibitory influence of the medial pallidal globe and substantia nigra to the thalamus. Lesions of thalamic nucleus reticularis itself can render the thalamus more sensible for sensory input (Demirkiran and Jankovic 1995). Thalamic neuronal hyperactivity is causally associated with idiopathic paroxysmal dyskinesias. Possibly faulty proprioceptive input into the thalamus alone provokes paroxysmal movement disorders, as shown by emergence of symptomatic PKD with demyelinating plaques in cervical spinal cord or peripheral lesions (Lotze and Jankovic 2003).

All kinds of paroxysmal dyskinesias may be symptomatic in origin. Twenty-two percent of one series of patients with paroxysmal movement disorders had underlying causative diseases. Clinical appearance is more variable than in idiopathic cases. Nearly 30% of symptomatic patients show an overlap between different forms. Dystonia is the most important movement. Age at onset ranges from 2.5 to 79 years, and the male preponderance of idiopathic diseases is not present (Blakeley and Jankovic 2002).

Multiple sclerosis is the most common cause of symptomatic paroxysmal dyskinesias. Painful hemidystonic spells following hyperventilation or rarely movement (kinesigenic) have been observed for decades in patients with multiple sclerosis. They last for seconds to minutes, appear several times per day and resolve within weeks to months, like other relapses in multiple sclerosis.

The second-most common underlying pathology is cerebrovascular disease. Metabolic disorders rank in line third, especially diabetic hyper- and hypoglycemia, thyrotoxic crisis and (pseudo-) hypoparathyroidism. PKD, PED and PNKD were observed after head and peripheral injury. Latency between causative event and first manifestation of the movement disorder (contralateral to the lesion side)

Table 9.3 Etiology of the paroxysmal dyskinesias

Idiopathic
  Familial
  Sporadic

Symptomatic
  Multiple sclerosis
  Vascular diseases (TIA, ischemic or hemorrhagic stroke)
  Carotid artery occlusive disease ("orthostatic paroxysmal
    dystonia" by intermittent cerebral ischemia with
    postural change)
  Hypoxic-ischemic encephalopathy
  Perinatal hypoxic encephalopathy
  Cortical vascular malformations
  Moyamoya disease
  Head trauma
  Peripheral trauma
  Inflammatory
    Human immunodeficiency virus infection
    CMV encephalitis
    SSPE infection
    Late-stage syphilis
  Metabolic
    (Pseudo-) hypoparathyroidism
    Thyrotoxicosis
    Hypo- and hyperglycemia
  Basal ganglia calcifications / Fahr's disease
  Kernicterus
  Migraine aura
  Lupus erythematosus
  Hemiatrophy/cortical dysgenesis
  Orbito-frontal dysplasia
  Maple syrup disease
  Succinic semialdehyde dehydrogenase deficiency (good
    response to vigabatrin)
  Steele-Richardson-Olszewski Syndrome
  Cerebral lymphoma
  Primary antiphospholipid syndrome
  Drugs
    methylphenidate
    fluoxetine

has been up to years after a stroke and days to months after traumatic brain lesions. Rare conditions with mostly single case reports are referred to in Table 9.3. Treatment results are mostly similar to the idiopathic disease (Blakeley and Jankovic 2002).

Animal models of paroxysmal dyskinesias

The dt^{sz} mutant hamster represents an animal model of PNKD. Episodes of generalized dystonic movements can age-dependently be induced by stress and last 5 to 8 hours (Richter and Loscher 1998). Attacks start with ear flattening and facial contortions, followed by stiffening of the hind limbs, gait abnormalities and frequent falling, and culminate with limb hyperextension and severe truncal torsion and flexion. At age 30 to 40

days, the dystonic movements reach their peak intensity, at age of more than 10 weeks they cease. At the age of most marked expression of dystonia, the density of GABAergic medium spiny interneurons which co-express calcium binding proteins are significantly reduced in the neostriatum of dystonic hamsters. Additionally, an age-related deficit of NOS-reactive interneurons in part contributes to the abnormal activity of striatal GABAergic projection neurons, but may be less important. Dystonic episodes are associated with temporary increases of striatal extracellular dopamine up to 6.5-fold, and the disappearance of paroxysmal dystonia is preceded by a normalization of dopamine to basal levels. Openers of the potassium K_v7 channels (KCNQ) and GABA transporter subtype 1 (GAT-1) inhibitors were found to potently reduce dystonic activity in this animal model. Blocking of striatal glutamatergic overactivity via kynurenine 3-hydroxylase inhibitor significantly ameliorates paroxysmal movements at well-tolerated doses. Involvement of cannabinoid and noradrenergic systems was studied in this model and excluded as a significant modulating factor.

Fibroblast growth factor (Fgf) 14 is widely expressed in the developing CNS and in the adult brain of mice. Wang et al. disrupted the Fgf14 gene expression. At one month of age, Fgf14$^{N-\beta-Gal/N-\beta-Gal}$ mice developed paroxysmal forelimb clonic spasms with hyperextended hindlimbs often accompanied by forelimb tremor. The symptoms occurred several times a day and lasted 7 to 12 minutes. The most frequently observed movements corresponded to the third and fourth dystonia stages in the dt^{sz} hamster. These symptoms became less severe in older mice (more than 3 months). Increased net inhibitory striatal output has been suggested as an etiology of the paroxysmal dyskinesia in the Fgf14$^{N-\beta-Gal/N-\beta-Gal}$ mouse similar to the dt^{sz} hamster model.

The mutation of the P/Q-type voltage-dependent calcium channel (VDCCs) in the leaner (tg^{la}/tg^{la}) mouse model leads to cerebellar ataxia, absence epilepsy and paroxysmal dyskinesia. The increased α1G subunit expression in Purkinje cells is localized in the anterior cerebellum, which may be related to the paroxysmal dyskinesia phenotype in leaner mice. Mutations affecting different parts of the α1A subunit of the P/Q-type calcium channel have also been associated with paroxysmal movement disorders but also with epilepsy, paroxysmal ataxia and hypoactivity in the tottering and the lethargic mouse model.

Assessment and laboratory work-up in general practice

History and neurologic examination are the cornerstones on the way to the diagnosis of paroxysmal dyskinesias. Trigger factors, detailed description of the attacks, and medical and family history are of paramount importance. Perinatal period, infantile development, previous seizures, CNS trauma, infection or stroke should be assessed. Whenever possible, an attack should be provoked and videotaped. Well-treated patients without actual signs, rare frequency of attacks or affected but absent family members may hinder this approach, but the ubiquitous spread of video equipment can help to overcome this obstacle. The first clinical test should comprise a brain MRI to exclude symptomatic disease at least in atypical presentation. In idiopathic and hereditary patients, the scan will be unremarkable. EEG with provocation methods during times of symptoms and times without symptoms will be normal. In unclear cases, long-term video-augmented EEG monitoring may help to distinguish movement disorders from epileptic seizures. Up to now, all laboratory examinations have been unremarkable in patients with idiopathic or familial paroxysmal dyskinesias. Additional laboratory tests should include electrolytes, including calcium and phosphate, serum glucose, erythrocyte sedimentation rate, liver function tests, ammonia, lactate, pyruvate, blood count and smear for acanthocytes, TSH, antinuclear antibodies, and serum and urine protein immunofixation. Wilson disease should be ruled out through measurements of copper concentration in serum and 24-hour urine specimens and serum ceruloplasmin level, and a slit-lamp examination of the eyes. Some laboratories offer commercial gene testing for PNKD (www.genetests.org). Symptomatic patients attract attention because of their atypical historical presentation or clinical examination (Bressman et al. 1988). Further assessment follows the supposed underlying disease.

No consistent neuropathologic findings have been reported until now. One PKD patient had slight asymmetry of the substantia nigra, and one had melanin in macrophages of locus coeruleus. One patient developed PNKD during severe HIV-encephalitis verified by autopsy. In comparison with non-dyskinetic HIV patients, a histology revealed reduced and dysmorphic calbindin-D28K-positive neurons in basal ganglia. A

Table 9.4 Differential diagnosis of paroxysmal movement disorders

Epileptic seizures
Psychogenic movement disorders
Hyperekplexia
Alternating hemiplegia of childhood
Benign dystonia of childhood
Benign paroxysmal tonic upgaze of childhood
Sandifer syndrome
Shuddering attacks
Hyperventilation, tetanic seizures
Drug-induced acute dystonic reaction
Tic disorders
Stereotypies
Dopa-responsive dystonia
Wilson's disease
Parkinson's disease, levodopa-induced dyskinesias
Westphal variant of Huntington's disease
Pantothenate kinase associated neurodegeneration (PKAN)
Myoclonic diseases
Myotonia
Drop attacks
Focal/segmental/generalized dystonia
Paroxysmal periodic paralysis
Paroxysmal ataxias

21-month-old toddler with dystonic fits from the second month of life died suddenly. Autopsy of the brain showed no distinctive features. Another patient dying of bladder carcinoma had normal brain in macroscopic examination (case IV.2 and case II.5; Lance 1977).

Differential diagnosis of paroxysmal dyskinesias

Paroxysmal dyskinesia, epilepsy and ion channels

The affiliation of paroxysmal dyskinesias to basal ganglia disorders or to epilepsy was disputed for a long time (Guerrini et al. 2002). Basal ganglia disease is assumed because of types of movement, lack of stereotypy and the mostly normal ictal and interictal EEG-pattern. Consciousness is unaffected and no postictal reorientation is necessary (Table 9.4).

Table 9.5 Association between paroxysmal dyskinesias, epilepsy and other paroxysmal neurological diseases (according to Guerrini et al. 2002)

Epilepsy and paroxysmal dyskinesias	Epilepsy and other paroxysmal neurological diseases	Paroxysmal dyskinesias and other paroxysmal neurological diseases
Autosomal dominant dystonic choreoathetosis with benign infantile convulsions Pericentromeric region of chromosome 16 Autosomal recessive Rolandic epilepsy, PED and graphospasm Chromosome 16p12–11.2	Episodic ataxia type 1 and infantile convulsions Gene: Potassium channel *KCNA 1* Hereditary hemiplegic migraine and seizures Chromosome 1p31	Autosomal dominant paroxysmal choreoathetosis and episodic ataxia Chromosome 1p Autosomal dominant paroxysmal dystonic choreoathetosis with migraine (Hofele et al. 1997) Chromosome 2q
Autosomal dominant PKD, migraine, hemiplegic migraine, generalized epilepsy (Singh et al. 1999)	Hereditary hemiplegic migraine and infantile convulsions	Autosomal dominant PED and migraine (Münchau et al. 2000)
Autosomal dominant PED and epilepsy	Infantile convulsions, idiopathic generalized epilepsy, episodic ataxia, migraine (Singh et al. 1999)	
PKD and ICCA (see Table 9.1)		
Autosomal dominant PKD and grand mal epilepsy with linkage to the pericentromeric region of chromosome 16		
PKD and absence epilepsy		

Functional imaging also points to basal ganglia disorders. Symptomatic (ictal) ^{99m}Tc-ECD-SPECT of one PKD patient showed increased blood flow in both basal ganglia and posterolateral thalamus. Two PKD patients had hyperperfusion in the basal ganglia and thalamus contralateral to their movements. Confusingly, another PKD patient had hypoperfusion in the contralateral basal ganglia. Interictally, the cerebral perfusion in the posterior parts of bilateral caudate nuclei was found to be reduced (Joo et al. 2005). In one PNKD patient, the ictal ^{99m}Tc-ECD-SPECT perfusion pattern has indicated increased blood flow in the caudate nucleus and thalamus contralateral to the forceful movement as well, and hypoperfusion over the ipsilateral inferior dorsal frontal area. Two patients with PED had ictal hypoperfusion of frontal cortex and basal ganglia and hyperperfusion of the cerebellum indicating a reduced thalamic influence on the frontal cortex. This kind of perfusion pattern has also been observed in symptomatic hemidystonia and idiopathic dystonia and, therefore, is regarded as proof for the basal ganglia nature of paroxysmal dyskinesias. Symptomatic paroxysmal dyskinesias show bilateral hypometabolism in the ventral striatum by ^{18}FDG-PET (Lombroso and Fischman 1999). MRI spectroscopy found reduced choline concentration contralateral to the movements in two patients with PKD, and a dysfunctional cholinergic system of the basal ganglia has been discussed.

The paroxysmal nature and predominantly short duration of the attacks, the aura symptoms and the response to even low doses of anticonvulsant drugs suggest that paroxysmal dyskinesias closely resemble epilepsy. Several familial syndromes feature both paroxysmal dyskinesia and overt epilepsy (Guerrini et al. 2002; see Tables 9.2 and 9.5). Some patients with paroxysmal dyskinesias have interictal EEG-abnormalities (Nagamitsu et al. 1999). An Italian group studying a girl with movement-induced dystonic posturing recorded ictal spikes in the supplementary motor area and anterior caudate nucleus in long-term invasive EEG-monitoring. They concluded that PKD is a kind of focal epilepsy, an opinion not generally accepted because the girl did not suffer from typical PKD and had major abnormal neurological findings between the attacks. A later publication by the same group reported a PNKD patient with caudate nucleus discharges and distinctive dopaminergic features in PET scanning (Lombroso and Fischman 1999). The distinction between movement-induced epileptic seizures, startle epilepsy and PKD may be subtle (Fish and Marsden 1994; Guerrini et al. 2002). PHD is currently classified as an epileptic disorder (Fish and Marsden 1994).

With the utmost probability, the link between the two groups are common mutations of ion channel genes in epilepsy, paroxysmal dyskinesias and other paroxysmal neurological disorders like periodic paralyses, ataxias or hemiplegic migraine (Guerrini et al. 2002; Table 9.5). All of these share the features of episodic attacks, normal results in interictal neurological examination and triggering factors like stress, fatigue, movement after rest and certain foods (Bhatia et al. 2000). Some families express several episodic disorders in concert (Singh et al. 1999). Anticonvulsant drugs and acetazolamide act in numerous ways and may cross the classification borders if defined by drug responsiveness. Epilepsy and paroxysmal dyskinesias may be the result of a common disturbance of ion channels in the motor cortex and the basal ganglia, in which the seizures usually manifest earlier than the movement disorder. The age-dependent expression of different sub-units of the ion channels may lead to changes in disease phenomenology during different times in one's lifetime (Guerrini et al. 2002).

Further differential diagnoses of paroxysmal movement disorders

The most common differential diagnostic possibility for the idiopathic sporadic paroxysmal dyskinesias is dissociative (psychogenic) movement disorder (Fahn 1994b). Blakeley and Jankovic proposed this diagnosis in 21 of their 76 patients with paroxysmal movement disorders (Blakeley and Jankovic 2002). Bressman et al. (1988) found dissociative disorders in 11 of 18 patients with paroxysmal dyskinesias (61% of their series), 8 of the 11 being female. Their age at onset ranged from 11 to 49 years. The functional movements were highly complex in some cases, including vocalization, dancing and running. In most instances, the distinction between paroxysmal dyskinesia and psychogenic movement disorder was extremely challenging. There are no pathognomonic findings for either diseases, and criteria for psychogenic movement disorders are not always conclusive (Table 9.6).

Hyperekplexia is a rare hereditary disorder with onset in infancy. Startle leads to movement storm with the affected persons sometimes jumping wildly, hence the name "jumping Frenchmen of Maine." Myoclonic

Table 9.6 Clues that suggest dissociative (psychogenic) movement disorder (reproduced with permission from Fahn 1994b)

Abrupt onset, maybe following adequate triggering event
Multiple different movements, bizarre gait disorders, rhythmical shaking, extensive slowness, excessive startle, varying tremors
Incongruous patterns or distribution of disordered movements
Highly variable expression
Increase of movement disorder during demonstration or focused attention
Pronounced distractibility
Pronounced decrease or termination of the movement during concentration on other examination procedures
Termination of the movement disorder in (seemingly) unobserved situation
Remissions
Inconsistent paresis
Inconsistent disturbance of sensibility
Multiple somatic complaints
Pronounced fatigability
Obvious psychiatric disturbances
Self-inflicted injuries
Response to placebo, suggestion, psychotherapy
Health system worker
Pending claims for litigation or compensation

or choreatic extremity movements can last for minutes. In abortive cases, the patients only have marked jerks. Increased muscle tone, gait disorder, nocturnal leg movements and increased sensibility to a sinister atmosphere can aid diagnosis.

Alternating hemiplegia of childhood starts before the age of 18 months. Bouts of hemiplegia with a change of the affected side between the attacks or even tetraplegia develop. Consciousness is preserved. Other movements like dystonia, chorea, tonic fits, nystagmus, dyspnea and autonomic features (paleness, flush) may accompany the attacks or emerge on their own. Muscle tone is flaccid except for concomitant dystonia. Attacks last from minutes to several days and abate in sleep. Intellectual impairment, long-lasting choreatic and dystonic movements and ataxia become manifest during the progression of this disorder. Achievement of developmental milestones is delayed or missed, and children will eventually lose already achieved abilities. Laboratory and imaging workup will render normal results.

Benign dystonia of childhood shows up with paroxysmal cervical dystonia or rarely with dystonic posturing of one arm or leg. The disease starts at age 2 to 30 months and ends at the age of 2 to 3 years. Attacks occur 2 to 3 times per month and last 10 minutes to 14 days. Between the attacks, the children move normally. The parents usually are more disturbed than the children. Exclusion of a mass lesion in the posterior fossa is important (Fahn 1994a).

Benign paroxysmal tonic up-gaze of childhood starts at 5 months (1 week to 26 months) and usually remits spontaneously within the following one or two years. Attacks last 15 to 30 seconds and appear in clusters. Tonic conjugate upward deviation of the eyes with neck flexion (chin down) may be accompanied by slight ataxia and dystonia of the trunk. During episodes, a downward gaze is difficult to maintain and the attempt may result in downbeat nystagmus. Consciousness is not disturbed. Between episodes, the children show normal neurological examinations. Patients respond well to low doses of levodopa, but treatment is rarely necessary. Nearly 40% of the patients will keep slight residual ataxia, ocular movement disorders or learning disabilities, and 10% develop moderate to severe intellectual impairment after cessation of the up-gaze spells. The disease occurs sporadically or is autosomal dominant. Some symptomatic cases have been described. The main differential diagnosis is absence seizures (Guerrini et al. 1998; Ouvrier and Billson 2005).

Sandifer syndrome is a rare movement disorder in toddlers. During or immediately after feeding, affected children exhibit severe dystonic movements or postures of the head and neck. They often vomit and are malnourished. Iron deficiency anemia may develop. The underlying cause is a phrenic hernia. Presumably, the children take the positions voluntarily to avoid awkward sensations from the hernia. After surgical closure, the movement and diet problems resolve.

Shuddering attacks represent shivering body movements lasting several seconds and are variably associated with dystonic posturing (flexion or stretching of the arms, squeezing hands, opisthotonic neck extension, clenching teeth). Consciousness is not disturbed. The spells appear up to 100 times a day. Age of onset is infancy or early childhood, and remission in the first decade is common. Most patients will have no developmental delay, but some expect borderline abnormal development. Parents may be far more embarrassed by these movements than the child. Parents often suspect epilepsy, especially West's syndrome. EEG and MRI findings are mostly normal. Family history is frequently positive for essential tremor, and shuddering attacks may represent an early manifestation of essential tremor in the immature brain. A different hypothesis lumps shuddering attacks and benign myoclonus of early infancy into the same nosologic entity. Kanazawa expressed his opinion that shuddering attacks may involve a problem related to nervous system development, which may be caused by stressful intrauterine conditions such as imminent preterm delivery (Kanazawa 2000).

Hyperventilation may lead to intermittent tingling around the mouth and at the tips of fingers/toes. Then muscle spasms form the hands into paws and the lips can be protruded. Blurred vision, vertigo and weakness may ensue. ECG shows prolongation of the QT-interval, and serum calcium is reduced during the attack. Very rarely, tremor or chorea may become visible in prolonged hypocalcemia and normalize after increase of serum calcium.

Tics are sudden, brief, irregular twitches mainly of facial muscles. Blinking, movements of the corners of the mouth, head-turning or bending, throat-clearing or vocalization and twiddling finger movements are most common. Dystonic tics run much more slowly. Sensory tics will lead to a movement in response to a tight feeling. Tics are semi-involuntary. Inhibition is possible but increases an inner tension which will resolve in a "storm" of several consecutive tics. Fear, anger and staring at the subject increase frequency of tics, whereas individual concentration or distraction will reduce them. Tics are very common. Males are much more susceptible than females. At least 10% of school boys (mean age 4–17 years) will display one or several tics at least for a certain period of time. After 20 years of age, the frequency drops quickly but re-increases in again in the elderly. In Tourette's syndrome, which starts before age 21 and lasts for more than one year, multiple motor and at least one vocal tic in varying expression over time and obsessive compulsive disorder are prominent. Treatment with dopamine antagonists, tetrabenazine or clonidine is only necessary when tics interfere with school success or social relations (Lees and Tolosa 1993).

A coordinated, repetitive, patterned, non-reflexive, rhythmical, senseless or ritualistic movement, posture or vocalization is called a stereotypy. It is regarded as self-generated sensible stimulus or expression of an underlying inner tension or fear. Disturbance of the dopaminergic basal ganglia system may be the underlying pathology. Movements are simple such as leg-wiggling, clapping hands, body-rocking or grunting, or complex like sitting/standing up and rituals, and can involve all body parts. The disorder is common in a variety of psychiatric disorders such as mental retardation, autism, Rett syndrome, schizophrenia, catatonia, mania, obsessive-compulsive disorder, psychosis from amphetamines or cocaine, and psychogenic movement disorders. They are also common in neurological diseases such as akathisia, tardive dyskinesia, Tourette's syndrome and neuroacanthocytosis. In fearful or incriminating situations also, otherwise healthy people may exhibit stereotypies. Twenty percent of children may develop stereotypies for a certain period during their development (Jankovic 1994).

Early disease onset, marked involvement of the legs, induction by movement and heredity are common in PED and dopa-responsive dystonia (DRD). However, PED has no diurnal fluctuations and does not or only minimally responds to levodopa. Cerebrospinal fluid homovanillic acid levels are low in DRD but there are no data about this in PED.

Idiopathic Parkinson's disease may start with movement-induced (foot) dystonia (Poewe et al. 1988). The age of onset, the clinical course and the emerging additional signs will set the diagnosis. The levodopa-induced dyskinesias in later stages of Parkinson's disease will give no reason for confusion with paroxysmal movement disorders. Delineation to Huntington's disease and its juvenile Westphal variant starting with bradykinetic and rarely dystonic movements will be easy considering family history and observing the progress.

In the first decades of life, Wilson's disease can emerge with fluctuating dystonic posturing at onset. A delay in diagnosis may lead to severe and often lasting damage in liver and brain function. Therefore, in every movement disorder starting before age 50, serum copper, serum ceruloplasmin and 24-hour copper excretion should be analyzed.

Dystonic and choreatic movements in infancy may be induced by pantothenate kinase associated neurodegeneration (PKAN, formerly Hallervorden-Spatz disease). The movements are not paroxysmal, and additional dysarthria and mental retardation, rigidity, spasticity and retinitis pigmentosa occur during the course of disease. Brain MRI is pathognomonic.

Focal dystonias may vary in intensity during the day and according to the surrounding situation. Usually, they will not subside totally, and neurological examination will help to differentiate from paroxysmal dyskinesias. The history will lead to the accurate diagnosis in task-specific dystonia (writing, playing instruments or sports).

Drug-induced acute dystonic reaction can easily be diagnosed by the history and response to biperiden. Orofacial dystonia and oculogyric crisis are very distinctive. Myotonia causes muscle cramps after movement or exposure to cold. History, clinical findings and the typical EMG pattern will enable the discrimination. The same is true for the paroxysmal dyskalemic paralyses.

Myoclonus is defined as a brief, sudden, shock-like involuntary movement caused by muscular contraction (positive myoclonus) or inhibition (negative myoclonus, asterixis). Confusion with paroxysmal dyskinesia is unlikely because of their more complex and long lasting movements. The falls during very short-lasting PKD may be confused with drop attacks. Trigger factors and accompanying movements may lead to the correct diagnosis.

Case presentations

Example of PKD is a case for kinesigenic dyskinesia (Case 2, Nardocci et al. 1989): At age 13 to 14 months, the now six-year-old boy developed episodes of sudden abduction and inner rotation of legs and arms, leading to frequent falls. Dystonic postures of trunk and extremities were added. Consciousness was always preserved. Triggers could not be identified. The attacks lasted up to 5 minutes and emerged once a week to once a month. Neurological examination detected no abnormalities between the attacks. Pregnancy and delivery were unremarkable. Family history gave no further neurologic or psychiatric diseases. Motor and intellectual development of the child was normal. Clonazepam reduced the frequency of the attacks.

Example of PNKD (Case IV.2, Schloesser et al. 1996): A 56-year-old lady suffered from fits since the age of 7 years. She feels an aura of stiffness and tightness in her extremities and rarely pain in hips and back for several minutes. The dyskinesia begins with a dystonic elevation of one arm and stiffening of the same-sided leg, accompanied by a painful constricted feeling in these extremities. Some minutes later, these extremities start involuntary choreatic and dystonic movements. The arm bends at the elbow and wrist, hand posture is dystonic and the distal parts of the leg move in a choreatic fashion. The attack can affect one or both sides of the body; in severe attacks, the face is involved and the speech becomes dysarthric. Duration is 3 minutes to 7 hours, frequency three times daily to twice weekly. Involvement of both sides of the body renders the patient immobile. In a half-sided attack she walks "like a drunkard" but can drive a car. Attacks are uniform besides the different propagation. Consciousness is not disturbed, and there is no postictal confusion. During menstruation or pregnancy, the attack frequency increased, and after menopause the intensity decreased. Trigger factors are alcohol, coffee, tea, chocolate, excitement and stress. If the patient rests for several minutes at the beginning of the attack, or even takes 5 mg of diazepam, the attack shortens and gets less intense.

The lady has been diagnosed previously as suffering from epilepsy, conversion disorder or anxiety disorder. Neurological examination between the attacks showed no abnormalities, and interictal EEGs and MRI imaging were normal. Anti-epileptic drugs were of no help, but diazepam reduced frequency to one fit every third day. Levodopa/carbidopa (5 × 125 mg Nacom) further downsized the attacks to three times a month. Clonazepam brought down the attacks to 1 to 4 in 6 months in mild intensity.

Example of a PED (Case II.4, Lance 1977, himself posted this case as "intermediate form" between the paroxysmal dystonic choreoathetosis and the paroxysmal kinesigenic choreoathetosis): Since his second year, a 56-year-old man has suffered from unilateral tonic flexion spasms affecting changing sides of his body. The first episode was observed shortly after he learned to walk. In childhood, the attacks repeated every several months and increased during adulthood to a frequency of up to 15 per month during phases of intense labor. The attack starts with bending of the fingers of one hand, and then the elbow is flexed. At the same time, the foot will drop down and the knee and hip deflect. The foot looses contact with the ground. All these flexion movements appear slowly, and the attack lasts 5 to 50 minutes. The patient has time to sit or lie down and has never fallen during an attack. Speech gets dysarthric, and at the peak of the attack the patient can only groan or is completely mute. He can see, listen and move the eyes but not the head. Consciousness is preserved. The mouth is open, saliva will drip down, swallowing or tongue movements are not possible. Passing water is unaffected. For some time the attacks have been milder, and athetotic movements have been observed. Until now the patient has never had epileptic seizures. Attacks start during rest after exercise, excitement or exhaustion, especially following alcohol ingestion. Interictal neurological examination and EEG are unremarkable, and skull x-ray was normal.

Example of a PHD (Case 10, Lugaresi et al. 1986): A 38-year-old lady reported multiple night time attacks in 4 to 5 nights per week since the age of 26 years. She awakes with a tight feeling around the head, screams, sits up in bed, stares and performs dystonic arm and leg movements for 15 seconds. After some years daytime seizures evolved where she shouts out loud, bends the arms and has a feeling of immobility. These attacks stopped without any action, and the nocturnal fits were completely controlled by daily use of 200 mg of carbamazepine.

References

Auburger G, Ratzlaff T, Lunkes A, et al. A gene for autosomal dominant paroxysmal choreoathetosis/spasticity (CSE) maps to the vicinity of a potassium channel gene cluster on chromosome 1p, probably within 2 cM between D1S443 and D1S197. *Genomics* 1996; **31**(1):90–94.

Bennett LB, Roach ES, Bowcock AM. A locus for paroxysmal kinesigenic dyskinesia maps to human chromosome 16, *Neurology* 2000, **54**:125–130.

Bhatia KP. Familial (idiopathic) paroxysmal dyskinesias: an update, *Semin Neurol* 2001, **21**:69–74.

Bhatia KP, Griggs RC, Ptacek LJ. Episodic movement disorders as channelopathies, *Mov Disord* 2000, **15**:429–433.

Blakeley J, Jankovic J. Secondary paroxysmal dyskinesias, *Mov Disord* 2002, **17**:726–734.

Bressman SB, Fahn S., Burke RE. Paroxysmal non-kinesigenic dystonia, *Adv Neurol* 1988, **50**:403–413.

Bruno MK, Hallett M, Gwinn-Hardy K et al. Clinical evaluation of idiopathic paroxysmal kinesigenic dyskinesia: new diagnostic criteria, *Neurology* 2004, **63**:2280–2287.

Bruno MK, Lee HY, Auburger GW et al. Genotype-phenotype correlation of paroxysmal nonkinesigenic dyskinesia, *Neurology* 2007, **68**:1782–1789.

Cuenca-Leon E, Cormand B, Thomson T et al. Paroxysmal kinesigenic dyskinesia and generalized seizures: clinical and genetic analysis in a Spanish pedigree, *Neuropediatrics* 2002, **33**:288–293.

Demirkiran M, Jankovic J. Paroxysmal dyskinesias: clinical features and classification, *Ann Neurol* 1995, **38**:571–579.

Du W, Bautista JF, Yang H, et al. Calcium-sensitive potassium channelopathy in human epilepsy and paroxysmal movement disorder. *Nat Genet* 2005; **37**(7):733–738. Epub 2005 Jun 5.

Fahn S. The paroxysmal dyskinesias. In: *Movement Disorders 3*, Marsden CD, Fahn S. (eds.). Oxford, London, Boston, Munich, New Delhi, Singapore, Sydney, Tokyo, Toronto, Wellington: Butterworth-Heinemann Ltd., 1994a, pp. 310–45.

Fahn S. Psychogenic movement disorders. In: *Movement Disorders 3*, Marsden CD, Fahn S. (eds.). Oxford, London, Boston, Munich, New Delhi, Singapore, Sydney, Tokyo, Toronto, Wellington: Butterworth-Heinemann Ltd., 1994b, pp. 359–372.

Fish DR, Marsden CD. Epilepsy masquerading as a movement disorder. In: *Movement Disorders 3*, Marsden CD, Fahn S. (eds.). Oxford, London, Boston, Munich, New Delhi, Singapore, Sydney, Tokyo, Toronto, Wellington: Butterworth-Heinemann Ltd., 1994, pp. 346–358.

Fouad GT, Servidei S, Durcan S, et al. A gene for familial paroxysmal dyskinesia (FPD1) maps to chromosome 2q. *Am J Hum Genet* 1996; **59**(1):135–139.

Guerrini R, Belmonte A, Carrozzo R. Paroxysmal tonic upgaze of childhood with ataxia: a benign transient dystonia with autosomal dominant inheritance, *Brain Dev* 1998, **20**:116–118.

Guerrini R, Bonanni P, Nardocci N, et al. Autosomal recessive rolandic epilepsy with paroxysmal exercise-induced dystonia and writer's cramp: delineation of the syndrome and gene mapping to chromosome 16p12-11.2. *Ann Neurol* 1999; **45**(3):344–352.

Guerrini R, Parmeggiani L, Casari G. Epilepsy and paroxysmal dyskinesia: co-occurrence and differential diagnosis, *Adv Neurol* 2002, **89**:433–441.

Hattori H, Fujii T, Nigami H et al. Co-segregation of benign infantile convulsions and paroxysmal kinesigenic choreoathetosis, *Brain Dev* 2000, **22**:432–435.

Hofele K, Benecke R, Auburger G. Gene locus FPD1 of the dystonic Mount-Reback type of autosomal-dominant paroxysmal choreoathetosis, *Neurology* 1997, **49**:1252–1257.

Jankovic J. Stereotypies. In: *Movement Disorders 3*, Marsden CD, Fahn S. (eds.). Oxford, London, Boston, Munich, New Delhi, Singapore, Sydney, Tokyo, Toronto, Wellington: Butterworth-Heinemann Ltd., 1994, pp. 503–517.

Jankovic J, Demirkiran M. Classification of paroxysmal dyskinesias and ataxias, *Adv Neurol* 2002, **89**:387–400.

Joo E, Hong S, Tae W et al. Perfusion abnormality of the caudate nucleus in patients with paroxysmal kinesigenic choreoathetosis, *Eur J Nucl Med Molecular Imaging* 2005, **32**:1205–1209.

Kanazawa O. Shuddering attacks-report of four children, *Pediatr Neurol* 2000, **23**:421–424.

Lance JW. Familial paroxysmal dystonic choreoathetosis and its differentiation from related syndromes, *Ann Neurol* 1977, **2**:285–293.

Lees AJ, Tolosa E. Tics. In: *Parkinson's Disease and Movement Disorders*, Jankovic J, Tolosa E. (eds.). Baltimore, Hong Kong, London, Munich, Philadelphia, Sydney, Tokio: Williams and Wilkins, 1993, pp. 329–335.

Lombroso CT, Fischman A. Paroxysmal non-kinesigenic dyskinesia: pathophysiological investigations, *Epileptic Disord* 1999, **1**:187–193.

Lotze T, Jankovic J. Paroxysmal kinesigenic dyskinesias, *Semin Pediatr Neurol* 2003, **10**:68–79.

Lugaresi E, Cirignotta F, Montagna P. Nocturnal paroxysmal dystonia, *J Neurol Neurosurg Psych* 1986, **49**:375–380.

Münchau A, Valente EM, Shahidi GA et al. A new family with paroxysmal exercise induced dystonia and migraine: a clinical and genetic study, *J Neurol Neurosurg Psych* 2000, **68**:609–614.

Nagamitsu S, Matsuishi T, Hashimoto K et al. Multicenter study of paroxysmal dyskinesias in Japan–clinical and pedigree analysis, *Mov Disord* 1999, **14**:658–663.

Ouvrier R, Billson F. Paroxysmal tonic upgaze of childhood–a review, *Brain Dev* 2005, **27**:185–188.

Poewe WH, Lees AJ, Stern GM. Dystonia in Parkinson's disease: clinical and pharmacological features, *Ann Neurol* 1988, **23**:73–78.

Richter A, Loscher W. Pathology of idiopathic dystonia: findings from genetic animal models, *Prog Neurobiol* 1998, **54**:633–677.

Schloesser DT, Ward TN, Williamson PD. Familial paroxysmal dystonic choreoathetosis revisited, *Mov Disord* 1996, **11**:317–320.

Singh R, Macdonell RA, Scheffer IE et al., Epilepsy and paroxysmal movement disorders in families: evidence for shared mechanisms, *Epileptic Disord* 1999, **1**:93–99.

Spacey SD, Adams PJ, Lam PC, et al. Genetic heterogeneity in paroxysmal nonkinesigenic dyskinesia. *Neurology* 2006; **66**(10):1588–1590.

Spacey SD, Valente EM, Wali GM et al. Genetic and clinical heterogeneity in paroxysmal kinesigenic dyskinesia: evidence for a third EKD gene, *Mov Disord* 2002, **17**:717–725.

Steinlein OK, Mulley JC, Propping P, et al. A missense mutation in the neuronal nicotinic acetylcholine receptor alpha 4 subunit is associated with autosomal dominant nocturnal frontal lobe epilepsy. *Nat Genet* 1995; **11**(2):201–203.

Szepetowski P, Rochette J, Berquin P, et al. Familial infantile convulsions and paroxysmal choreoathetosis: a new neurological syndrome linked to the pericentromeric region of human chromosome 16. *Am J Hum Genet* 1997; **61**(4):889–898.

Chapter

10

Cramps, spasms, startles and related symptoms

Hans-Michael Meinck

Introduction

Since antiquity, medical terminology has used the word "spasm" – which comes from the Greek word σπασμός, meaning semiologically distinct phenomena, cramp or convulsion – to signify a transient, unwilled, often violent and painful muscle contraction. Moreover, both patients and their doctors subsume under the term "cramps" medically different entities such as a diffuse or circumscribed muscular pain, for example, fibromyalgia, myogelosis; disorders of muscle relaxation, such as myotonia; painful contracture of a muscle, like muscle glycogenosis; a variety of muscle cramps in a proper sense, such as benign cramps of the calves, hemifacial spasm; dystonia, such as blepharospasm, writer's cramp; and focal or even generalized seizures (Rowland 1985). Taking the patient's history and physical examination in the interictal state may therefore lead to an erroneous diagnosis. Provocation and, if possible, neurophysiologic analysis of symptoms is often essential.

Spasms or cramps may occur in all striated or smooth muscles. However, considering the neurological focus of this book, this chapter will deal with cramps and spasms of striated muscles. The purpose of this article is to provide readers with a diagnostic track through a terrain with common and uncommon neurologic symptoms of which some are poorly understood and therefore vaguely defined.

Cramps

Definition

Involuntary contraction of muscles may be generated in the central or peripheral nervous system, or in the muscle itself. However, differentiation between central and peripheral sources is regarded essential for diagnosis. Therefore, the terms spasm and cramp will be used here to describe profoundly different entities. Spasm describes a particular type of centrally generated motor hyperactivity (see following). In contrast, the term cramp will be confined here to muscular hyperactivity that is generated in the peripheral nervous system or in the muscle itself. However, it should be emphasized that the author's intention is by no means to propose a new classification of symptoms or diseases but didactically to sharpen terminology. Therefore, previously well-known medical terms such as hemifacial spasm, carpopedal spasm or writer's cramp will be preserved (Table 10.1).

In the aforementioned narrow sense, cramp describes an unwilled, transient, maximal and thus usually painful contraction of a single muscle or even parts of it, typically with a visible or palpable knotting (Layzer 1994). An "explosive" onset is not a regular feature according to personal experience and reported evidence. The painful involuntary contraction can be "broken" by passively stretching or massaging the muscle.

Epidemiology and general manifestations

Cramps are common complaints. They are not specifically associated with a few circumscribed causes but are frequently observed in peripheral neurogenic diseases. From a pragmatic point of view, cramps may be classified into three groups: common cramps, cramping disorder and symptomatic cramps (Layzer 1994; Parisi et al. 2003; Table 10.2).

Common cramps afflict otherwise healthy people, usually involve a few (typically distal) muscles and occur in a few characteristic situations. Cramps always in one and the same muscle, for example, the triceps surae on one side, may hint at chronic irritation of the local nerve supply, such as a Baker cyst. Provocative

The Paroxysmal Disorders, ed. Bettina Schmitz, Barbara Tettenborn and Donald L. Schomer. Published by Cambridge University Press. © Cambridge University Press 2010.

Table 10.1 Manifestation of cramps, spasms and other motor paroxysms

	Cramp	Spasm	Paroxysmal dystonia	Focal epilepsy
Manifestation	single muscles mono-/polytopic	group of neighboring muscles spread, generalization		
Intensity	intense	mild to moderate, occasionally intense		
Pain	mandatory, intense	facultative, mild to moderate	occasionally, mild	
Myoclonic components	no		occasionally	frequent
Reflex elicitation	no	exteroceptive (proprioceptive)	no	occasionally
Syndromal association	neuromuscular	spastic paresis	extrapyramidal	(spastic paresis)
Suppression by	muscle stretch, massage	(repositioning of the limb)	not known	

( ) = partially valid

mechanisms of common cramps comprise forceful contraction over a long time, maintenance of abnormal postures of the body or even a limb, or accidental dehydration. Common cramps are not a disorder in a proper sense. However, if they occur frequently, such as nocturnal cramps of the calves in the elderly, they can be a real torture and require treatment.

Cramping disorders constitute a small group of diseases, most of them with familial occurrence, where frequent cramps afflict various muscles, often without precipitating factors, for example, familial nocturnal cramps, hereditary cramping disease. In spite of their polytopic distribution, cramps are the only relevant symptom in "idiopathic cramps." Frequent cramps, particularly of the hands or feet, may induce transient bizarre and painful posturing resembling dystonia (Jusic et al. 1972; Tuite et al. 1996).

The group of symptomatic cramps comprises neuromuscular, endocrine, metabolic and toxic causes of cramps and thus a wide spectrum of differential diagnoses (Table 10.2). Diseases belonging to this group have in common frequent cramps with a polytopic pattern and only a loose association to specific precipitating factors. Stereotyped occurrence of cramps in always the same few muscles suggests a local cause such as residuals of nerve or nerve root entrapment. On physical examination, the characteristics of a nerve or nerve root lesion will be identified almost regularly.

Owing to the nature of cramps, electromyography (EMG) is particularly suited not only for their detection but also their analysis. EMG during a cramp usu-

Table 10.2 Differential diagnosis of symptomatic cramps

NEUROMUSCULAR DISORDERS

Muscle diseases
Glycogenosis (usually painful contracture)
Myotonia, Schwartz-Jampel syndrome (usually painless)

Motoneuron diseases
Amyotrophic lateral sclerosis/spinal muscle atrophy
Poliomyelitis residuals, post polio syndrome

Neuropathies
Mononeuropathy/radiculopathy
Polyneuropathy
Neuromyotonia

SYSTEMIC DISEASES

Endocrine/metabolic

Hypothyroidism
Hyper-/hypoparathyroidism, tetany
Uremia
Pregnancy
Acute dehydration (diaphoresis, diarrhea, vomiting, diuretic treatment, hemodialysis)

Intoxication
Drugs
Pesticides
Toxic oil syndrome
Malignant hyperthermia

ally shows a dense interference pattern that changes into irregular high-frequency discharges of single motor unit potentials (Auger 1994; Denny-Brown and Foley 1948; Layzer 1994). Before and after the cramp, fasciculations may be recorded from the same muscle, often in salvos with a high internal frequency (Fig. 10.1).

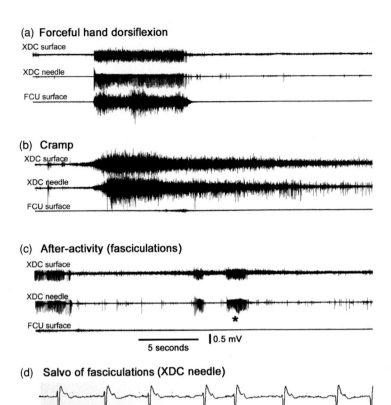

(a) Forceful hand dorsiflexion

XDC surface

XDC needle

FCU surface

(b) Cramp

XDC surface

XDC needle

FCU surface

(c) After-activity (fasciculations)

XDC surface

XDC needle

FCU surface

5 seconds | 0.5 mV

(d) Salvo of fasciculations (XDC needle)

20 ms | 0.5 mV

Fig. 10.1. Polygraph recording of cramps and, for comparison, EMG activity during voluntary innervation from patient with multifocal motor neuropathy (Case 1). EMG activity was recorded from the right extensor digitorum communis (XDC) and flexor carpi ulnaris (FCU) muscles with surface or concentric needle electrodes. (a) Forceful volitional hand dorsiflexion: synergistic activation of finger extensors and flexors. Note neurogenic reduction of the interference pattern in the XDC (needle recording). (b) Selective activation of the XDC in a spontaneous cramp. During the cramp, both the EMG amplitude and interference exceed voluntary forceful hand dorsiflexion. (c) As the cramp subsides, fasciculations discharge as single potentials and in salvos. Salvo labeled by an asterisk is shown at expanded horizontal and vertical calibrations in panel (d). Horizontal and vertical calibrations in panel (c) apply to panels (a–c). Reproduced from Veltkamp et al. 2003, with permission.

Case report: A 40-year-old waitress began to suffer from nocturnal cramps in her right forearm muscles in 1992. In the following years, wrist drop gradually developed without sensory loss, pain nor wasting. However, painful cramps were provoked when using the hand and, in spite of weakness, induced forceful involuntary ulnar deviation of the hand and unequal extension of the fingers. Physical examination revealed dense paresis of the finger and ulnar hand extensors without sensory loss, suggestive of radial nerve entrapment in the passage through the supinator muscle. However, deep tendon reflexes of the right arm were attenuated or even lost. EMG revealed chronic neurogenic changes in the wrist and finger extensors without fibrillations or positive sharp waves (Fig. 10.1). Several extensive work-ups, including MRI of the cervical spine and the brachial plexus, myelography, spinal tap and immunological tests did not solve the diagnostic enigma. It was not until 1999 that a conduction block of the brachial plexus was identified between Erb's point and axilla. Tests for serum auto-antibodies against myelin sheath proteins were negative.

With the tentative diagnosis of multifocal motor neuropathy with atypical unifocal manifestation, the patient received 30 g immunoglobulin (IgG) i.v. on five successive days. Symptoms and signs completely resolved within 10 days, the remission lasting for 3 months (Veltkamp et al. 2003). During the subsequent years, repeated i.v. IgG infusions with a reduced dosage yielded similar effects which, however, gradually lessened over time, necessitating co-medication with methotrexate.

In the last 8 years, we identified another four patients with wrist drop of the type seen in nerve entrapment within the supinator canal, three of them with and one without auto-antibodies against myelin sheath proteins. They all promptly responded to i.v. IgG. Multifocal motor neuropathy presenting with unifocal conduction block in the brachial plexus should be considered a differential diagnosis in such cases before surgery is initiated.

Selected diseases

Patients with myotonia may refer to the characteristically disordered relaxation of a forcefully activated muscle as a cramp. However, specific inquiry reveals that the myotonic relaxation disorder per se is not painful. Patients with dystrophia myotonica type 1 and 2 frequently complain of muscle pain resembling sore muscles rather than cramps, which are a long-lasting pain that preferentially afflicts certain regions such as the shanks. Obviously, myotonia induced by voluntary contraction, percussion or electric stimulation is not forceful enough to provoke the characteristic contraction pains of cramps hence, muscle fibers afflicted by myotonic runs contract individually and not as synchronized motor unit discharges.

In certain metabolic myopathies, in particular McArdle or Pompe diseases of glycogen storage, forceful long-time activation of a muscle, that is, loading under poor oxygenation, may provoke muscle contracture. Contractures last much longer than cramps and cannot be broken by passively stretching the afflicted muscle. Moreover, in spite of the maximally forceful mechanical contraction the characteristic EMG feature of muscle contracture is electrical silence. In cases with suspected metabolic myopathy, the forearm ischemic work test helps the diagnosis. Subsequent to a muscle contracture, substantial elevations of the creatine kinase with myoglobinuria may develop as a consequence of damage to muscle fibers, rhabdomyolysis and the EMG of such muscles displays fibrillations and positive sharp waves.

The particular relationship between muscle fasciculations and cramps is obvious in diseases of the motoneurons or their axons. Fasciculations not only frequently precede and follow a cramp (Fig. 10.1; Layzer 1994), they both are also provoked by similar conditions, and physiological investigations suggest that the majority of both arise from the distal arborization of the motor axons. Fasciculation and cramps occasionally are the initial manifestation of motor neuron diseases, long before muscle fatigue and progressive weakness and wasting develop. However, fasciculation and cramps may occur isolated but syndromatically linked in Denny-Brown's and Foley's syndrome of benign fasciculations and cramps (see neuromyotonia).

Another four distinct clinical syndromes have in common attacks of cramps and, on EMG, a particular type of repetitive spontaneous activity as the dominant finding. These disorders are tetany, hemifacial spasm, neuromyotonia and, with some reservations, myokymia.

In tetany, the axonal membrane is hyperexcitable. This is most often due to hypocalcemia, but disequilibrium of other electrolytes and/or serum pH may contribute. Hypocalcemia is commonly provoked by hypercapnia and results in paresthesias around the mouth and in the hands and feet and in a characteristic unpleasant cramping of distal muscles on both sides, carpal-pedal spasm, that lasts over minutes. On physical examination between attacks, the Trousseau test or Chvostek sign hint at an increased neuromuscular excitability, and EMG shows the characteristic duplets, triplets or multiplets. EMG recording from a hand muscle during the Trousseau test where there is an induction of forearm ischemia by inflating a sphygmomanometer cuff to suprasystolic pressure for 3 minutes (Fig. 10.2) is diagnostic by demonstrating the development of characteristic spontaneous activity (Deecke et al. 1983).

Hemifacial spasm involves almost all muscles of one side of the face supplied by the seventh cranial nerve including the platysma. However, it may start in the periorbital muscles. It is a strictly unilateral disorder, which distinguishes it from blepharospasm. This is another movement disorder of the face that is of central origin and may also start in the periorbital muscles on one side (see following). The muscles supplied by the seventh cranial nerve are subject to involuntary, brief and strictly synchronous contractions which repetitively persist for a short time. Such series of twitch-like contractions can be provoked by a short voluntary innervation of the facial musculature and may pause with relaxation of the face. In spite of severe hemifacial spasm, signs of facial nerve palsy are usually mild, for example, signe des cils, or even absent. However, as in many patients who recovered from Bell's palsy, a blink of the eye spreads to the perioral muscles producing a synkinesia. Neurophysiology suggests a defective insulation between facial nerve axons to different

Tetany   Hemifacial Spasm   Neuromyotonia

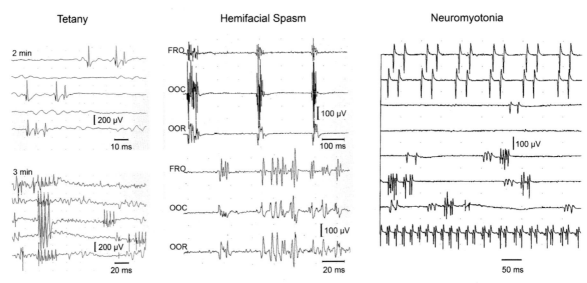

Fig. 10.2. Neuromuscular disorders with multiplet on EMG. Left panel: Tetany (Trousseau test), EMG from the first dorsal interosseous muscle (needle electrode, continuous recording). Forearm ischemia for 2 min induces spontaneous single motor unit discharges with a tendency to repeat ("singlets," duplets; top registration). After 3 min of ischemia (bottom recording), profuse spontaneous multiplet discharges are recorded and the ischemic hand develops carpal spasm. Middle panel: EMG in hemifacial spasm. Needle EMG recorded with three channels simultaneously from the frontalis (FRO), orbicularis oculi (OOC) and orbicularis oris (OOR) muscles at a slow (top registration) and fast (bottom registration) sweep speed. Notice strict synchrony and similarity between muscles of both, burst discharges and multiplet patterns within bursts. Left panel: Polymorphic spontaneous activity in immunogenic neuromyotonia (reproduced with permission from Meinck 2001). Pseudomyotonic discharges, duplets, triplets and multiplets. The position of the needle electrode remained unchanged throughout registration.

muscles to cause a pathological "ephaptic" spread of excitation. Needle EMG recorded simultaneously from representative face muscles demonstrates concomitant bursts of duplet, triplet or multiplet potentials with close similarity between muscles even in detailed analysis (Auger 1994; Fig. 10.2). In most cases, the nature of ephaptic current spread between axons remains obscure. Presently, and in analogy to trigeminal neuralgia, vascular compression of the seventh cranial nerve root is discussed. Occasionally, a tumor is identified. Differential diagnosis of hemifacial spasm comprises myokymia of the seventh cranial nerve. Facial myokymia is usually caused by brain stem lesions located close to the seventh nerve nucleus such as multiple sclerosis, or glioma of the pons. The main phenomenological difference between hemifacial spasm and facial myokymia is that myokymia does not occur with attacks and pauses but persists continuously over weeks or even months or years as an undulating mild contraction of the facial muscles. The treatment of choice for hemifacial spasm is the partial chemo-denervation of the orbicularis oculi and other muscles with botulinum toxin. Anticonvulsants

are effective too, but refractoriness to treatment develops more often.

Often described as continuous muscle fiber activity syndrome or the Isaac's syndrome, neuromyotonia is an uncommon manifestation of predominantly motor polyneuropathies of various etiologies. The chief complaint is a delayed muscular relaxation after voluntary contraction resembling myotonia, hence the name. As in tetany, the main symptoms and signs are usually symmetric and predominantly involve the hands, the feet and the face. Neuromyotonia begins insidiously with paraesthesias of electric or pulsating character, cramps of individual distal muscles and disturbed muscle relaxation after a forceful contraction. Symptoms gradually spread to involve the limbs and trunk. Even trivial movements, such as bending forward to pick something up or even yawning, triggers painful cramps of the rectus abdominis or pterygoid muscles, respectively. Disordered muscle relaxation combines with frequent fasciculations or myokymia; this may cause fluctuating muscle rigidity. Moreover, many patients complain of profuse sweating. Whether this is due to permanent excess activity of muscles or to ectopic excitation of sudomotor nerve fibers remains unsolved. Sensory, motor and autonomic symptoms disturb sleep, which causes daytime sleepiness. Symptoms and signs of a mild sensorimotor polyneuropathy may add on with distal muscle wasting and weakness, numbness of toes and fingers, and loss of the ankle jerks. EMG displays an abundance of variable spontaneous activity patterns even at the same needle position: frequent and polymorphic fasciculations, duplets, triplets, multiplets and, less frequently, also pseudomyotonic discharges (Mertens and Zschocke, 1965; Fig. 10.2). Distal muscles may show fibrillations and positive sharp waves and neurogenic alterations of motor unit potentials. Electric stimulation of a motor nerve may induce afterdischarges in the indirectly excited muscle. About 40% of patients harbor auto-antibodies against voltage-gated potassium channels of peripheral nerves (VGKC-abs). VGKC-abs are considered to specifically cause primary immunogenic neuromyotonia, hence their elimination results in immediate relief (Vincent 2000). It is discussed whether Denny-Brown and Foley's syndrome of benign fasciculations and cramps is a variant of neuromyotonia.

Myokymia describes an irregular undulation of the muscle surface that often continuously persists days or even weeks, and is perceived unpleasant but not painful. Physiologically, myokymia is due to involuntary and disorganized continuous activation of motor units within the muscle that does not induce a movement of the depending limb. Another type of involuntary muscle undulation that is shortlasting, regular like waves and electrically silent is the "harp phenomenon" in rippling muscle disease due to mechanical alterations of caveolin-deficient muscle fibers. Myokymia is relevant as a differential diagnosis, hence the spectrum of causes includes a variety of peripheral and central nervous system lesions such as acute or chronic polyradiculitis or polyneuropathy, bacterial or neoplastic meningoradiculopathy, radiogenic lesions, multiple sclerosis, or intramedullary or pontine lesions. Clinically, myokymia arising from the nerves or nerve roots may be associated with cramps but otherwise phenomenologically resembles myokymia in CNS disorders. However, EMG in peripheral causes discloses fasciculations and duplets, triplets or multiplets well known from tetany (see previous).

Electrical stimulation of the nerve supplying a myokymic muscle may cause multiplet-like discharges

Table 10.3 Cramps and spasms of the pericranial muscles

	One side	Both sides
Peripheral neuropathies/ neuronopathies		
Hemifacial spasm	+	
Myokymia (V[th] or VIIth nerves)	+	
Hemimasticatory spasm	+	
Tetany		+
Neuromyotonia		+
Satoyoshi disease		+
Central motor disorders		
Blepharospasm		+
Cephalic tetanus		+
Strychnine poisoning		+
Focal motor epilepsy	+	+
Tonic spasm	+	
Dystonia, dyskinesia	+	+
Whipple disease	+	+
Myokymia (pontine lesion)	+	(+)

to follow the MSAP. In CNS disorders such as multiple sclerosis, myokymia suggests a lesion in close vicinity to the motor nucleus of the respective muscle. EMG in such cases shows profuse fasciculation potentials instead of multiplets, often with a regular, low-frequency repetition. Possibly, this type of myokymia is due to an abnormal "bi-stability" of the α-motoneuron membranes that leads to a self-sustained repetitive discharge of anterior horn cells with a regular moderate frequency (Baldissera et al. 1994).

Differential diagnosis of paroxysmal excess muscle activity occasionally is a challenge, particularly in the face, comprising rare syndromes and uncommon manifestations of common diseases (Table 10.3; Thompson et al. 1986).

Treatment

Many cramps can be broken instantaneously by passive stretch or massage of the muscle. In cases with frequent cramps without treatable cause, membrane-stabilizing drugs such as quinine or quinidine, carbamazepine, diphenyl-hydantoin, magnesium citrate or lactate may reduce both frequency and intensity of cramps (Diener et al. 2002; McGee 1990; Roffe et al. 2002; Young and Jewell 2002). It should be remembered that not only carbamazepine or diphenyl-hydantoin but also quinine, even in minor dosages, may cause toxic side-effects (Brasic 2001). Neuromyotonia usually responds to anticonvulsants in moderate to high dosages. In primary immunogenic neuromyotonia, elimination of VGKC-abs by means of a standard series of plasmaphereses or immuno-modulation with i.v. IgG infusion causes distinct clinical improvement corresponding to a reduction or even abolition of the abnormal EMG spontaneous activity (Newsom-Davis and Mills 1993).

Spasms

Definition

The term spasm will be used here to describe a certain type of involuntary, complex but usually stereotyped motor pattern that is generated in the CNS (Table 10.1). In distinction to the peripherally generated cramps which, as a rule, involve isolated muscles or only parts of muscles, spasms usually afflict groups of neighboring muscles instead, such as a limb segment or a whole limb, and may even generalize. Spasms may occur spontaneously with a tendency to recur at regular or irregular intervals. However, they can often easily be provoked in a reproducible manner by cutaneous stimulation. Intensity of muscular contraction during a spasm is variable and usually below maximal. Correspondingly, pain is usually not a chief complaint. The course of a spasm is often characterized by a rapid crescendo reaching its maximum within 1 to 2 seconds followed by a slow decrescendo within seconds or even minutes (Table 10.1). Occasionally, spasms have a brisk and violent, that is, myoclonic onset and may cause serious falls.

Epidemiology and general manifestation

As compared to cramps, spasms are clearly less common. Spasms represent an excess motor activity due to a defective central motor control. Spasms per se are unspecific with regard to the nature of the underlying disease. However, they gain diagnostic significance through the syndromic company they share. These include pyramidal tract disorders with central weakness and/or positive Babinski signs, flexor or extensor spasms; monosymptomatic or complex basal ganglia disorders, for example, blepharospasm and multiple system atrophy; characteristic types of epileptic seizures, such as focal seizures with tonic posturing; exaggerated startle, lockjaw and autonomic dysregulation, such as tetanus; or trunk stiffness, gait disorder and task-specific phobia in the stiff-man syndrome.

Selected diseases

Blepharospasm defines an unwilled forceful activation of the orbicularis oculi muscles on both sides that may persist the whole day, thereby rendering the patient functionally blind. To the examiner, abnormal eye closure may appear jerky or tonic, or a mixture of both. In many cases, the feeling of a foreign body in one or both eyes precedes the development of blepharospasm by weeks or months, and bright light or emotional stress may reinforce the spasm. Blepharospasm is considered a focal form of dystonia. However, excess activity may spread to the perioral region (Meige syndrome), and larynx and neck muscles (segmental dystonia). Not infrequently, blepharospasm is a constituent of complex movement disorders such as multiple system atrophy, cortico-basal ganglionic degeneration, or drug-induced acute or tardive dyskinesia. In a minor variant, blepharospasm may be confined to the pretarsal parts of the orbicularis oculi muscles whose contraction is difficult to identify. Particularly, the isolated pretarsal form of blepharospasm may be difficult to discriminate clinically from other forms of isolated bilateral lid-drop such as senile ptosis, myasthenia or true eyelid apraxia. Simultaneous EMG recordings from the orbicularis oculi and levator palpebrae or frontalis muscles may show paradoxical excess activation of the orbicularis oculi when the patient attempts to open the eyes. Moreover, the orbicularis oculi blink reflex in patients with blepharospasm often displays a stable R3 component and poor habituation with repeated stimulation (Berardelli et al. 1999). In clinically equivocal cases, the treatment of choice helps diagnostically and the injection of small doses of botulinum toxin into the orbicularis oculi muscle or into its pretarsal part relieves symptoms.

Flexor spasms describe spontaneous and involuntary flexion movements of one or both legs, which stereotypically recur at long and irregular intervals. The motor pattern of flexor spasms resembles the flexor reflex with dorsiflexion of the big toe and the foot combined with flexion of the hip and knee joints, and is occasionally associated with intense pain. Flexor spasms may also radiate into the muscles of the bladder or bowel. In turn, a full bladder or bowel may provoke flexor spasms. Occurrence of flexor spasms in a given patient often follows a circadian rhythm with increase of both intensity and frequency during the night, which may considerably interfere with the patient's sleep.

Flexor spasms predominantly involve patients with spinal cord diseases, and are usually associated with hyperreflexia, spasticity, central weakness and positive Babinski signs. However, hyperreflexia and spastic increase of muscle tone are not prerequisites for development of flexor spasms as evidenced from patients with co-existing polyneuropathy. This suggests that flexor spasms relate to abnormalities of exteroceptive rather than proprioceptive input processing. Close phenomenological and physiological similarity to abnormal flexor reflexes elicited by mechanical stimulation of the foot sole has led to the opinion that flexor spasms represent abnormal responses of a spinal cord neuronal network that is deprived of supraspinal control due to a rostral lesion. The network is driven by a continuous normal background activity from skin or visceral receptors, or both, mediated via intact afferent fibers to the cord. EMG recordings show that during flexor spasms not only the flexors but also the extensor muscles are activated (Shahani and Young 1980; Fig. 10.3a, b) but the flexors dominate. However, in certain spastic patients extensor activity exceeds flexor activity, thus resulting in extensor thrusts with transient extension of the hip, knee and ankle joints. The reason for such a differential patterning is not clear. Nevertheless, both flexor spasms and extensor thrusts usually respond to treatment with antispastic drugs such as baclofen, tizanidine or benzodiazepines. Because these drugs in greater dosages unmask central weakness and may cause sedation, the main dosage should be taken in the evening.

Tonic spasms describe an uncommon motor disorder that is characteristically associated with, and occasionally is the presenting symptom of, multiple sclerosis. Tonic spasms last long and, in a given patient, have a tendency to spontaneously recur at a low frequency, typically a few times per hour, with a specific motor pattern. Often the feeling of an increasing tension in the afflicted body parts precedes onset of motor activity like an aura preceding an epileptic seizure. Muscle contraction during a spasm slowly develops, reaches a maximum and gradually subsides. The contraction is usually forceful and thus often associated with pain. However, the range of the movement is narrow due to co-contraction of antagonistic groups of muscles.

Tonic spasms involve regions such as the face or the hand and forearm, and often spread over one side, paroxysmal hemidystonia, or even generalize. The face or limbs, or both, perform involuntary bizarre and stereotyped movements. Many patients report trigger mechanisms such as physical exertion. Tonic spasms are usually observed in a clinical setting with a pyramidal tract lesion between capsula interna and lower thoracic spinal cord (Tranchant 1995).

Clinical differential diagnosis of tonic spasms and flexor spasms/extensor thrusts is often impossible without provocation of the ictus. In flexor spasms/extensor thrusts, the face and arms are usually not involved. If pyramidal tract signs are absent, paroxysmal kinesigenic choreoathetosis, paroxysmal dyskinesia, atypical dystonia and focal epileptic seizures with tonic posturing are the differential diagnoses. Tonic spasms may disappear spontaneously, but may also recur. In cases with an established diagnosis of multiple sclerosis, de novo manifestation of tonic spasms can be regarded equivalent to an exacerbation. Correspondingly, tonic spasms may disappear after a high-dosage methylprednisolone treatment. Anticonvulsants in standard oral dosages such as carbamazepine (600–1200 mg/day) or gabapentin (600–1200 mg/day) are usually effective as symptomatic medication.

Case report: A 43-year-old speech therapist was admitted with recurring intense muscle contractions in her right leg. Contractions evolved slowly, involved almost all leg muscles concomitantly, lasted for minutes and recurred up to 150 times per day but not during the night. They were excruciatingly painful, valued at 9/10 on a visual analogue scale. Spasms were not provoked but showed some association to a forced use of the leg. If a spasm developed, the leg showed freezing of the respective position due to co-contraction of almost all muscles, which became as hard as a board. Between spasms, she was free of complaints. She had a history of autoimmune thyroiditis with latent hypothyroidism and had suffered a three-month episode with similar, but less intense, right-leg muscle spasms 5 years ago. Her family history was unremarkable. Clinical examination between spasms and conventional neurophysiologic studies yielded normal results, as did laboratory tests including antineuronal auto-antibodies and cerebrospinal fluid analysis. MRI displayed a normal brain and degenerative changes of the C5 and C6 vertebrae with mild

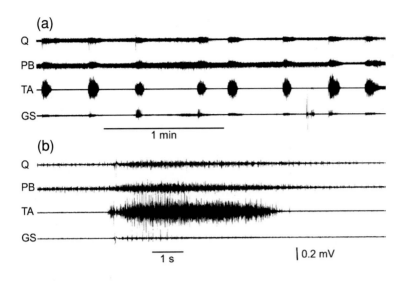

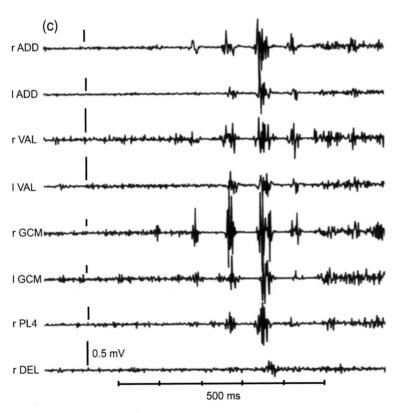

Fig. 10.3. Spontaneous spasms in spasticity (a, b) and in the stiff-man syndrome (c). Flexor spasms in a patient with cervical spondylotic myelopathy. Simultaneous EMG recording with surface electrodes from leg muscles on one side (Q = quadriceps, PB = posterior biceps, TA = tibialis anterior, GS = gastrocnemius-soleus). Registration at a slow sweep speed (a) shows spontaneous spasms at fairly regular long intervals. At a fast sweep speed (b), a spindle-shaped in and decrease of EMG activity and transient clonus activity in the GS muscle becomes visible. Vertical calibration in (b) is valid for all registrations in (a) and (b). (c) Spontaneous myoclonic spasm in a patient with SMS. Simultaneous EMG registration with surface electrodes from the adductor magnus (ADD), vastus lateralis (VAL), gastrocnemius medius (GCM), paraspinal L4 (PL4) and deltoid (DEL) muscles on the right (r) and left sides (l). Spasm begins with a series of five hypersynchronous myoclonic bursts that start in the rGCM, increase and spread into the other muscles, and are followed by long-lasting desynchronized activity. Please notice variable vertical calibration, with each bar representing 0.5 mV.

retrolisthesis, bulging of the disc and some deformation of the spinal cord but without signal abnormality within it. Incipient cervical spondylotic myelopathy with tonic spasms was diagnosed. However, antispastic treatment with high doses of oral baclofen (150 mg/day), carbamazepine (2000 mg/day), clonazepam

(20 mg/day) and levetiracetam (4000 mg/day) did not significantly improve the patient's condition, but did cause distinct sedation and other side-effects. Clinical and neurophysiologic re-evaluation yielded unchanged results. Considering complete refractoriness to antispastic and anti-myoclonic treatment,

dystonia appeared a reasonable differential diagnosis. Molecular genetic analysis for mutations of the DYT1 gene was negative, and an oral trial of levodopa was interrupted after 2 days because of severe diarrhea, vomiting and metabolic disequilibrium with confusion. However, after some weeks another trial of levodopa was tolerated well. She became symptom-free since being on 200 mg/day of the levodopa plus carbidopa. Tests for mutations of genes encoding cyclohydrolase 1 or tyrosine hydroxylase were negative. Preliminary diagnosis is levodopa-sensitive dystonia.

Stiff-man or stiff-person syndrome (SMS) is clinically characterized by fluctuating stiffness, that is, rigidity, of the trunk and proximal limb muscles superimposed by painful muscle spasms. Symptoms develop insidiously over months or years and may remain stable thereafter over years or even decades. Firm neurological signs are absent. However, a spectrum of uncommon symptoms frequently combine with the aforementioned core features comprising exaggerated startle, attacks of autonomic dysregulation particularly profuse sweating, skeletal deformities such as hyperlordosis, awkward disturbance of gait that distinctly improves with minor help, and a particular type of anxiety that resembles agoraphobia but is specifically confined to standing and walking without support, so-called task-specific phobia. Occasionally, patients present with the symptoms of SMS but confined to one limb, usually a leg, thus the so-called stiff-limb syndrome (SLS). However, more frequent is the combination of SMS with firm neurological signs such as myoclonus, ocular motor disturbance, ataxia, epilepsy, central or peripheral weakness, positive Babinski signs or the progressive encephalomyelitis with rigidity and myoclonus (PERM) syndrome.

About 70% of patients with SMS, SLS or PERM harbor antineuronal serum auto-antibodies that are directed against glutamic acid decarboxylase (GAD). GAD decarboxylates glutamic acid to γ-aminobutyric acid, a major inhibitory transmitter in the brain and spinal cord. Moreover, many of these patients have one or more organ-specific autoimmune diseases such as type 1 diabetes mellitus, Hashimoto thyroiditis or pernicious anemia (Meinck and Thompson 2002). A minority of patients develops SMS or its variants as an autoimmune paraneoplastic disease. Cases so far reported had neoplasms of the lung or breast, and manifestation of motor disorder preceded diagnosis of the tumor by up to 5 years. Presence of antineuronal serum autoantibodies directed against amphiphysin 1, a synaptic vesicle protein, in such cases may serve as a biochemical marker for the paraneoplastic nature. Taken together, these features suggest that SMS and its variants are manifestations of a chronic autoimmune encephalomyelitis. Indeed, cerebrospinal fluid studies revealed elevated IgG levels, oligoclonal bands and intrathecal de novo synthesis of GAD autoantibodies.

In patients with SMS, SLS and PERM, spasms may vary between a slowly developing, regional and transient increase of muscle tone that lasts seconds or minutes to violent generalized spasms with a jerky (i.e., myoclonic) onset and slow cessation. The characteristic motor pattern of such myoclonic spasms comprises forceful retropulsion of the trunk, that is, opisthotonus, and hyperextension and slight abduction of the legs with inward rotation of the feet. In Figure 10.3c, the EMG shows the onset of a violent spasm with a series of hypersynchronous, that is, myoclonic, bursts that spread over both legs and transition into bilateral tonic decrescendo activity. Spasms may be violent enough to cause subluxation of joints, spontaneous fracture or bending of implanted Smith-Peterson nails, and they may cause excruciating pain. Although many spasms occur spontaneously, they are as a rule to be provoked by a variety of external triggers such as touch and electrical stimulation but also startle, anger or fright. Spasms elicited by exteroceptive stimulation habituate rapidly, which may suggest to the naïve observer that their elicitation lacks reliability. When elicited with sufficiently long intervals (more than 30 seconds), they usually are to be provoked in a stereotypical fashion and may be subject to EMG analysis. They are characterized by a short latency (less than 80 ms) and a hypersynchronous onset in all muscles recorded, and often show repetition of the myoclonic bursts at short intervals, from around 100 ms. Desynchronized tonic activity follows and slowly subsides over seconds or even minutes. Such myoclonic reflex spasms are a characteristic of SMS and its variants. We have found them in more than 80% of untreated patients regardless of their antibody status, and we have never seen them in normal subjects or in patients with other disorders of muscle tone. Not only myoclonic reflex spasms but also their response to benzodiazepines may help diagnosis. Subhypnotic doses of diazepam (5 mg applied i.v. within 5 minutes; if required, this may be repeated

139

after another 5 minutes) effectively suppress sponta-neous and reflex spasms and normalize muscle tone (Meinck 2001).

A distinct rigid increase of muscle tone, which usu-ally begins in the face as risus sardonicus or masseter spasm, violent spasms of the trunk and limb muscles, and exaggerated startle, characterize tetanus. Except for rare forms where symptoms remain focal such as in cephalic tetanus, muscle rigidity and spasms general-ize within days or even hours. Soon after onset, spasms may involve the respiratory or laryngeal muscles, and liability to acute autonomic disturbance may develop. Moreover, generalized spasms are often linked with acute autonomic disturbance, and both can be eas-ily triggered by minor external stimuli. A noise, a jolt to the bed or routine activities of the nursing staff may provoke massive spasms and life-threatening increase of heart rate and blood pressure, or both. Systematic physiological investigations of spasms in tetanus are lacking. However, as symptoms almost regularly begin in the pericranial muscles, investiga-tion of electrophysiological brain stem reflexes, par-ticularly of the masseter inhibitory reflex, helps early diagnosis. Reflex inhibition of the jaw-closing mus-cles is to be elicited by a gentle tap with a reflex hammer to the chin, or by electrical stimulation of the lips. EMG recordings from the voluntarily inner-vated masseter or temporalis muscles in normal sub-jects display a biphasic inhibition with onset latency around 15 ms after stimulation and an overall dura-tion of some 80 ms. In tetanus, masseter inhibition is lost but masseter spasms are elicited instead with a latency around 30 ms (Fig. 10.4c). Once the diagnosis is suspected, instantaneous admission to an intensive care unit including preventive, that is, early intubation is necessary to secure vital functions. Passive immu-nization with human tetanus immunoglobulin (3.000–6.000 I.U. i.m.), antibiotic treatment with penicillin ($10–12 \times 10^6$ I.U. per day), cut-out of wounds sus-pected to serve as microbial entrance for *Clostridium tetani* and sedation with high-dosage benzodiazepines are essential.

Exaggerated startle

Epidemiology and general manifestation

Although a prominent feature in the stiff-man syn-drome and in tetanus, exaggerated startle is gener-ally considered an uncommon neurologic sign. In other neurological diseases, exaggerated startle typ-ically occurs in the company of brain stem lesions. Occasionally, it may present as an isolated disorder. A key feature of startle disorders is the startle reflex to acoustic or tactile stimulation. This reflex has a stereotyped motor pattern with brief retropulsion and subsequent anteflexion of the head or trunk, or both, accompanied by elevation and flexion of the arms. The exaggerated startle reflex is profoundly sensitized by stress, and poorly habituates with repeated elicitation. EMG recordings demonstrate bursts with a latency of 20 to 60 ms in the head, neck and trunk muscles resem-bling reflex myoclonus. Indeed, certain types of exag-gerated startle are considered a manifestation of retic-ular reflex myoclonus.

Definition

Exaggerated startle has been reported in various dis-eases but has been further characterized so far in only a few. Phenomenologically, two types of exaggerated startle may be distinguished (Matsumoto and Hallett 1996; Table 10.4). In the first type, a trivial, weak and not surprising stimulus startles the patient, usually even when repeated or after a pre-warning, that is, a stimulus that would be ineffective in a normal per-son reproducibly evokes an inadequate, abnormally frequent and often violent startle. Among such cases a group of diseases share specific clinical and neu-rophysiologic abnormalities of an exaggerated star-tle reflex, namely the hyperekplexias (Matsumoto and Hallett 1996). The second type of exaggerated startle is actually characterized by what immediately follows startle rather than by the startle itself. In such cases, startle appears normal, that is, adequate with respect to both stimulus and subsequent jerk, and with rapid habituation. However, the apparently normal startle, but not the stimulus without startle, induces complex and stereotyped motor or behavioral abnormalities, or both, that last several seconds. Some of these motor and/or behavioral patterns can be classified as epilep-tic, that is, startle epilepsy. In most of these cases, a star-tle reflex normal in all respects provokes a complex-partial or generalized epileptic seizure, usually with a delay of one or more seconds (Aguglia et al. 1984; Manford et al. 1996). Others are currently considered stimulus-sensitive tics, or culture-bound stereotypic behavior, for example, Latah, jumping Frenchmen of

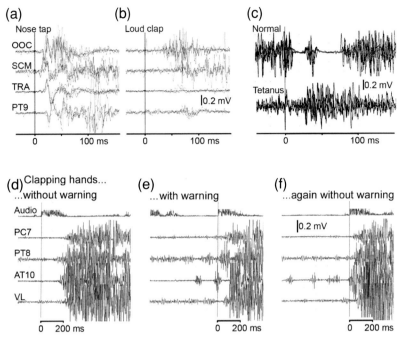

Fig. 10.4. Abnormal reflex patterns in patients with exaggerated startle. EMG pattern of the head retraction reflex (a) and the exaggerated acoustic startle reflex (b) in a patient with progressive encephalomyelitis with rigidity and myoclonus ("jerking stiff-man syndrome"). Each panel represents four superimposed registrations. Stimulus (0 ms) is marked by a vertical line. The reflex jerk is clearly stronger with tactile stimulation and occurs with shortest latency in the sternocleidomastoideus (SCM), followed by the orbicularis oculi (OOC), trapezius (TRA) and paraspinal T9 (PT9) muscles. Acoustic stimulation evokes only the late reflex components. Calibration bars are valid for all channels. Re-arranged from Meinck 2006, with permission. (c) Abnormal masseter inhibitory reflex in a patient with tetanus and in a normal subject. Surface EMG from the masseter muscle during forceful pre-innervation, four sweeps superimposed for each registration. Electrical stimulation of the lips normally induces a biphasic exteroceptive inhibition, which in tetanus is replaced by a short-latency (about 30 ms) reflex spasm. Vertical calibration is valid for both recordings. (d, e, f) EMG polygraph recording of startle in a patient with psychogenic startle disorder. Surface electrodes were placed on one side over the paraspinal muscles (P) at the C7 and T8 levels, the rectus abdominis (A) at the T10 level, and over the vastus lateralis (VL). The audio channel (top registration) was rectified to avoid overlap with the EMG channels. Patient rests supine on couch with the instruction to keep the eyes closed. (d) Surprising loud clap (onset marked by a vertical line). (e) Loud clap with previous warning (end of warning instruction is visible on the audio channel). (f) Repeat loud clap without pre-warning.

Maine, Myriachit or Goosey (Howard and Ford 1992). For the sake of clarity, this chapter focuses on hyperekplexia.

Selected diseases

Hyperekplexia as an inherited disorder, mostly with an autosomal dominant trait, and manifests shortly after birth (Brown et al. 1991; Matsumoto et al. 1992). Babies with hereditary hyperekplexia are usually delivered as stiff as a board, hence the nickname "stiff-baby syndrome." They are in vital danger due to apneic spells and laryngospasm. Sleep attenuates or even abolishes muscle stiffness. Emotions and acoustic or tactile, particularly perioral, stimulation provoke massive startle and subsequent stiffness with opisthotonus of the head and trunk and a characteristic stereotyped flexion pattern of the limbs. Usually, the first diagnostic suspicion is spasticity and epileptic seizures due to perinatal brain damage. However, muscle tone normalizes within the first year, and psychomotor development in most cases is not significantly delayed except for standing and walking. However, startle reflexes remain exaggerated and frequently cause paroxysmal falls described as "like a log," that is, without reaction of the arms to break the fall. Furthermore, a particular fear of free standing and walking persists, in some patients even in adolescence, with a protective, broad-based and hesitating gait pattern that improves immediately and distinctly with minor support. In contrast, emotional stress significantly augments all symptoms (Tijssen 1997).

Table 10.4 Clinical syndromes with abnormal startle

Type 1: Primary exaggerated startle
  Hyperekplexia
    Genetic
    Symptomatic
      Brain stem disorders (encephalitis, hemorrhage)
      Stiff-man syndrome
      Tetanus
      Strychnine intoxication
    Idiopathic

Type 2: Primary normal startle with secondary abnormalities
  Startle epilepsy
  Culture-bound abnormal startle behaviors
  (e.g., jumping Frenchmen of Maine, Myriachit, Latah, Goosey)
  Psychogenic startle

Unclassified
  Thalamic lesions (e.g., inflammatory, vascular)
  Posttraumatic stress disorder
  Tourette's disease
  Drug intoxication or withdrawal
  Dementia

The characteristic neurologic sign associated with hyperekplexia is the head retraction reflex (Fig. 10.4a, b). Slight taps with a finger to the center of the face, for example, glabella, bridge of nose, upper lip and chin, evoke a brisk retraction of the head that habituates poorly with repeated taps (Tijssen 1997). The head retraction reflex belongs to the group of facial withdrawal reflexes, and is not to be elicited in normal subjects. However, the reflex is not specific for hyperekplexia but may also be present, though less brisk and with rapid habituation, in a variety of brain disorders such as Parkinsonian syndromes or amyotrophic lateral sclerosis. In subjects with hereditary hyperekplexia, the head retraction reflex persists throughout life which, in cases with unremarkable family history, occasionally allows one to identify a seemingly normal parent as affected and thus helps diagnose hereditary hyperekplexia. EMG recordings in hyperekplectic patients show that the startle reflex in the pericranial and neck muscles is to be recorded with abnormally high amplitude, irradiates into muscles normally not involved and habituates poorly with repeated elicitation (Brown and Thompson 2001; Thompson et al. 1992). Molecular genetic testing in a considerable proportion of patients reveals an inherited or (less common) spontaneous point mutation of the gene encoding the α1-subunit of the glycine receptor on chromosome 5q31.2 (Shiang et al. 1993).

Exaggerated startle in familial hyperekplexia may manifest itself with two distinct phenotypes, the major and minor forms, even in the same family (Bakker et al. 2006). As compared to the previously described major form, the minor form manifests itself later usually between infancy and puberty and is less severe with startles but without stiffness. Within the same family, relatives presenting with the major form were tested positive for the aforementioned gene mutation, however relatives afflicted with the minor form tested negative. A simple explanation of such a rather complex relationship is not available.

Hyperekplexia as an acquired disorder is a feature of encephalopathy. Symptomatic hyperekplexia in adulthood has been reported with various etiologies including alcohol and drug withdrawal and with a variety of lesions in the brain stem and midbrain, and is associated with respective neurological signs in addition to exaggerated startle and the head retraction reflex (Brown et al. 1991). Both spontaneous course and prognosis of symptomatic hyperekplexia are determined by the underlying disease. However, hyperekplexia may present without a detectable cause. Both idiopathic and symptomatic hyperekplexia are not well-characterized (Brown et al. 1991). Clinical manifestations of idiopathic hyperekplexia in many instances resemble symptomatic hyperekplexia with exaggerated startle, positive head retraction reflex, awkward gait disorder with startle-induced falls and task-specific phobia. However, its spontaneous course has been reported stable over several years. The symptomatic treatment of choice in hereditary or symptomatic hyperekplexia is clonazepam (Tijssen et al. 1997). Other anticonvulsants or myorelaxants as well as behavioral therapy or forced physiotherapy are poorly effective.

Spasms and exaggerated startle may also occur as a psychogenic movement disorder. Distinction from organic diseases may be difficult, hence unequivocal neurological signs are often also lacking in the stiff-man syndrome, hyperekplexia or dystonia. Moreover, augmentation of disordered movements by emotional stress, the presence of autonomic disturbance or phobic avoidance, specifically of free stance and gait, may dominate the clinical picture. According to the author's impression, which admittedly is not scientifically validated, patients with organic disease often experience emotional augmentation of symptoms as a particular torment and unreservedly talk about it. In contrast, patients with somatoform disorder often deny a significant emotional influence on their symptoms, which may relate to the strategies underlying conversion. EMG analysis of evoked spasms or startle reflexes in patients with organic disease reveals abnormal reflex patterns with a short latency that are exactly reproducible. In contrast, patients with psychogenic disorders produce responses with inconsistent patterns and a wide scatter of latencies (Brown and Thompson 2001; Thompson et al. 1992). Occasionally, EMG allows the identification of patients who simulate disordered startle (Fig. 10.4d–f).

References

Aguglia U, Tinuper P, Gastaut H. Startle-induced epileptic seizures. *Epilepsia* 1984, 25:712–720.

Auger R. Diseases associated with excess motor unit activity. *Muscle Nerve* 1994, 17:1250–1263.

Bakker M et al. Startle syndromes. *Lancet Neurol* 2006, 5:513–524.

Baldissera F, Cavallari P, Dworzak F. Motor neuron 'bistability'. A pathogenetic mechanism for cramps and myokymia. *Brain* 1994, 117:929–939.

Berardelli A et al. The orbicularis oculi reflexes. The International Federation of Clinical Neurophysiology. *Electroencephalogr Clin Neurophysiol Suppl* 1999, 52:249–253.

Brasic J. Quinine-induced thrombocytopenia in a 64-year old man who consumed tonic water to relieve nocturnal leg cramps. *Mayo Clin Proc* 2001, 76:863–864.

Brown P, Thompson P. Electrophysiological aids to the diagnosis of psychogenic jerks, spasms, and tremor. *Mov Disord* 2001, 16:595–599.

Brown P et al. The hyperekplexias and their relationship to the normal startle reflex. *Brain* 1991, 114: 1903–1928.

Deecke L, Müller B, Conrad B. Standardisierung des elektromyographischen Tetanietests in der Diagnose der normokalzämischen Tetanie: 10-minütiger Trousseau bei Patienten und gesunden Kontrollen. *Arch Psychiatr Nervenkr* 1983, 233:23–37.

Denny-Brown D, Foley J. Myokymia and the benign fasciculation of muscle cramps. *Trans Assoc Am Phys* 1948, 61:88–96.

Diener H et al. Effectiveness of quinine in treating muscle cramps: a double-blind, placebo-controlled, parallel-group, multicentre trial. *Int J Clin Pract* 2002, 56:243–246.

Gutman L. Facial and limb myokymia. *Muscle Nerve* 1991, 14:1043–1049.

Howard R, Ford R. From the jumping Frenchmen of Maine to posttraumatic stress disorder: the startle response in neuropsychiatry. *Psychol Med* 1992, 22:695–707.

Jusic A, Dogan S, Stojanovic V. Hereditary persistent distal cramps. *J Neurol Neurosurg Psych* 1972, 35:379–384.

Layzer R. The origin of muscle fasciculations and cramps. *Muscle Nerve* 1994, 17:1243–1249.

Manford M, Fish D, Shorvon S. Startle provoked epileptic seizures: features in 19 patients. *J Neurol Neurosurg Psych* 1996, 61:151–156.

Matsumoto J, Hallett M. Startle syndromes. In: *Movement disorders 3*, Marsden CD, Fahn S. (eds). Butterworth Heinemann: London, 1996, p. 418–433.

Matsumoto J et al. Physiological abnormalities in hereditary hyperekplexia. *Ann Neurol* 1992, 32:41–50.

McGee S. Muscle cramps. *Arch Intern Med* 1990, 150:511–518.

Meinck H. Stiff man syndrome. *CNS Drugs* 2001, 15:515–526.

Meinck H. Startle and its disorders. *Neurophysiologie Clinique* 2006, 36:357–364.

Meinck H-M, Thompson P. Stiff man syndrome and related conditions. *Mov Disord* 2002, 17:853–866.

Mertens H, Zschocke S. Neuromyotonie. *Klin Wschr* 1965, 43:917–925.

Newsom-Davis J, Mills K. Immunological associations of acquired neuromyotonia (Isaacs' syndrome). Report of five cases and literature review. *Brain* 1993, 453–469.

Parisi L et al. Muscular cramps: proposals for a new classification. *Acta Neurol Scand* 2003, 107:176–186.

Roffe C et al. Randomised, cross-over, placebo controlled trial of magnesium citrate in the treatment of chronic persistent leg cramps. *Med Sci Monit* 2002, 8:CR 326–330.

Rowland L. Cramps, spasms and muscle stiffness. *Rev Neurol* 1985, 141:261–273.

Shahani B, Young R. The flexor reflex in spasticity. In: *Spasticity: disordered motor control*. Feldman R, Young R, Koella W. (eds). Symposia Specialists, Inc.: Chicago, 1980, p. 287–300.

Shiang R, Ryan S, Zhu Y, Hahn A, O'Connell P, Wasmuth J. Mutations in the alpha 1 subunit of the inhibitory glycine receptor cause the dominant neurologic disorder, hyperekplexia. *Nat Genet* 1993, 5:351–358.

Thompson P et al. Voluntary stimulus-sensitive jerks and jumps mimicking myoclonus or pathological startle syndromes. *Mov Disord* 1992, 7:257–262.

Thompson PD et al. Focal dystonia of the jaw and the differential diagnosis of unilateral jaw and masticatory spasm. *J Neurol Neurosurg Psych* 1986, **49**:651–656.

Tijssen M. Hyperekplexia – startle disease. In: *Neurology*. Rijksuniversiteit Leiden: Leiden/N, 1997, p. 1–173.

Tijssen M et al. The effects of clonazepam and vigabatrin in hyperekplexia. *J Neurol Sci* 1997, **149**:63–67.

Tranchant C, Bhatia K, Marsden C. Movement disorders in multiple sclerosis. *Mov Disord* 1995, **10**:418–423.

Tuite P et al. Idiopathic generalized myokymia (Isaacs' syndrome) with hand posturing resembling dystonia. *Mov Disord* 1996, **11**:448.

Veltkamp R et al. Progressive nonatrophic arm weakness and tonic spasm: isolated manifestation of multifocal motor neuropathy in the brachial plexus. *Muscle Nerve* 2003, **28**:242–245.

Vincent A. Understanding neuromyotonia. *Muscle Nerve* 2000, **23**:655–657.

Young G, Jewell D. Interventions for leg cramps in pregnancy. *Cochrane Database Syst Rev* 2002(1): CD000121.

Definition

Myoclonic jerks are sudden, brief, involuntary simple movements caused by a pathological increased excitation of motor neurons. Myoclonus can be puzzling for physicians, and its clinical recognition and phenomenology has been confused by the use of historical terms and conventions that often conflict with the notion of modern physiological findings. Myoclonus, a frequent clinical sign and one of the most common abnormal movements, consists of simple, brief, jerky, shock-like, involuntary muscular contractions or inhibitions (Marsden et al. 1981) involving the extremities, face and trunk without loss of consciousness (Fahn et al. 1986). These features make myoclonic jerks different from most other involuntary movements. Myoclonic jerks are either caused by muscle contraction (positive myoclonus) or by a sudden inhibition during a voluntary tonic muscle contraction (negative myoclonus), causing insteadiness or a loss of movement control. Myoclonic jerks may occur spontaneously but may also be brought up by muscle activation (action-myoclonus) or sensory (i.e., tactile or acustic) stimuli (reflex-myoclonus). If rhythmical, myoclonic jerks may resemble tremor (van Rootselaar et al. 2004). Rarely, myoclonus can be caused by lesions of the spinal cord, nerve roots (Brown et al. 1994) or peripheral nerves (Assal et al. 1998).

Myoclonic jerks may be one or the only symptom of an underlying neurological condition, that is, they may be present in isolation or be combined with other neurological symptoms. The etiology of the underlying disease is variable (Table 11.3). In principle, myoclonus may affect any part of the body. Myoclonic jerks may be restricted to a limited group of muscles or they may be generalized or multifocal, affecting different groups of muscles independently. Disability therefore varies according to the clinical picture. They may be minor and only affect certain movements or impair walking or standing. In severe cases, even food intake can be affected.

Epidemiology

Like myoclonus at sleep onset or during awakening, physiological myoclonus are frequent and do occur in most subjects. Another very common form of physiological myoclonus is singultus (hiccups), a manifestation of diaphragmatic myoclonus, which when persisting as with spinal pathology, brain stem lesions or drug-induced may be pathological (Launois et al. 1993). Data on the epidemiology of myoclonus is sparse. In a retrospective study (Caviness et al. 1999), the mean annual incidence of persisting, pathological myoclonus of any kind was 1.3 per 100,000 person-years, and the lifetime prevalence 8.6 per 100.000. Incidence correlated with age. In subjects over the age of 70 years, the mean incidence was 7.2 per 100.000. It was higher in men than in women (Caviness et al. 1999). Symptomatic myoclonus was the most frequent etiology, followed by epileptic and hereditary or sporadic myoclonus. The most frequent etiology was Alzheimer's dementia. Compared to other movement disorders, myoclonus was 1.3 times less frequent than idiopathic Parkinson's desease, half as frequent as dystonia and four times more frequent than Huntington's disease.

Diagnosis, differential diagnosis and classification

On clinical grounds, myoclonic jerks can easily be distinguished from other phenomenologically similar movement disorders (Table 11.1). Myoclonic jerks are brief, shock-like and are usually accompanied by a visible movement. In contrast, fasciculations involve

Table 11.1 Clinical-phenomenological distinction between myoclonus and other motor disturbances/types of ataxia

	Clinical characteristics	Myoclonus
tics	can at least temporarily be suppressed voluntarily, complex motoric patterns (except for "simple tics"), urge to carry out the movements and relief afterward	cannot be suppressed voluntarily, stereotypical twitches of muscle groups not present
chorea	continuous sequence of motions, randomly distributed and not predictable regarding the time and place of their occurrence	stereotypical short twitches of one or a few similar patterns of extension and distribution
dystonia	predominantly longer-lasting tonic muscle contractions that lead to malposition of the extremities or the head	of shorter duration, abrupt
tremor	rhythmic, sinusoidal muscle contractions that occur in an alternating pattern in agonistic and antagonistic muscles	abrupt muscle twitches that are often accompanied by simultaneous contractions of agonistic and antagonistic muscles

only part of a muscle and are not accompanied by movements. Dystonic movements are tonic postures and choreatic movements are complex, random in location and time, and are of longer duration. Simple motor tics might be the phenomenologically most resembling abnormal movements, which can be distinguished by their historical suppressibity, the urge to perform movement relief afterward. Myoclonic jerks might be difficult to differentiate from epilepsia partialis continua, an epileptic status of clonic epileptic seizures. Clinically, it may be difficult to distinguish myoclonic jerks from other clonic movements, particularly when jerks occur repetitively. Usually, clonic jerks due to focal epilepsy are longer lasting (more than 30 seconds), whereas myoclonic jerks are shorter in duration or dependent on an external trigger or voluntary muscle activation.

Myoclonic jerks of high frequency may be confused with tremor, in particular essential tremor brought about by action. The movements are characterized by rhythmic EMG bursts lasting less than 50 ms synchronously appearing in agonist and antagonist muscles at a rate of 9 to 18 Hz (Toro et al. 1993). Families with cortical myoclonic tremor and epilepsy (FCMTE) have also been reported (van Rootselaar et al. 2005). Finally, patients in addition to myoclonus may also present with a combination of different abnormal movements like dystonia, even in the same muscle. This makes a distinction difficult (Quinn et al. 1988).

A classification is obligatory for prognosis and impacts on treatment (Marsden et al. 1981). Myoclonic jerks may be classified according different criteria, that is, presentation, cause, examination findings and clinical neurophysiology testing. Myoclonus should be characterized by presentation, neurophysiology

and etiology because different etiologies might present with the same clinical features. In addition, all three aspects are important. Description of the clinical features is important to judge the degree of disability, the location influences the choice of symptomatic treatment, and the etiology is crucial for prognosis. A useful basic distinction based on etiology differentiates physiological, essential, epileptic and symptomatic myoclonus (Marsden et al. 1981). A detailed clinical classification already helps to localize the orgin within the nervous system as a clinical picture and the origin of myoclonus often correlate. The neurophysiological classification of myoclonus serves to summarize the information regarding the neuroanatomical localization of myoclonus within the nervous system (Caviness 2003).

Myclonic jerks are a clinical sign due to overexcitation of nervous elements, which may be physiological or be caused by a variety or inherited or acquired conditions. Myoclonus may be a minor sign as with progressive myoclonic epilepsies or Alzheimer's disease. They can also be the dominant clinical sign defining the degree of disability, as with chronic post-hypoxic myoclonus. What follows is a brief description of the diseases that have myoclonus as a major clinical sign (see Table 11.2).

Physiological myoclonus in healthy individuals

Physiological myoclonus most often is not disturbing and does not need to be treated. They can be brought up by sleep, anxiety or exercise. In rare cases, if persisting and severe, that is, with persisting hiccups, symptomatic causes need to be excluded. Sleep (hypnic) jerks or jerks on awakening do occur in

Table 11.2 Clinical descriptive classification of types of myoclonus

Distribution	focal	(cortical, spinal myoclonus)
	multifocal	(cortical myoclonus)
	generalized	(reticular reflex myoclonus of the brain stem)
Occurrence	spontaneous	
	in motion	(cortical myoclonus)
	continuous	(epilepsia partialis continua, spinal myoclonus)
	reflex	(cortical myoclonus, reticular reflex myoclonus of the brain stem and others)
	acoustic	(hyperekplexia, pathological fright reaction)
	visual	
	pain stimuli	
	touch	
	muscle stretching	
	stimulation of peripheral	
	nerves	

most people and may be accompanied by arousal or disturb sleep partners. Myoclonus often occurs during syncope where more than 80% of young healthy individuals with orthostatic syncope have it during the syncope (Lempert et al. 1994), and may therefore be confused with generalized tonic-clonic seizures. They are typically arrhythmical, multifocal, come in brief series and are more prominent in proximal muscles. Although they occur in healthy individuals, they might not be called physiological because they occur during the syncope, a state of transient hypoxia of the brain. Sensitive individuals startle with a sudden stimulus. This reaction habituates usually rapidly in healthy individuals. A startle reaction that occurs with weak subthreshold stimuli or does not habituate is termed pathological startle-response.

Essential myoclonus

In essential myoclonus, myoclonus is an almost isolated or essential phenomenon, from which a mild disability might result. Essential myoclonus is idiopathic or genetic, with no or only minor progression and no other disability like dementia, epileptic seizures or ataxia. The EEG, imaging and laboratory findings are normal. Sporadic and hereditary forms of this type of myoclonus exist. Hereditary essential myoclonus is characterized by an autosomal-dominant inheritance, onset before the age of 20 years and a benign course compatible with an active life and normal life expectancy in the absence of ataxia, spasticity, dementia and epileptic seizures (Mahloudji and Pikielny 1967). Myoclonic jerks are generalized or multifocal, more prominent in the upper body and present at rest and in action, and are greatly abated by alcohol ingestion. Myoclonus is usually non-stimulus sensitive and dystonia might coincide frequently in these cases, hence introducing the term myoclonus-dystonia (Vidailhet et al. 2001) for some of these cases. The phenotype in families with hereditary essential myoclonic syndromes is heterogenous, some familiy members presenting with essential tremor and some with dystonia. The tremor might be more prominent in the older generation, whereas myoclonus prevails in the young. A delineation of hereditary essential and hereditary essential myoclonic dystonia often is impossible (Quinn et al. 1988). However, one needs to differentiate patients with hereditary torsion-dystonia, in whom myoclonus is present in only 3% of cases.

Advances have been made in the genetics of the myoclonus-dystonia syndrome, giving insights into pathophysiology. Mutations in the ε-sarcoglycan gene have an association with the myoclonus-dystonia syndrome (Asmus and Gasser 2004). Epsilon-sarcoglycan dysfunction seems to interfere with normal GABA inhibitory receptors. There is a large and increasing number of mutations reported, and most loss-of-function mutations and paternal expression have been associated with reduced penetrance (Muller et al. 2002). Other reported mutations involve the dopamine D2-receptor and torsin A in combination with a ε-sarcoglycan mutation. Families with no ε-sarcoglycan mutation and linkage to chromosome 18 or with unknown linkage have also been described, yet other studies report no clear relationship between mutation type and phenotype in myoclonus-dytonia (Han et al. 2003; Hjermind et al. 2003). Two thirds of patients exhibit dystonia, mostly but not invariably of neck and arm. Other features like obsessive-compulsive or anxiety disorders, cognitive slowing and alcohol dependence have been associated with ε-sarcoglycan mutation (Hess et al. 2007).

Epileptic myoclonus

Epileptic myoclonus is usually defined by the presence of myoclonus in the setting of epilepsy. Myoclonus can occur as its own seizure type or be part of seizure semiology, or it may be generalized or restricted to a certain body region in focal epilepsy. In fact, if lateralized epileptic clonus is a classical feature of focal epilepsy already described more than 100 years ago by Hughlings Jackson and point to the contralateral motor strip. Cortical myoclonus and epilepsy with myoclonus share similar pathophysiological mechanisms. Symptomatic therapy is also comparable, and the transition from myoclonus to epileptic myoclonus is blurred. What follows is a brief description of epileptic seizures and syndromes that often present with myoclonus.

The earliest life expression of symptomatic generalized epilepsy is early myoclonic encephalopathy (Aicardi 1992), characterized clinically by irregular ("erratic") generalized or multifocal myoclonus, focal epileptic seizures, tonic seizures with severe mental delay, marked hypotonia, disturbed alertness and rarely signs of peripheral neuropathy occurring even as early as a few hours after birth. Myoclonic seizures occur in different idiopathic generalized epilepsies (IGE). The earliest life expression of IGE is benign (Dravet et al. 1992) and severe (Lombroso 1990) infantile myoclonic epilepsy (Dravet), thought to be a sodium channelopathy with mutation in SCN1A (Claes et al. 2001). The benign form is characterized by brief, 1 to 3 seconds, generalized non-stimulus sensitive myoclonus during the first and second year of life in normal children who often have a family history of epilepsy. In the severe variant, seizures begin during the first year of life as generalized or unilateral febrile clonic seizures, myoclonus occurring later as do partial seizures, psychomotor development is retarded and there is ataxia, pyramidal signs and interictal myoclonus.

Epileptic seizures consisting of myoclonus are a characteristic of juvenile myoclonic epilepsy (JME; Dreifuss 1989; Janz and Christian 1957), the most frequent adult form of IGE. Here, myoclonus is accompanied by generalized epileptiform EEG discharges, either spike-waves or poly-spike-wave, although the myoclonic jerks may affect only the upper body part, typically proximal muscles of the shoulder, or

even somewhat lateralized clinically. This may lead to confusion with clonic or myoclonic seizures in patients with frontal lobe epilepsy which originates from perirolandic areas of the contralateral cortex. These seizures are unilateral and typically present in distal extremity muscles or the face. Some progress has been made on the genetics of JME, although it is clinically and genetically heterogeneous. Although several major genes for JME have been identified and pathogenetic mechanisms suggested based on these findings, as these genes account for only a small proportion of JME cases, suggesting multifactorial or complex inheritance in most (Durner et al. 2005; Zifkin et al. 2005).

It is sometimes difficult to grasp the difference between IGE syndromes because some features are also occurring in the same patient in an age-dependent fashion or clinical features may vary from seizure to seizure in the same individual. In "classical" absence seizures, there may be myoclonus of the eyelid as a typical sign. In epilepsy with myoclonic absence (Tassinari et al. 1970), loss of consciousness is combined with continuing, bilateral, synchronous and rhythmical contractions of about 3 Hz, mainly in the arms and shoulders. Characteristically, prior to myoclonus a tonic elevation of the arms may be seen. Although myoclonus with absence (dialeptic) seizures are more proximal in neck and face, bilateral myoclonus in JME occurs in the shoulder and proximal parts of the upper body but may also affect the arm and hand. Myoclonic seizures prevail in adolescence, whereas later in adult life generalized tonic-clonic seizures are more prominent.

Severe jerks in axial muscles may lead to falls, and in some cases the succession of negative and positive myoclonus in proximal joints may cause disequilibrium. If jerks occur in the hands, patients may report dropping of objects with negative and throwing of items or spilling liquids with positive myoclonus, particularly in the morning after awakening. Generalized tonic-clonic seizures are usually preceded by a series of myoclonic jerks that might not be remembered later, hence one should always ask for isolated myoclonus in young people with a first generalized tonic-clonic seizure.

Similar to stimulus-senitive myoclonus, photosensitivity is a form of cortical reflex-hyperexcitability. In patients with photoparxysmal reactions myoclonus is present in 20% to 30%, usually as jerking eyelids and facial muscles. In severe cases, jerks might involve the shoulders or the whole body. In atypical benign epilepsy of childhood (Aicardi and Chevrie 1982), usually starting before age 10 years in mentally normal children, negative myoclonus is combined with atypical absences and atonic seizures.

The frequency of myoclonus in the Lennox-Gastaut syndrome (LGS) is between 10% and 30% (Aicardi and Levy 1992; Blume 1987) with a broad clinical spectrum. Jerks might be followed by atonic symptoms, hence the term myoclonic-astatic seizures. It has been debated whether it makes sense to differentiate LGS from myoklonic-astatic epilepsy as described by Doose (1992) or just assume the latter as a myoclonic form of LGS with a more benign course (Doose 1992). Patients with myoclonic-astatic epilepsy differ from LGS in that tonic seizures during the day are uncommon and patients are usually mentally less retarded.

The term progressive myoclonus epilepsy (PME) summarizes a number of gentic conditions characterized by sponatenous, action- or reflex-induced myoclonic jerks, epileptic seizures with progressive course, dementia and ataxia (Berkovic et al. 1993). In PME, myoclonus and epileptic seizures can often be induced by photic stimulation. The most common cause of PME is Unverricht-Lundborg disease (Lehesjoki 2002), an autosomal recessive disorder the major mutation having been mapped on chromosome 21q22 (EPM1), the underlying gene encoding cystatin B, a cysteine protease inhibitor. In addition, five "minor" mutations have been described. Cystatin B mutations are now known to account for both Mediterranean myoclonus and for "Baltic" myoclonus, described mainly from Finland, thus solving a long-term controversy and proving that these two disorders are one single disease entity.

Clinically, the condition is characterized by onset between the ages of 6 to 17 years, irregular action and reflex myoclonus in proximal muscles, cerebellar ataxia, epileptic seizures and mild intellectual dysfunction (Chew et al. n.d.). The course usually may be rapidly progressive in the first 5 to 10 years to stabilize later in life, with many patients reaching a normal life span (Magaudda et al. 2006). With modern anticonvulsive therapy, the prognosis has improved significantly. Symptoms are nowadays relatively well-controlled and the disease may not always progress (Kinrions et al. 2003; Magaudda et al. 2004), although drugs like phenytoin and lamotrigine may aggrevate the myoclonus (Genton et al. 2006). The acronym PMA has been introduced for progressive myoclonus ataxia, in which the ataxia and myoclonus are the most prominent features, in which epileptic seizures are rare and there is no cognitive decline.

Epilepsia partialis continua is a form of focal spontaneous myoclonus occurring irregularly or regularly with intervals of less than 10 seconds and lasting for hours, days or even weeks. Apart from the duration of the myoclonus, its irregularity and variability in topography and intensity (even in the same patient) is a clinical hallmark. Jerks come and go, may be worsened by sensory triggers or be combined with focal motor seizures from the same body region that generalize. There is no consensus on terminology. The definition of the ILAE is ictal activity that is focal and motor and continuing. Some use the term focal cortical myoclonus, yet in some cases the origin is not cortical (Cockerell et al. 1996). Thomas et al. used the definition of regular or irregular clonic muscle jerks of a part of the body for at least one hour, occurring at intervals not longer than 10 seconds (Thomas et al. 1977). The etiology may vary, that is, Rasmussen's encephalitis, stroke, cerebral vasculitis, cerebral trauma, malignancy and in 25% etiology remains unclear (Cockerell et al. 1996).

Symptomatic myoclonus

Symptomatic myoclonus occurs in the setting of an identifiable underlying disorder. Myoclonus as a clinical sign can be seen in a great variety of neurological and non-neurological diseases. The etiological classification includes different categories, listed in Table 11.3. Often symptomatic myoclonus comes along with clinical evidence of diffuse nervous system involvement. Patients may present with a variety of different clincal symptoms, some of which might even be more prominent than myoclonus. Most frequently, myoclonus occurs with neurodegenerative disease like Alzheimer's disease and following cerebral hypoxia. Cognitive abnormalities, seizures, ataxia and other movement disoders are frequently associated with symptomatic myoclonus. The course is dependent on the underlying etiology, and if the causitive agent or mechnism can be corrected, that is, drug-induced myoclonus or caused by metabolic derangement, myoclonus is usually fully reversible. Chronic or subacute clinical progression is always suggestive for symptomatic myoclonus. A detailed description of all different diseases is out of the range of this chapter.

Table 11.3 Etiological classification of myoclonus and myoclonus syndromes

1. Physiological myoclonus
   a. singultus
   b. myoclonus when falling asleep or waking up
   c. myoclonus caused by strain, orgasm, fear
   d. syncopal myoclonus (myoclonic syncopes)
   e. feeding myoclonus in early childhood
   f. physiological fright reaction

2. Hereditary myoclonus syndromes
   a. hereditary hyperekplexia (startle disorder)
   b. hereditary essential myoclonus
   c. hereditary myoclonic dystonia

3. Sporadic myoclonus syndromes
   a. sporadic hyperekplexia (startle disorder)
   b. sporadic essential myoclonus (no further neurological deficits, no encephalopathy)
   c. sleeping myoclonus ("periodic movement of sleep") in the sense of a motoric parasomnia, often associated with restless legs

4. Myoclonic attacks associated with epileptic syndromes (seizures are more prominent, except for PME, see below)
   a. myoclonic epilepsies in newborns
   b. focal epilepsy (e.g., epilepsia partialis continua)
   c. generalized epilepsy
      Lennox-Gastaut syndrome
      Myoclonic astatic epilepsy (Doose)
      absence epilepsies (with myoclonic absences, absences with myoclonus of the eyelid)
      juvenile myoclonic epilepsy (Janz)
   d. progressive myoclonic epilepsies (PME), myoclonus and epileptic seizures dominating to the same extent, encephalopathies more or less pronounced
      Unverricht-Lundborg disease
      Lafora body disease
      myoclonic epilepsy with "ragged red fibers" (MERRF)
      neuronal ceroid lipofuscidosis
      sialidosis ("cherry-red spot")
      Gaucher disease

5. Symptomatic myoclonus syndromes (encephalopathy with myoclonus)
   a. progressive myoclonic ataxia (PMA)
      spinocerebellar degeneration
      Unverricht-Lundborg disease
      Lafora body disease
      myoclonic epilepsy with "ragged red fibers" (MERRF)
      neuronal ceroid lipofuscidosis
      sialidosis ("cherry-red spot")
      celiac disease
   b. degenerative diseases of the CNS
      dentato-rubro-pallido-luysian atrophy (DRPLA)
      corticobasal degeneration (CBD)
      multiple system atrophy (MSA)
      Alzheimer's disease
      Huntington's disease
      Streele-Richardson-Olszewski syndrome (progradient supranuclear paralysis)
   c. encephalopathies caused by infections
      viral types of encephalitis: herpes simplex, herpes zoster, Coxsackie, Arbor, HIV, subacute sclerosing panencephalitis (SSPE)
      isolated post-infectious myoclonus
      spongiform encephalopathies (prion diseases)

Table 11.3 (cont.)

   –Creutzfeld-Jacob disease
   –Gerstmann-Sträussler syndrome
   –Kuru
   impairment of movement with immunological causes (stiff-person-syndrome, PERM: "progressive encephalomyelitis with rigidity and myoclonus," Hashimoto encephalopathy)
   d. metabolic encephalopathies
      liver and kidney failure, dialysis encephalopathy (aluminum)
      hyposodiumaemia
      hypoglycaemia, non-ketonic hyperglycaemia
   e. toxic encephalopathies
      medications and drugs
      cocaine, LSD, cannabinoids, L-dopa, dopamine agonists, lithium, tricyclic antidepressants, MAO inhibitors, cyclosporines, penicillins, cephalosporines, ethomidates, opiates, Amiodarone, Propafenone, Clozapine, Propofol
      heavy metals, methyl bromide, DDT, bismuth
   f. paraneoplastic encephalopathies
      opsoclonus-myoclonus syndrome
   g. posthypoxic encephalopathies
      acute posthypoxic myoclonus syndrome (partially status myoclonicus)
      chronic posthypoxic myoclonus syndrome (Lance-Adams syndrome)
   h. encephalopathies caused by traumata
      heat stroke, electric shock, traumatic brain injuries, decompression sickness
   i. myoclonus caused by focal lesions of the CNS
      tumor, bleeding, stroke
      stereotactic thalamotomy (asterixis)

Psychogenic myoclonus

What follows will be a brief description of details on myoclonus in some conditions.

Myoclonus in autosomal recessive, rapidly progressive Lafora body disease (Minassian 2002) are usually mild and infrequent but worsen continously. Myoclonus is combined with apraxia, loss of vision and dementia. Most patients die within 2 to 10 years. In myoclonus epilepsy and ragged-red fibers on muscle biopsy (MERRF; Fukuhara 1991) cortical reflex-myoclonus may be accompanied by seizures, dementia, dysarthria, shortness of stature, hypacusis, optical atrophy, neuropathy and migraine (Berkovic et al. 1989). The neuronal ceroid-lipofucsinosis (Cooper 2003) is a group of diseases with evidence of multiple unsaturated fatty acids characterized by seizures, dementia, cortical blindness, spasticity and myoclonus that may start at different ages, the adult form (Kufs) having a more benign course. In sialidosis ("cherry-red spot myoclonus syndrome"; Thomas et al. 1979), there is accumulation of oilgosaccharides due to a genetic defect with degeneration of neuroaminidase and beta-galactosidase. Progressive generalized or multifocal myoclonus occurs spontaneously and may be triggerd by action and sensory stimuli. Patients typically present a cherry-red spot at the macula, loss of vision, generalized tonic-clonic seizures and dementia.

Myoclonus often occurs with neurodegenerative disorders (Thompson 2002). Cortical myoclonus can be present in all Lewy body disorders (Caviness et al. 2002). Small-amplitude, irregular, cortical myoclonus brought up by action may be found in pathologically proven idiopathic Parkinson's disease without dementia, whereas the myoclonus in Lewy body dementia is of larger amplitude and occurs more often at rest (Caviness et al. 2002). About half of patients with Alzheimer's disease have cortical or subcortical myoclonus before death (Hauser et al. 1986). Myoclonus, which is present in 30% of patients with corticobasal degeneration, is usually focal, distal, unilateral and of reflex character. SSEPs are not enlarged, and there is no EEG potential preceeding the jerks on back-averaging.

Generalized and multifocal cortical action myoclonus may be found in Huntington's disease. Symptomatic myoclonus can also present as negative myoclonus (Shibasaki 2002). Clinically, negative myoclonus is a shock-like involuntary jerky movement caused by a sudden, brief interruption of muscle activity, leading a loss of muscle tone and the inability to maintain tonic muscle activity. Therefore, it might be missed clinically if tonic muscle activation is not specially tested. On EMG, negative myoclonus is characterized by brief interruptions of a tonic EMG activity, not preceded by a positive myoclonus in the agonist and antagonist muscles of the affected limb. Negative myoclonus has been shown to be of cortical or subcortical origin (Rubboli and Tassinari 2006). Asterixis is a type of negative myoclonus that occurs typically in toxic-metabolic encephalopathies and was first been described with hepatic failure. Negative myoclonus of cortical origin can also be the main feature of focal epileptic seizures, even as epileptic status of negative myoclonus, and often does not have EMG evidence of an antecedent positive myoclonus in target muscles (Tassinari et al. 1995). Negative myoclonus might be induced by some antiepileptic drugs like lamotrigine, carbamazepine or oxcarbazepine (Cerminara et al. 2004; Hahn et al. 2004; Parmeggiani et al. 2004).

The opsoclonus-myoclonus syndrome is characterized by fast, multidirectional saccadic eye movements and multifocal or generalized myoclonus. Commonly, it is infectious or paraneoplastic, most often bronchial, ovarian or breast malignancies, or Hodgkin's lymphoma. Symptomatic myoclonus is often present following cerebral hypoxia and may be cortical or subcortical, as well as brain-stem generated. In severe hypoxia, a status of stimulus-sensitive jerks or status myoclonicus and generalized tonic-clonic seizures during coma with generalized spikes on EEG may be a fragment of generalized status epilepticus and have a particularly bad prognosis (Krumholz et al. 1988). Myoclonus occurs in 35% of patients who are comatose for at least 24 hours where the coma is caused by global hypoxia due a cardiac arrest (Krumholz et al. 1988). In 78%, they also have generalized tonic-clonic seizures.

Given the bad prognosis, it is suggested to differentiate between acute (during coma) and chronic post-hypoxic myoclonus with a much more favorable prognosis (Werhahn et al. 1997). In chronic post-hypoxic myoclonus (Werhahn et al. 1997), also called Lance-Adams syndrome, myoclonus triggered by acoustic or sensory stimuli mostly occurs already during coma. However, it is not in the foreground and there is no status of generalized myoclonus or epileptic seizures. Myoclonus may become more evident or is only noticed if the patient regains consciousness and starts to move (action myoclonus). Action myoclonus, multifocal or generalized, then becomes the most prominent clinical sign and may be present next to occasional spontaneous myoclonus and generalized tonic-clonic seizures. In rare cases, myoclonus may also start weeks and months after the onset of coma. The most common etiology of coma is complications during anesthesia or asthma attacks, but intoxication or myocardial infarction may also be the cause. In most cases, cardiopulmonary arrest leading to cerebral hypoxia was present. Patients are handicapped by action myoclonus, particularly in walking and fine motor tasks. Despite therapy, the ability to walk unaided is reached by only one third of patients even years after onset. However, optimal treatment may be beneficial even months after the initial event.

A number of different startle syndromes have been described. They include hereditary hyperekplexia, symptomatic hyperekplexia, startle epilepsy and the Latah syndrome (Brown 2002). In startle epilepsy, an unexpected stimulus causes a startle response and epileptic seizure. Hereditary hyperekplexia is an autosomal-dominant disorder caused by a mutation on the alpha-1 subunit of the glycine receptor (Shiang et al. 1993). The mutation leads to a disturbance of ligand binding or chloride-ion channels. Glycine is a inhibitory transmitter of spinal interneurons. Newborns with the disorder are stiff and present with an increased muscular tone and develop a pathological startle reaction in childhood, which may cause strategies of avoidance. The startle reaction shows some progression in adolescence and remains more stable or is even decreasing later in adulthood. Motor development might be somewhat delayed. A minority of patients might additionally have generalized tonic-clonic seizures.

Voluntary, that is, psychogenic myoclonus can only be diagnosed indirectly by exclusion of other forms of myoclonus using neurophysiological testing, and resembles voluntary movement in its organization. Clinically, jerks are less stereotypical, can be modulated by attention and may habituate with reflex jerks. It may be generalized, focal, stimulus-sensitive and may resemble pathological startle. Criteria that help find the diagnosis are:

- Variable onset latency, if elicited by external triggers. In addition, latency should be longer than in non-psychogenic myoclonus and be similar to normal reaction time
- Changing pattern of muscle recruitment on polymyography
- Tendency to habituate
- If possible, registration of a *Bereitschaftspotential* (readiness potential), a slow negative potential on EEG, over 1–2 sec before spontaneous or reflex jerks (Brown and Thompson 2001)

Evaluation and clinical neurophysiology

Neurophysiology helps to determine the origin of myoclonus. This serves to classify myoclonus in different pathophysiological entities with therapeutic consequences. Wherever possible, this should be done in addition to tests claryfing the etiology. A part of the evaluation can be done routinely, whereas some tests require special techniques that are not readily avaible. Tests should be ordered based on a clinical hypothesis. Following a full history and physical examination, one should determine the distribution of the myoclonus; focal, segmental, multifocal, hemi or generalized, the temporal profile; rhythmic, irregular, continous, intermittent and the activation profile; spontaneous, on action, following sensory stimuli like touch, sound, visual or muscle strech. With this information, one can determine the major clinical syndrome category: physiological, essential, epileptic, symptomatic. In a second phase of the evaluation, additional testing may include EEG, EMG and evoked potentials based on what cortical area is involved. A third phase of assessment inlcudes EMG with jerk-locked, back-averaging with simultaneous EEG, polymyography, long-latency EMG following peripheral stimuli and recording of pre-movement potentials if psychogenic myoclonus is assumed. A description of the neurophysiological findings with the different types of myoclonus is given following.

Cortical myoclonus (Ugawa et al. 2002) predominantly affects hands and face, given the large cortical representation, and is often lateralized. It is characterized by brief (mostly less than 75 ms on EMG) multifocal or focal jerks in circumscribed and mostly distal parts of a body region. It may occur spontaneously, be brought up by voluntary muscle activation or be triggered by external stimuli like touching or local pain to the affected body part, then referred to as reflex myoclonus (Ugawa et al. 2002) suggesting an abnormally increased sensory input to the motor cortex. If hyperexcitability of the somatosensory cortex is present, the second component (P1N2) of the somatosensory-evoked potentials are enlarged, giant SSEPs. Back-averaging the EEG time-locked to myoclonus reveals a postive cortical potential preceding the jerks by a latency compatible with motor conduction time, that is, measured by using transcranial magnetic stimulation (Fig. 11.1). With peripheral stimuli to mixed nerves, a long-loop response may be present (C-reflex).

A special form of myoclonus presents as a sudden loss of muscle tone on activation and is termed negative myoclonus (Shibasaki 2002). This sudden interruption of muscle activation leads to a loss of tonic motor control of the involved body part, and if axial muscles are involved may lead to falls. With focal postive or negative myoclonus, the precise site or distribution pattern should be noted because it has localizing significance similar to focal epileptic seizures. Cortical-subcortical myoclonus, that is, in generalized myoclonic seizures, is typically generalized or

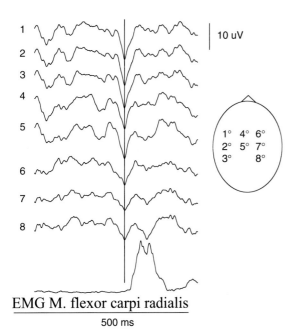

EMG M. flexor carpi radialis

500 ms

Fig. 11.1. Example of EEG back-averaging in cortical myoclonus. Back-averaging of EEG-traces ($n = 32$) relative to movement onset in a patient with myoclonus of the right lower arm. EEG shows a positive jerk-locked deflection 18 ms prior to EMG onset, confirming a cortical origin of myoclonus.

multifocal but otherwise has the same clinical characteristics as cortical myoclonus. With neurophysiology, EEG back-averanging is also positive, standard EEG may show generalized epileptiform discharges and SSEPs an enlarged cortical component. On EMG, bursts last less than 100 ms and a C-reflex may or may not be present.

Subcortical-supraspinal (brain stem) myoclonus (Hallett 2002) is generated by the reticular system of the brain stem. The myoclonus is usually generalized, especially axial, showing burts of variable duration and properties (up to 200 ms) and very sensitive to sound (Hallett 2002). In fact, auditory reflex jerks are a hallmark of hyperekplexia and brain stem reflex myoclonus (Brown 2002). There is no EEG correlate and standard EEG is often normal, as are SSEPs. Polymyography might show caudo-cranial recruitment pattern (i.e., muscles of lower cranial nerves, m. sternocleidomastoideus, are activated earlier than muscles innervated by upper cranial nerves, facial muscles). A C-reflex is usually missing. Palatale myoclonus or tremor (Deuschl and Wilms 2002) are rhythmical contractions of the soft palate. Myoclonus may also be present in the pharynx, chin or perioral muscles. This is a form of segmental myoclonus with

origin in the brain stem (triangle of Guillain-Mollaret: Olive-Ncl. dentatus-Ncl. ruber). Palatale myoclonus may be essential or symptomatic, the latter being characterized by the spread of myoclonus to axial muscles. In essential palatale myoclonus, 80% of patients report ear clicks synchronous to myoclonus, which is present in only 10% of symptomatic cases.

Myoclonus of spinal origin (Rothwell 2002) may present in two ways. Spinal segmental systems may become hyperexcitable due to spinal pathology (i.e., viral, syringomyelia, spinal ischemia or glioma). This may result in one or two contiguous spinal segments to generate myoclonus that is resistant to supraspinal influences, such as sleep or voluntary movements. The second type of spinal myoclonus is generated by the propriospinal system, a slow conducting intraspinal pathway that connects several segmental levels (Brown et al. 1994). Myoclonus generated here predominantly leads to axial jerks that, unlike brain stem myoclonus, spare the face and are not sensitive to acoustic stimuli. Polymyography may reveal EMG bursts of long duration that slowly spread up and down from the level of origin. EMG bursts are of longer duration (more than 100 ms), more rhythmical and in some cases of slower frequency. The EEG, EEG back-averaging and SSEPs are normal. If present, long-loop reflexes can be very short in latency, incompatible with a supraspinal loop. Myoclonus may persist in sleep and typically is unaffected by sensory stimuli.

Therapy

The best option for treatment is treating the underlying disease. If the etiology is metabolic, intoxication or due to an excisable lesion, myoclonus can be reversed partially or totally. However, in most cases treatment is symptomatic. Ideally, treatment of myoclonus can be based on its physiological classification. In general, treatment is started with a single drug based on the physiological type of myoclonus, starting slowly and increasing the dose according to the clinical benefit. Side-effects, particularly sedation, are commonly dose-limiting. Abrupt withdrawl of drugs should generally be avoided because it may precipitate a severe worsening of myoclonus or epileptic seizures. Multiple drugs are sometimes necessary in certain patients, and a combination may be more efficient than monotherapy at high doses, particularly when several different types of myoclonus are present. Some drugs used for epilepsy, with the important exception of carbamazepine, tiagabine, pregabalin and possibly lamotrigine, can also be used to treat myoclonus, particularly if of cortical origin. Studies using the anti-epileptic drugs of newer generation are sparse; some promising preliminary results have been reported for levetiracetam (Frucht et al. 2001), topiramate (Kutluay et al. 2007) and zonisamide (Kyllerman and Ben-Menachem 1998). Valproate and clonazepam are the drugs of first choice in cortical myoclonus. Piracetam and 5-HTP may be beneficial in chronic post-hypoxic myoclonus. Piracetam is limited to cortical myoclonus (Brown et al. 1993). Therefore, neurophysiological testing should indicate cortical myoclonus if piracetam is used. With essential and post-hypoxic myoclonus as well as in myoclonic ataxias and progressive myoclonus epilepsy, a positive effect of alcohol has been described and may even lead to alcohol abuse. The choice of drug can be based on neurophysiological classification of myoclonus. However, the majority of treatment recomendations are not evidence-based, instead based on case reports and empirical data. What follows is a brief discussion of treatment based on the physiological classification of the myoclonus origin.

In cortical myclonus, the aim is to enhance deficient inhibitory processes by reinforcing GABAergic mechanisms that represent a significant part of pathophysiology. GABAergic drugs are therefore the cornerstone of treatment, and of these drugs sodium valproate and clonazepam are the most effective. Sodium valproate can be titrated failrly rapidly if needed, but is usually started slowly to target doses of 1000 to 3000 mg per day. Limiting side-effects are tremor, gastric pain, hair loss, weight gain, hepatotoxicity and drowsiness. Clonazepam, starting with 3×0.5 mg and increasing the dose by 1 to 2 mg/day every week or fortnight, with consideration of administration on alternative days, is the most useful antimyoclonic drug. Large doses (up to 15 mg/day) are often needed for beneficial effects, and titration must be very slow to avoid sedative side-effects. Tolarance may develop that might be avoided by intake on alternative days (Suzuki et al. 1993).

Piracetam (2.4–21.6 g/day, initial target dose 7.2 g/day, increase by 4.8 g every third day; Brown et al. 1993) and levetiracetam (1000–3000 mg/day, start with 2×500 mg, increase by 500 mg/week) are increasingly used to treat myoclonus because of their favorable side-effect profile and lack of sedation. These drugs may become the initial treatment of choice for cortical myoclonus. The levetiracetam successor brivaracetam has been shown to be more efficient than levetiracetam in an animal model of posthypoxic myoclonus (Tai and Truong 2007). Other possible drugs are zonisamide (Kyllerman and Ben-Menachem 1998), and some patients might benefit from oxitriptane, 5-HTP, 4×100 mg, increase by 100 mg/day to 1000 to 3000 mg, or occasionally dopamine agonists or estrogen (Fahn 1986; Obeso et al. 1983; Pranzatelli 1994). 5-HTP has to be combined with a peripheral decarboxylase inhibitor, carbidopa 100 to 300 mg/day, to avoid gastrointestinal side-effects. Fluoxetine might help to reduce the 5-HTP dose. Other options include phenobarbital (50–200 mg daily, start low, can be given once at night) or primidone (500–750 mg, start low and go slow, has to given twice).

In cortical-subcortical myoclonus, drugs are sodium valproate or lamotrigine. The latter should be started with a low dosage of 25 mg/day slowly increasing up to 100–600 mg/day due to the increased incidence of drug allergy during rapid escalation. Other drugs of utility are clonazepam, levetiracetam and zonisamide.

In subcortical-supraspinal myoclonus, antiepileptic drugs are usually not helpful. Clonazepam should be tried first. In brain stem-reflex myoclonus, if polytheray is needed the combination of sodium valproate, with piracetam and 5-HTP, can be tried. The hyperekplexias are difficult to treat. Trials can be made using clonazepam and betablockers. Essential myoclonus and ballistic overflow myoclonus might benefit from trihexyphenidyl ($3–4 \times 1$ mg/day, increase by 2 mg every 3 to 4 days to a maximum dose of 35 mg) and benzatropine (3×1 mg/day, increase every 3–4 days by 2 mg to 4–9 mg/day). The benefit from these drugs is often less than from alcohol intake, and there is a significant danger of alcohol abuse.

Palatal myoclonus is also difficult to treat symptomatically. Anecdotal success has been reported for clonazepam, carbamazepine, baclofen, tetrabenanzine, sodium valproate, sumatriptan and piracetam. Attempts have been made to improve earclicking by tensor veli palatini tenotomy or botulinum toxin injections. In spinal myoclonus, treatment is usually disappointing. Clonazepam is the drug of first choice in propriospinal and spinal segmental myoclonus (Caviness and Brown 2004). Diazepam, tetrabenazine and levetiracetam have been used in a few cases. In hemifacial spasm, a form of peripheral myoclonus, botulinum toxin works quite well.

Carbamazepine might be an alternative if botulinum toxin does not work or is not possible. The childhood opsoclonus-myoclonus syndrome should be treated with steroids, plasmapheres or immunoglobulin therapy.

References

Aicardi J. Epileptic encephalopathies of early childhood. *Curr Opin Neurol Neurosurg* 1992, **5**(3):344–348.

Aicardi J, Chevrie JJ. Atypical benign partial epilepsy of childhood. *Dev Med Child Neurol* 1982, **24**:281–292.

Aicardi J, Levy G. Clinical and electroencephalographic symptomatology of the 'genuine' Lennox-Gastaut syndrome and its differentiation from other forms of epilepsy of early childhood. *Epilepsy Res Suppl* 1992, **6**:185–193.

Asmus F, Gasser T. Inherited myoclonus-dystonia. *Adv Neurol* 2004, **94**:113–119.

Assal F, Magistris MR, Vingerhoets FJ. Post-traumatic stimulus suppressible myoclonus of peripheral origin. *J Neurol Neurosurg Psych* 1998, **64**(5):673–675.

Berkovic SF, Carpenter S, Evans A, Karpati G, Shoubridge EA, Andermann F et al. Myoclonus epilepsy and ragged-red fibres (MERRF). 1. A clinical, pathological, biochemical, magnetic resonance spectrographic and positron emission tomographic study. *Brain* 1989, **112**(Pt 5):1231–1260.

Berkovic SF, Cochius J, Andermann E, Andermann F. Progressive myoclonus epilepsies: clinical and genetic aspects. *Epilepsia* 1993, 34 Suppl **3**:S19–S30.

Blume WT. Lennox-Gastaut syndrome. In: Lüders H, Lesser RP, Swash M. (eds.). *Epilepsy: Electroclinical Syndromes*. New York: Springer, 1987. p. 73–92.

Brown P. Neurophysiology of the startle syndrome and hyperekplexia. *Adv Neurol* 2002, **89**:153–159.

Brown P, Steiger MJ, Thompson PD, Rothwell JC, Day BL, Salama M et al. Effectiveness of piracetam in cortical myoclonus. *Mov Disord* 1993, **8**(1):63–68.

Brown P, Rothwell JC, Thompson PD, Marsden CD. Propriospinal myoclonus: evidence for spinal "pattern" generators in humans. *Mov Disord* 1994, **9**(5):571–576.

Brown P, Thompson PD. Electrophysiological aids to the diagnosis of psychogenic jerks, spasms, and tremor. *Mov Disord* 2001, **16**(4):595–599.

Caviness JN. Clinical neurophysiology of myoclonus. In: Hallett M (ed). *Handbook of clinical neurophysiology*. London: Elsevier, 2003. p. 521–548.

Caviness JN, Brown A. Myoclonus: current concepts and recent advances. *Lancet Neurol* 2004, **3**:598–607.

Caviness JN, Alving LI, Maraganore DM, Black RA, McDonnell SK, Rocca WA. The incidence and prevalence of myoclonus in Olmsted County, Minnesota. *Mayo Clin Proc* 1999, **74**(6):565–569.

Caviness JN, Adler CH, Beach TG, Wetjen KL, Caselli RJ. Small-amplitude cortical myoclonus in Parkinson's disease: physiology and clinical observations. *Mov Disord* 2002, **17**(4):657–662.

Cerminara C, Montanaro ML, Curatolo P, Seri S. Lamotrigine-induced seizure aggravation and negative myoclonus in idiopathic rolandic epilepsy. *Neurology* 2004, **63**(2):373–375.

Chew NK, Mir P, Edwards MJ, Cordivari C, Martino D, Schneider SA et al. The natural history of Unverricht-Lundborg disease: a report of eight genetically proven cases. *Mov Disord* 2007 Nov 9 [Available from: http://www.ncbi.nlm.nih.gov/entrez/query.fcgi?cmd=Retrieve&db=PubMed&dopt=Citation&list˙uids=17994572].

Claes L, Del-Favero J, Ceulemans B, Lagae L, Van Broeckhoven C, De Jonghe P. De novo mutations in the sodium-channel gene SCN1A cause severe myoclonic epilepsy of infancy. *Am J Hum Genet* 2001, **68**(6):1327–1332.

Cockerell OC, Rothwell J, Thompson PD, Marsden CD, Shorvon SD. Clinical and physiological features of epilepsia partialis continua. Cases ascertained in the UK. *Brain* 1996, **119**(Pt 2):393–407.

Cooper JD. Progress towards understanding the neurobiology of Batten disease or neuronal ceroid lipofuscinosis. *Curr Opin Neurol* 2003, **16**(2):121–128.

Deuschl G, Wilms H. Palatal tremor: the clinical spectrum and physiology of a rhythmic movement disorder. *Adv Neurol* 2002, **89**:115–130.

Doose H. Myoclonic-astatic epilepsy. *Epilepsy Res Suppl* 1992, **6**:163–168.

Dravet C, Bureau M, Roger J. Beningn myoclonic epilepsy in infants. In: Roger J, Bureau M, Dravet C, Dreifuss F, Perret A, Wolf P. (eds.). *Epileptic syndromes in infancy, childhood and adolescence*. 2nd edn. London: John Libbey & Company Ltd., 1992. p. 67–74.

Dreifuss FE. Juvenile myoclonic epilepsy: characteristics of a primary generalized epilepsy. [Review]. *Epilepsia* 1989, 30 Suppl **4**:S1–S7.

Durner M, Pal D, Greenberg D. Genetics of juvenile myoclonic epilepsy: faulty components and faulty wiring? *Adv Neurol* 2005, **95**:245–254.

Fahn S. Newer drugs for posthypoxic action myoclonus: observations from a well-studied case. *Adv Neurol* 1986, **43**:197–199.

Fahn S, Marsden CD, Van Woert MH. Definition and classification of myoclonus. *Adv Neurol* 1986, **43**:1–5.

Frucht SJ, Louis ED, Chuang C, Fahn S. A pilot tolerability and efficacy study of levetiracetam in patients with chronic myoclonus. *Neurology* 2001, **57**(6): 1112–1114.

Fukuhara N. MERRF: a clinicopathological study. Relationships between myoclonus epilepsies and mitochondrial myopathies. *Rev Neurol (Paris)* 1991, **147**(6–7):476–479.

Genton P, Gelisse P, Crespel A. Lack of efficacy and potential aggravation of myoclonus with lamotrigine in Unverricht-Lundborg disease. *Epilepsia* 2006, **47**(12):2083–2085.

Hahn A, Fischenbeck A, Stephani U. Induction of epileptic negative myoclonus by oxcarbazepine in symptomatic epilepsy. *Epileptic Disord* 2004, **6**(4):271–274.

Hallett M. Neurophysiology of brainstem myoclonus. *Adv Neurol* 2002, **89**:99–102.

Han F, Lang AE, Racacho L, Bulman DE, Grimes DA. Mutations in the epsilon-sarcoglycan gene found to be uncommon in seven myoclonus-dystonia families. *Neurology* 2003, **61**(2):244–246.

Hauser WA, Morris ML, Heston LL, Anderson VE. Seizures and myoclonus in patients with Alzheimer's disease. *Neurology* 1986, **36**(9):1226–1230.

Hess CW, Raymond D, de Carvalho Aguiar P, Frucht S, Shriberg J, Heiman GA et al. Myoclonus-dystonia, obsessive-compulsive disorder, and alcohol dependence in SGCE mutation carriers. *Neurology* 2007, **68**(7):522–524.

Hjermind LE, Werdelin LM, Eiberg H, Krag-Olsen B, Dupont E, Sorensen SA. A novel mutation in the epsilon-sarcoglycan gene causing myoclonus-dystonia syndrome. *Neurology* 2003, **60**(9):1536–1539.

Janz D, Christian W. Impulsiv-Petit mal. *Dtsch Z Nervenheilk* 1957, **176**:346–386.

Kinrions P, Ibrahim N, Murphy K, Lehesjoki AE, Jarvela I, Delanty N. Efficacy of levetiracetam in a patient with Unverricht-Lundborg progressive myoclonic epilepsy. *Neurology* 2003, **60**(8):1394–1395.

Krumholz A, Stern BJ, Weiss HD. Outcome from coma after cardiopulmonary resuscitation: Relation to seizures and myoclonus. *Neurology* 1988, **38**:401–405.

Kutluay E, Pakoz B, Beydoun A. Reversible facial myoclonus with topiramate therapy for epilepsy. *Epilepsia* 2007, **48**(10):2001–2002.

Kyllerman M, Ben-Menachem E. Zonisamide for progressive myoclonus epilepsy: long-term observations in seven patients. *Epilepsy Res* 1998, **29**(2):109–114.

Launois S, Bizec JL, Whitelaw WA, Cabane J, Derenne JP. Hiccup in adults: an overview. *Eur Respir J* 1993, **6**(4):563–575.

Lehesjoki AE. Clinical features and genetics of Unverricht-Lundborg disease. *Adv Neurol* 2002, **89**:193–197.

Lempert T, Bauer M, Schmidt D. Syncope: a videometric analysis of 56 episodes of transient cerebral hypoxia. *Ann Neurol* 1994, **36**(2):233–237.

Lombroso CT. Early myoclonic encephalopathy, early infantile epileptic encephalopathy, and benign and severe infantile myoclonic epilepsies: a critical review and personal contributions. *J Clin Neurophysiol* 1990, **7**(3):380–408.

Mahloudji M, Pikielny RT. Hereditary essential myoclonus. *Brain* 1967, **90**:669–674.

Magaudda A, Ferlazzo E, Nguyen VH, Genton P. Unverricht-Lundborg disease, a condition with self-limited progression: long-term follow-up of 20 patients. *Epilepsia* 2006, **47**(5):860–866.

Magaudda A, Gelisse P, Genton P. Antimyoclonic effect of levetiracetam in 13 patients with Unverricht-Lundborg disease: clinical observations. *Epilepsia* 2004, **45**(6):678–681.

Marsden CD, Hallett M, Fahn S. The nosology and pathophysiology of myoclonus. In: Marsden CD, Fahn S. (eds.). *Neurology 2 – Movement disorders*. London: Butterworth Scientific, 1981, p. 196–248.

Minassian BA. Progressive myoclonus epilepsy with polyglucosan bodies: Lafora disease. *Adv Neurol* 2002, **89**:199–210.

Muller B, Hedrich K, Kock N, Dragasevic N, Svetel M, Garrels J et al. Evidence that paternal expression of the epsilon-sarcoglycan gene accounts for reduced penetrance in myoclonus-dystonia. *Am J Hum Genet* 2002, **71**(6):1303–1311.

Obeso JA, Rothwell JC, Quinn NP, Lang AE, Thompson C, Marsden CD. Cortical reflex myoclonus responds to intravenous lisuride. *Clin Neuropharmacol* 1983, **6**(3):231–240.

Parmeggiani L, Seri S, Bonanni P, Guerrini R. Electrophysiological characterization of spontaneous and carbamazepine-induced epileptic negative myoclonus in benign childhood epilepsy with centro-temporal spikes. *Clin Neurophysiol* 2004, **115**(1):50–58.

Pranzatelli MR. Serotonin and human myoclonus. Rationale for the use of serotonin receptor agonists and antagonists. *Arch Neurol* 1994, **51**(6):605–617.

Quinn NP, Rothwell JC, Thompson PD, Marsden CD. Hereditary myoclonic dystonia, hereditary torsion dystonia and hereditary essential myoclonus: an area of confusion. *Adv Neurol* 1988, **50**:391–401.

Rothwell JC. Pathophysiology of spinal myoclonus. *Adv Neurol* 2002, **89**:137–144.

Rubboli G, Tassinari CA. Negative myoclonus. An overview of its clinical features, pathophysiological mechanisms, and management. *Neurophysiol Clin* 2006, **36**(5–6):337–343.

Shiang R, Ryan SG, Zhu YZ, Hahn AF, O'Connell P, Wasmuth JJ. Mutations in the alpha1 subunit of the inhibitors glycine receptor cause the dominant neurologic disorder, hyperekplexia. *Nat Genet* 1993, **5**:351–357.

Shibasaki H. Physiology of negative myoclonus. *Adv Neurol* 2002, **89**:103–113.

Suzuki Y, Edge J, Mimaki T, Walson PD. Intermittent clonazepam treatment prevents anticonvulsant tolerance in mice. *Epilepsy Res* 1993, **15**(1):15–20.

Tai KK, Truong DD. Brivaracetam is superior to levetiracetam in a rat model of post-hypoxic myoclonus. *J Neural Transm* 2007, **114**(12):1547–1551.

Tassinari CA, Lyagoubi S, Santos V, Gambarelli F, Roger J, Dravet C et al. Studies on spike and wave discharges in man. II. Clinical and EEG aspects of myoclonic absences. *Electroencephalogr Clin Neurophysiol* 1970, **29**(1):103.

Tassinari CA, Rubboli G, Parmeggiani L, Valzania F, Plasmati R, Riguzzi P et al. Epileptic negative myoclonus. In: Fahn S, Hallett M, Lüders HO, Marsden CD. (eds). *Negative Motor Phenomena*. Philadelphia: Lippincott-Raven, 1995, p. 181–198.

Thomas JE, Reagan TJ, Klass DW. Epilepsia partialis continua. A review of 32 cases. *Arch Neurol* 1977, **34**(5):266–275.

Thomas PK, Abrams JD, Swallow D, Stewart G. Sialidosis type 1: cherry red spot-myoclonus syndrome with sialidase deficiency and altered electrophoretic mobilities of some enzymes known to be glycoproteins. 1. Clinical findings. *J Neurol Neurosurg Psychiatry* 1979, **42**(10):873–880.

Thompson PD. Neurodegenerative causes of myoclonus. *Adv Neurol* 2002, **89**:31–34.

Toro C, Pascual-Leone A, Deuschl G, Tate E, Pranzatelli MR, Hallett M. Cortical tremor. A common manifestation of cortical myoclonus. *Neurology* 1993, **43**(11):2346–2353.

Ugawa Y, Hanajima R, Okabe S, Yuasa K. Neurophysiology of cortical positive myoclonus. *Adv Neurol* 2002, **89**:89–97.

van Rootselaar AF, Aronica E, Jansen Steur EN, Rozemuller-Kwakkel JM, de Vos RA, Tijssen MA. Familial cortical tremor with epilepsy and cerebellar pathological findings. *Mov Disord* 2004, **19**(2):213–217.

van Rootselaar AF, van Schaik IN, Van Den Maagdenberg AM, Koelman JH, Callenbach PM, Tijssen MA. Familial cortical myoclonic tremor with epilepsy: a single syndromic classification for a group of pedigrees bearing common features. *Mov Disord* 2005, **20**(6):665–673.

Vidailhet M, Tassin J, Durif F, Nivelon-Chevallier A, Agid Y, Brice A, et al. A major locus for several phenotypes of myoclonus–dystonia on chromosome 7q. *Neurology* 2001, **56**(9):1213–1216.

Werhahn KJ, Brown P, Thompson PD, Marsden CD. The clinical features and prognosis of chronic post hypoxic myoclonus. *Mov Disord* 1997, **12**(2):216–220.

Zifkin B, Andermann E, Andermann F. Mechanisms, genetics, and pathogenesis of juvenile myoclonic epilepsy. *Curr Opin Neurol* 2005, **18**(2):147–153.

Chapter 12

Paroxysmal memory loss

Peter P. Urban

Paroxysmal memory loss is a frequent cause for consultation of a neurologist in the emergency room of a general hospital. In the majority of cases, the reason for presentation is the presence of transient global amnesia (TGA), characterized by a temporary loss of anterograde and recent retrograde memory at preserved consciousness and self-awareness.

Transient global amnesia

Definition and clinical presentation

The term "transient global amnesia" was introduced by Fisher and Adams in 1958 in a study describing 12 patients with acute onset of temporary memory loss. Transient global amnesia (TGA) is characterized by temporary loss of anterograde and recent memory affecting all memory contents – visual, tactile, and verbal – with preserved consciousness and self-awareness. During the attack, the memory span for retaining new information is reduced to 30 to 180 seconds, which leads to the inability to store new information over a longer period of time (anterograde amnesia). In parallel, there is impaired recall of older memory contents which were obtained prior to the development of TGA (retrograde amnesia). This affects the contents of recent history (days to years). Very old memories and the knowledge of facts regarding personal and public life remain unaffected. The patients are therefore not oriented regarding the present time and situation but remain oriented regarding their own person.

The accompanying persons frequently report repeated questions on the part of the patients, even after these have previously been answered, for example, "How did I get here?" "What I am doing here?" "What time is it?" They describe the patients as helpless and insecure. Thus, the impression of general disorientation and confusion arises, which is most probably due to the sudden onset of the memory loss. The repetitive questioning represents a very frequently observed accompanying feature in TGA and is, in our experience, present in about 90% of patients. In contrast to patients with Korsakoff syndrome, confabulations are absent in TGA. Although the patients do not remember how they came to the hospital, they are nevertheless able to perform complex learned activities like driving a car, riding a train to the correct destination, cooking, and so on. Some patients complain of associated symptoms like headache (40%), dizziness (25%), nausea (21%), chills and flushes (16%), fear of dying (14%), paraesthesia (12%), cold extremities (12%) and a number of additional symptoms (Quinette et al. 2006). The neurological examination is otherwise unremarkable and other cognitive functions like language or intellectual function are not impaired.

Several studies have suggested that TGA attacks occur primarily in the morning (e.g., Pantoni et al. 2005). Although amnesia is obviously not detectable during sleep, no patient was reported to have been awakened in a "TGA state," or to have started TGA while awake between midnight and 6 A.M.

The exact duration of TGA is often difficult to measure accurately. Although the onset of the attack is usually easy to determine when it is witnessed because it is so sudden, the recovery is gradual or during the night and there is no criterion to determine the time when TGA comes to an end. However, in the majority of studies the duration of TGA has been reported to range from 1 to 8 hours. The maximal duration of TGA is thought to be 24 hours. During the recovery period, patients are able to form new memories. When patients are found to be oriented in time and space, and when they are able to explain the reasons for

The Paroxysmal Disorders, ed. Bettina Schmitz, Barbara Tettenborn and Donald L. Schomer. Published by Cambridge University Press. © Cambridge University Press 2010.

their hospitalization and recall the neurologist's name, the episode is generally considered to be over. Out of 145 attacks for which the duration of TGA was estimated, 3% of the episodes lasted less than 1 hour, with the majority persisting 1 to 10 hours. For one episode, a duration of 16 hours was reported (Quinette et al. 2006).

Retrograde amnesia diminishes in parallel to the increasing ability to form new memories; however, permanent amnesia persists for the duration of TGA. Although TGA does not affect daily life, in psychological studies a significant impairment of verbal long-term memory, visual attention, visual short-term memory and logical memory has been described (Gallassi et al. 1988). Other authors found changes in the results of the Wechsler Memory Scale only after recurrent episodes of TGA (Mathew and Meyer 1974).

Case Report

A 59-year-old woman had arranged to meet her husband for an evening concert, which both had been looking forward to for some time. Her husband reported that they agreed to meet in the foyer of the concert hall because he had a prior job-related appointment. The woman did not appear at the agreed time, although they had spoken on the phone only two hours earlier. He was concerned and called home. During the phone call his wife repeatedly asked the same questions: "Where are you?" "What time is it?" "What happened?" She also did not remember the appointment at the concert hall. After driving home, he found that she also did not remember certain events which occurred in the last few days and weeks. The husband then called the ambulance and when they arrived at the hospital, she was still not oriented regarding time and space. She continued to ask the same questions but remembered the names of the last heads of state. Neither the neurological examination nor the additional EEG and CT scan showed any abnormalities. The next morning, the patient was oriented and had recovered anterograde and recent retrograde memory but had no memory of events which occurred during the attack.

Precipitating events

In approximately 50% of patients, TGA episodes occur spontaneously. In the remaining patients, a variety of circumstances present immediately prior to TGA have frequently been reported as precipitating factors. As early as 1964, Fisher and Adams described several physical activities as precipitating events, including swimming in cold water, taking a hot shower, sexual intercourse and pain. In a retrospective study of 142 patients (Quinette et al. 2006), TGA-precipitating events included physical effort (31%), emotional stress (28%), water contact or temperature change (14%), sexual intercourse (12%), acute pain (2%) and other factors (13%).

In several case-control studies, migraine was identified as the only factor significantly associated with an increased risk for TGA compared with healthy subjects (Melo et al. 1992) and TIA patients (Hodges and Warlow 1990a). However, the headache observed to precipitate TGA in some patients is not typically noted for migraine.

Epidemiology

The incidence of TGA, which is distributed similarly between men and women, is about 8.5 per 100,000 inhabitants per year. The vast majority of attacks occur between the ages of 50 and 80 years, with the maximum incidence noted in the sixth decade (Hodges 1991). TGA is found in only a very small number of patients aged less than 40 years.

In the majority of patients, TGA occurs only once in a lifetime. Although recurrences have been reported, several authors have shown that compared with TIA, the recurrence rate is very low. About 3.5% to 14% of patients have been found to suffer a second TGA attack (Agosti et al. 2006; Quinette et al. 2006). The annual recurrence rate ranges at 5.8%. Similar findings have been reported in 1.75% of a series of 114 TGA patients (Hodges and Warlow 1990b).

Diagnosis

The diagnosis of TGA is based on the neurological examination and neuropsychological findings. After exclusion of results from other differential diagnoses, the diagnosis of TGA can be made clinically with consideration of the criteria established by Caplan (1985) and Hodges and Warlow (1990b):

- TGA must be observed by another person
- Acute onset of a profound impairment of anterograde and retrograde memory
- Duration of amnesia between 1 and 24 hours

- Absence of focal neurological deficits and additional cognitive impairments
- Absence of precipitating trauma or epilepsy

Unequivocal focal neurological signs are exclusion criteria for TGA. Additional criteria for the exclusion of TGA include severe headache, vomiting, profound disorientation and an incomplete recovery after more than 24 hours.

Specific examination techniques

The following bedside memory tests are useful diagnostic tools.

Anterograde amnesia

TGA represents an anterograde disturbance of the explicit (declarative) memory. Declarative memory function is the conscious memory, including free recall or recognition.

Anterograde memory for verbal material

Anterograde memory for verbal material can be tested using word lists or a short story. Free recall has to be demonstrated by the patient after a list of words or a story has been presented once or several times. Free recall after 1 minute should show results in the normal range, whereas delayed recall after 10 minutes is regarded as incomplete or a possible failure. A well-established test for memory performance on verbal material is the Rey Auditory Verbal Learning Test (AVLT; Rey 1964), which is standardized for different age groups from 16 to 70+ years. Further tests of memory function can be done with the Wechsler Memory Scale (Wechsler 1987); the Subtest Pair Recognition offers two versions, allowing progress examination. A test created for short-term memory performance without being based on verbal material is the Corsi Block-Tapping Test (Corsi 1972), which was designed to assess the visual memory span. The test material consists of ten small wooden blocks randomly arranged on a board; the examiner then taps on different groups (varying from two up to eight blocks). After each trial the patient is asked to recall and reproduce the tapping sequence.

Anterograde memory for nonverbal material

To examine the memory span for visual clues, the subject is shown the Rey-Osterrieth figure (Osterrieth 1944) and asked to prepare a copy. The production of an accurate copy serves as the basis for evaluation.

Similar to the verbal material tests, recall after 1 minute is considered to be within the normal range, whereas the results of subjects who are not able to remember elements of the Rey-Osterrieth figure 10 minutes later range from incomplete to failure. An additional instrument to assess the visual memory span is the Recurring Figure Test (Kimura, 1963), which presents a number of unfamiliar geometric figures that have to be memorized by the subject and should be retrieved after a specific time interval.

Retrograde amnesia

The retrieval of episodic memories is also impaired in TGA. For example, the patient is not able to remember certain events, such as their last birthday or vacations. Furthermore, current television or radio broadcasts of political or sports events are not remembered. However, the semantic memory is not affected, and previously learned dates of world wars, names of the heads of states or presidents, capitals, important public persons and so on are retained. Famous faces and events can be remembered.

Diagnostic imaging

In patients with typical TGA, no further diagnostic measures are required (Schmidtke et al. 1999). The EEG may show theta and delta waves in the temporal leads but demonstrates normal results in the majority of cases. Patients with an atypical clinical presentation or focal signs require additional neuroimaging (CCT/MRT), and further diagnostic measures are necessary in some cases (Table 12.1).

Treatment

Owing to the spontaneous and full recovery, there is no need for treatment. The patient should be observed until the end of the attack. Both the patients and their relatives should be informed of the benign course of the disease. Preventive therapeutic measures are not required, although prophylactic treatment with metoprolol has been reported (Berlit 2000).

Lesion localization

The memory deficit as defining criterion of the disease implies a transient dysfunction of the mediobasal portions of the temporal lobe, including the hippocampus. This assumption is further substantiated by the findings of SPECT studies during TGA,

Table 12.1 Differential diagnoses of acute memory disturbances

Diseases	Clinical hallmarks
transient global amnesia (TGA)	complete anterograde amnesia, repetitive questioning, retrograde amnesia regarding recent events, preserved consciousness
commotio cerebri	trauma, vomiting, precipitating loss of consciousness
Intoxication	clinical history, indications of ingestion of drugs (especially benzodiazepines), somnolence, profound disorientation, ß-EEG, toxicological screening
complex-partial seizures ("epileptic amnesia")	aura, additional impairment of consciousness or behavioral abnormalities (automatisms, absence of repetitive questioning), short duration (minutes), recurrent episodes
herpes encephalitis	fever, frequently with aphasia and confusion, additional focal signs, pathological MRI and EEG, cerebrospinal fluid abnormalities
ischemia/intracranial hemorrhage/cerebral thrombosis affecting thalamus or hippocampus	disorientation, somnolence, longer duration of amnesia, additional focal signs
psychogenic amnesia	younger persons following emotional trauma, especially with retrograde amnesia, disorientation regarding personality, agitation or apparent emotional indifference, no repetitive questioning
angiography-induced amnesia	complication following cerebral angiography, especially of the vertebrobasilar arteries

demonstrating a bilateral temporal hypoperfusion. PET studies have only rarely been performed, showing hypoperfusion of the amygdala and left hippocampus ($n = 2$; Guillery et al. 2002) and in the right frontal cortex ($n = 1$; Baron et al. 1994), as well as in the left prefrontotemporal cortex and nucleus lentiformis ($n = 1$; Eustache et al. 1997). Diffusion-weighted magnetic resonance imaging (DWI) has demonstrated small punctate signal intensity increases in the mediobasal temporal lobe, including the hippocampus and the neighbored entorhinal cortex in up to 84% of patients during and until several hours after the attack (Ay et al. 1998; Sander and Sander 2005; Strupp et al. 1998). However, other authors who performed additional examinations of the apparent diffusion coef-

ficient (ADC) did not observe any changes on MRI ($n = 8$, Gass et al. 1999; $n = 10$, Huber et al. 2002). Furthermore, MRI spectroscopy during TGA showed no abnormalities (Zorzon et al. 1998).

In a recent DWI study, the topography of hippocampal DWI lesions was been investigated in 41 TGA patients using 3T high-resolution MRI (Bartsch et al. 2006). Twenty-nine patients of this group showed unilateral (left or right) or bilateral DWI lesions in the hippocampus within a period of 48 hours after onset. In contrast to the DWI lesions, lesions in the T2-weighted images were not detectable in the periacute phase (less than 6 hours after onset of symptoms) but were frequently observed later than 24 hours after onset. Almost all lesions (94%) were selectively found in the CA-1 sector (Sommer sector) of the hippocampal cornu ammonis. These findings have recently been confirmed by another group of researchers (Lee et al. 2007). A follow-up study in 16 patients 4 to 6 months after the TGA episode did not show a transition of the DWI/T2-leisons into residual cavities. In TGA following vertebrobasilar angiography, DWI and T2-abnormalities have been observed in the right hippocampus and both occipital lobes (Woolfenden et al. 1997).

Etiology and pathomechanisms of TGA

The etiology of a TGA episode is still unknown, and several hypotheses have been put forward thus far.

Migraine hypothesis

Owing to similar precipitating events, the transient and fully reversible symptomatology, and a significant coincidence with migraines, a connection between the two disorders has been suspected. However, against this hypothesis speaks the greater patient age in TGA compared with migraine. "Spreading depression" was assumed to be a common pathophysiological correlate of TGA and migraines, although other focal neurological signs which might be expected to occur have never been reported in conjunction with TGA. Furthermore, the duration of TGA does not lend support to the spreading depression hypothesis.

Vascular ischemic hypothesis

The temporal evolution of the apparent diffusion coefficient (ADC) changes in the hippocampus shows a time course previously described for ischemic lesions in human stroke patients (Bartsch et al. 2007). This might imply a vascular origin of the diffusion changes described previously. Following consideration of preceding Valsalva maneuvers, the possibility of crossed cardiac embolization has been discussed. In 55% of a series of 53 TGA patients, atrial septum defect was identified, demonstrating a greater prevalence than in the general population (25%; Klötzsch et al. 1996). However, in a subsequent study with an age-matched control group, no difference was observed between TGA patients ($n = 48$) and controls regarding a patent foramen ovale (Maalikjy Akkawi et al. 2003). Furthermore, it seems unlikely that crossed emboli might be responsible for the described monomorphous symptomatology.

Vascular venous hypothesis

In view of the fact that TGA is frequently associated with a Valsalva-like mechanism, increased intrathoracic pressure might temporarily reduce the cerebral venous outflow (Lewis 1998). Retrograde intracranial venous flow caused by insufficient valvular closure has been identified by duplex sonography in significantly more TGA patients compared to controls (Sander et al. 2000). Using time-of-flight (TOF) magnetic resonance angiography (MRA), a retrograde intracranial venous flow due to occlusion of the left brachiocephalic vein by the sternum and aorta during regular breathing was found in 5 out of 10 TGA patients, but in none of the 50 did age and gender match normal individuals (Chung et al. 2006). However, if venous reflux is assumed to be the reason for TGA, it would need to be explained why, in the majority of patients, TGA occurs only once during a lifetime and does not represent a frequent sign in cerebral venous thrombosis.

Epileptic hypothesis

Several patients have been reported with transient amnesia as the sole manifestation of temporal lobe epilepsy (Mendes 2002). In a follow-up study of 114 TGA patients, 7% developed epilepsy, presenting as temporal lobe epilepsy in seven patients and generalized tonic-clonic seizures in one patient (Hodges and Warlow 1990a). However, TGA was not witnessed in any of these patients. Against the assumption of an epileptic origin of TGA episodes speak the single occurrence in most patients, the absence of additional demonstrable seizures, the focused semiology with amnesia only in the absence of other features of complex-partial seizures, the longer duration of TGA

and the absence of epileptic EEG abnormalities during the attack (Gallassi 2006).

Benzodiazepine hypothesis

Another hypothesis suggests that an increased excretion of endogenous benzodiazepines might be responsible for transient amnesia. However, the intravenous application of the benzodiazepine antagonist flumazenil did not exert an effect on amnesia (Danek et al. 2002).

References

Agosti C, Akkawi NM, Borroni B, Padovani A. Recurrency in transient global amnesia: a retrospective study. *Eur J Neurol* 2006, **13**:986–989.

Ay H, Furie KL, Yamada K, Koroshetz WJ. Diffusion-weighted MRI characterizes the ischemic lesion in transient global amnesia. *Neurology* 1998, **51**:901–903.

Baron J-C, Petit-Taboue MC, Le Doze F, Desgranges B, Ravenel N, Marchal G. Right frontal cortex hypometabolism in transient global amnesia. A PET study. *Brain* 1994, **117**:545–552.

Bartsch T, Alfke K, Stingele R, Rohr A, Freitag-Wolf S, Jansen O, Deuschl G. Selective affection of hippocampal CA-1 neurons in patients with transient global amnesia without long-term sequelae. *Brain* 2006, **129**:2874–2884.

Bartsch T, Alfke K, Deuschl G, Jansen O. Evolution of hippocampal CA-1 diffusion lesions in transient global amnesia. *Ann Neurol* 2007, **62**:475–480.

Berlit P. Successful prophylaxis of recurrent transient global amnesia with metoprolol. *Neurology* 2000, **55**:1937–1938.

Caplan LB. Transient global amnesia. In: Frederiks JAM (ed.). *Handbook of clinical neurology*. Vol. 1. Amsterdam: Elsevier, 1985, 205–218.

Chung CP, Hsu HY, Chao AC, Chang FC, Sheng WY, Hu HH. Detection of intracranial venous reflux in patients with transient global amnesia. *Neurology* 2006, **66**:1873–1877.

Corsi PM. *Human memory and the medial temporal region of the brain*. Montreal: McGill University Montreal, Department of Psychology, 1972.

Danek A, Uttner I, Straube A. Is transient global amnesia related to endogenous benzodiazepines? *J Neurol* 2002, **249**:628.

Eustache F, Desgranges B, Petit-Taboue M-C, de la Syaette V, Piot V, Sable C, Marchal G, Baron J-C. Transient global amnesia: implicit/explicit memory dissociation and PET assessment of brain perfusion and oxygen metabolism in the acute stage. *J Neurol Neurosurg Psych* 1997, **63**:357–367.

Fisher CM, Adams RD. Transient global amnesia. *Trans Am Neurol Ass* 1958, **83**:143–146.

Fisher CM, Adams RD. Transient global amnesia. *Acta Neurol Scand* 1964, **40** (Suppl. 9):1–83.

Gallassi R, Stracciari A, Moorelae A, Lorusso S, Ciussi G. Transient global amnesia follow-up: a neuropsychological investigation. *Ital J Neurol Sci* 1988, (Suppl. 9):33–34.

Gallassi R. Epileptic amnesic syndrome: an update and further considerations. *Epilepsia* 2006, **47** (Suppl. 2):103–105.

Gass A, Gaa J, Hirsch J, Schwartz A, Hennerici MG. Lack of evidence of acute ischemic tissue change in transient global amnesia on single-shot echo-planar diffusion-weighted MRI. *Stroke* 1999, **30**: 2070–2072.

Guillery B, Desgranges B, de la Sayette V, Landeau B, Eustache F, Baron J-C. Transient global amnesia: concomitant episodic memory and positron emission tomography assessment in two additional patients. *Neurosci Lett* 2002, **325**:62–65.

Hodges JR. *Transient amnesia. Clinical and Neuropsychological aspects.* London: WB Saunders, 1991.

Hodges JR, Warlow CP. The aetiology of transient global amnesia. A case-controlled study of 114 cases with prospective follow-up. *Brain* 1990a, **113**:639–657.

Hodges JR, Warlow CP. Syndrome of transient global amnesia: towards a classification. A study of 153 cases. *J Neurol Neurosurg Psych* 1990b, **53**:834–843.

Huber R, Aschoff, Ludolph AC, Riepe MW. Transient global amnesia. *J Neurol* 2002, **249**:1520–1524.

Kimura D. Right temporal lobe damage: Perception of unfamiliar stimuli after damage. *Arch Neurol* 1963, **89**:264–271.

Klötzsch C, Sliwka U, Berlit P, Noth J. An increased frequency of patent foramen ovale in patients with transient global amnesia. *Arch Neurol* 1996, **53**:504–508.

Lee HY, Kim JH, Weon YC, Kim SY, Youn SW, Kim SH. Diffusion-weighted imaging in transient global amnesia exposes the C1 region of the hippocampus. *Neuroradiology* 2007, **49**:481–487.

Lewis SL. Aetiology of transient global amnesia. *Lancet* 1998, **352**:397–399.

Maalikjy Akkawi N, Agosti C, Anzola GP, Borroni B. Transient global amnesia: a clinical and sonographic study. *Eur Neurol* 2003, **49**:67–71.

Mathew NT, Meyer JS. Pathogenesis and natural history of transient global amnesia. *Stroke* 1974, **5**:303–311.

Melo T, Ferro JM, Ferro H. Transient global amnesia. *Brain* 1992, **115**:261–270.

Mendes MHF. Transient epileptic amnesia: an under-diagnosed phenomenon? Three more cases. *Seizure* 2002, **11**:238–242.

Osterrieth PA. Le test de copie d'une figure complexe. *Arch Psychol* 1944, **30**:206–356.

Pantoni L, Bertini E, Lamassa M, Pracucci G, Inzitari D. Clinical features, risk factors and prognosis in transient global amnesia: a follow-up study. *Eur J Neurol* 2005, **12**:350–356.

Quinette P, Guillery-Girard B, Dayan J, Del la Sayette V, Marquis S, Viader F, Desgranges B, Eustache F. What does transient global amnesia really mean? Review of the literature and thorough study of 142 cases. *Brain* 2006, **129**:1640–1658.

Rey AL. *L'examen clinique en psychologie.* Paris: Presses Universitaires de France, 1964.

Sander D, Winbeck K, Etgen T, Knapp R, Klingelhöfer J, Conrad B. Disturbance of venous flow patterns in patients with transient global amnesia. *Lancet* 2000, **356**:1982–1984.

Sander K, Sander D. New insights into transient global amnesia: recent imaging and clinical findings. *Lancet Neurol* 2005, **4**:437–44.

Schmidtke K, Strupp M, Brüning R, Reinhardt M. Transiente globale Amnesie. *Dt Ärztebl* 1999, **96**:2602–2606.

Strupp M, Brüning R, Wu RH, Deimling M, Reiser M, Brandt T. Diffusion-weighted MRI in transient global amnesia: elevated signal intensity in the left mesial temporal lobe in 7 of 10 patients. *Ann Neurol* 1998, **43**:164–170.

Wechsler D. WMS-R: Wechsler Memory Scale – Revised. San Antonio, TX: The Psychological Corporation, 1987.

Woolfenden AR, O'Brien M, Schwartzberg RE, Norbash AM, Tong DC. Diffusion-weighted MRI in transient global amnesia precipitated by cerebral angiography. *Stroke* 1997, **28**:2311–2314.

Zorzon M, Longo R, Mase G, Biasutti E, Vitrani B, Cazzato G. Proton magnetic resonance spectroscopy during transient global amnesia. *J Neurol Sci* 1998, **156**:78–82.

Chapter 13

Dissociative seizures

Bettina Schmitz*

Introduction

Dissociative seizures present with a very variable semiology. They may mimic any type of organic seizure, and therefore play an important role in the differential diagnostic work-up of any paroxysmal disorder. However, the diagnosis of dissociative seizures should not simply be based on the exclusion of an organic etiology. There are positive diagnostic criteria, and the etiological differentiation is crucial for treatment and prognosis.

Psychogenic seizures are often misdiagnosed as epilepsy. In Germany, the mean interval between first manifestation and correct diagnosis is 7.2 years (Reuber et al. 2002a). About 75% of patients are initially treated with anticonvulsants, with risks of side-effects (Benbadis 1999; Reuber et al. 2003). Lancman et al. (1995) calculated that for patients with dissociative seizures a mean of $15,000 was spent on inappropriate medical resources.

If considered, the diagnosis is in many cases not difficult, and also non-neurological medical staff and emergency personnel can easily learn the main diagnostic criteria. However, in some cases the differentiation between dissociative and organic, particularly epileptic, seizures can be very challenging, and knowledge of the most common pitfalls is useful (Table 13.1). The main reason for misdiagnosis is incomplete or superficial history-taking. Single symptoms may be over-interpreted, for example, a tongue bite, "generalized" convulsions or enuresis are not necessarily indicative of epilepsy.

On the other hand, organic seizure disorders can present with bizarre symptoms, such as some forms of frontal lobe epilepsy, or be triggered by emotions such as cataplexy. Other paroxysmal disorders such as the channelopathies are often misdiagnosed as psychogenic. Early concerns that the diagnosis of non-organic or psychogenic disorders carried a high risk of missing organic disease (e.g., Marsden 1986) have not been supported by more recent studies. In a meta-analysis, the rate of misdiagnosis was only 4% according to studies published since 1970 (Stone et al. 2005).

Definition and classification

Dissociative seizures are paroxysmal disorders of behavior, perception or experience which have a psychological etiology and resemble somatic seizures, in particular epileptic seizures, without an underlying organic disorder of function which is typical for these disorders. The psychodynamic mechanism is believed to be the psychological attempt to cope with internalized conflicts, psychological trauma or external psychosocial stress.

"Dissociative seizures" is the preferred and internationally more broadly accepted term. Nevertheless, terminology remains confusing. Names such as hysteria, pseudoseizures or psychogenic disorders are criticized for being etiologically misleading, illogical or discriminatory. Many epileptologists use the term psychogenic non-epileptic seizure (PNES), which can also be criticized because of its exclusive reference to epilepsy.

Modern psychiatric terminology distinguishes psychogenic seizures according to the level of consciousness and underlying motivation (Table 13.2). However, seizures in the context of simulation,

* I am grateful to John Moriarty for his constructive comments.

Fig. 13.1. Psychogenic seizures: terminology.

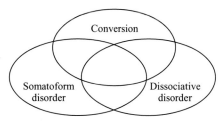

Transformation of a psychological conflict into a somatic expression

Conversion

Somatoform disorder

Dissociative disorder

Symptoms suggest an organic disorder, without organic signs

Disintegration of identity, memory consciousness

Table 13.1 Diagnostic challenges and pitfalls in the differentiation between dissociative and epileptic seizures

Epileptic seizures
- Psychogenic triggers
- Bizarre automatisms
- Normal surface ictal EEG
- Normal EEG/MRI
- Psychiatric comorbidity

Dissociative seizures
- Seizures during pseudo sleep
- Injuries, tongue biting
- Ictal EEG artifacts
- Pathological EEG/MRI
- Positive family seizure history

Table 13.2 Dissociative seizures: A continuum of consciousness

	Symptom production	Motivation
Simulation/malingering	conscious	conscious
Factitious disorder	conscious	unconscious
Conversion/dissociation	unconscious	unconscious

Table 13.3 Classification of psychogenic seizures in the ICD-10

	Dissociative (conversion) disorder	Somatoform disorder
Diagnostic	No somatic problem	Recurrent presentation of multiple symptoms
Criteria	Evidence for psychological etiology	Refusal to accept non-somatic etiology
Subforms	Amnesia, fugue Stupor, trance Movement disorders Seizures Somatosensory problems Ganser syndrome Multiple personality	Somatization Hypochondriasis Autonomic disorder Pain disorder

malingering or factitious disorder, such as Munchausen syndrome, are rare compared to those seizures which are dissociative.

The three psychiatric terms which are commonly used to describe psychogenic seizures are conversion, somatoform disorder and dissociation (Fig. 13.1). Conversion according to Freud relates to the somatization of an unconscious, unbearable, inner psychic conflict. The diagnosis of conversion requires the identification of the underlying responsible conflict. The term dissociation describes a mental process with disintegration of identity, memory or consciousness.

Somatoform disorder simply means that, although symptoms suggest an organic disorder, organic signs are lacking.

These three terms cannot be strictly distinguished. In fact, they may describe identical problems on different levels or from different perspectives. Therefore, it is not easy to integrate them in a classification system. Unfortunately, the two main international diagnostic systems have come to different solutions.

The ICD-10 (Table 13.3) does not differentiate between conversion and dissociation disorders. Both terms are used and define one diagnostic group comprising relatively discrete symptoms in one sphere, for example, motor disorder, memory disorder or convulsions. Somatoform disorders describe repeated presentation of physical symptoms and include somatization disorder and hypochondriasis.

The system of the American DSM-IV is different. Conversion disorder and somatization are two separate variants of somatoform disorders. Depending

165

Reuber *Neurology* 2002a

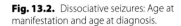
Fig. 13.2. Dissociative seizures: Age at manifestation and age at diagnosis.

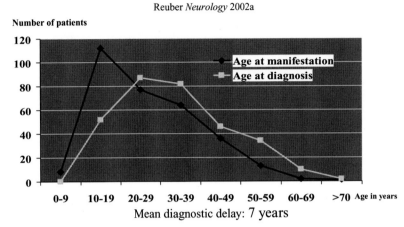

Mean diagnostic delay: 7 years

Table 13.4 Classification of psychogenic seizures in DSM-IV

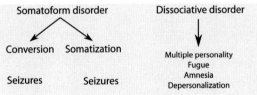

on associated features, psychogenic seizures can be classified in either category. The American definition of somatoform disorder is based on the exclusion of organic signs, perhaps related to the relative importance of legal issues in the United States, whereas the diagnosis of conversion/dissociation in the ICD-10 is positively defined by a psychological etiology.

In the DSM-IV system (Table 13.4), dissociative disorder is an independent group comprising pure mental disorders of memory, personality or consciousness. Pseudoneurological symptoms with primary motor manifestations such as convulsive psychogenic seizures cannot be classified in this category. Thus, in the DSM-IV psychogenic seizures belong to different categories according to their semiology. When the dominating symptoms are negative these are classified as dissociation, and when they are positive (convulsions) they are classified as conversion.

Epidemiology

About 25% of patients who present with seizures in specialized epilepsy clinics have dissociative seizures. More than 20% of patients who undergo video-EEG telemetry are diagnosed with non-epileptic seizures (Blumer et al. 1995), and pseudo status epilepticus is the most common explanation for pharmacore-

sistent status epilepticus (Shorvon 1994). In contrast to the frequency of dissociative seizures from a clinical perspective, according to epidemiological studies the prevalence is only 2 to 33 per 100,000, the incidence 1.4 to 3 per 100,000 persons (Gates et al. 1985; Sigurdatottir and Olafsson 1998), suggesting that epileptic seizures are 25 times more common.

However, the discrepancy between clinical and population based studies can easily be explained because the larger epidemiological studies have used a very restrictive definition of dissociative seizure based on a video-EEG confirmed diagnosis. Therefore, benign cases who never seek professional advice are not included as well as those patients who are incorrectly diagnosed.

In most cases, psychogenic seizures manifest after puberty (Fig. 13.2). They are most common among young adults (50% of patients are between 15 and 25 years old), and women are affected three times more commonly than men. Onset before the age of five is reported to be rare; however, benign seizures in children which are clearly identified as psychogenic by parents (e.g., breath-holding spells) are usually not considered in epidemiological studies. Also elderly patients with psychogenic seizures are often not included in case series from epilepsy centers because they are rarely referred for video-EEG monitoring. In elderly patients, there is no gender difference and the etiology is more often related to health-related traumatic experiences (Duncan et al. 2006).

A combination of both epileptic and dissociative seizures is not uncommon. Ten percent of all patients who are treated in epilepsy centers suffer from both seizure types with epileptic seizures preceding dissociative seizures in almost all cases.

Diagnosis

The diagnosis of dissociative seizures should be made with care and never on the basis of a single sign or symptom. Not only epileptic seizures but also other medical and neurological paroxysmal disorders need to be excluded, and disentangling organic and psychogenic seizures may be extremely difficult if patients suffer from both seizure types. It is not rare that epileptic seizures are triggered by stressful events, and some patients develop dissociative seizures as an immediate reaction to epileptic auras, such as ictal fear. Taking a history can be difficult, for example, in patients with learning disabilities, and seizure descriptions by eyewitnesses should always be sought.

Nevertheless, seizure history is the main tool for diagnosis. Ideally, this is complemented by the simultaneous registration of a video and an EEG. Video-EEG telemetry should be performed in all patients with a doubtful diagnosis. Even an amateur video which can be recorded with most modern mobile phones can be very helpful for the diagnosis.

Although video-EEG recordings are considered the diagnostic gold standard, they also have limitations and shortcomings, for example, when only a single seizure is recorded, when the video quality is not perfect, when patients are not tested during their seizure and when the EEG is disturbed by movement artifacts. Some patients with epilepsy develop de novo dissociative seizures during the monitoring due to the stressful and highly suggestive situation. Therefore, it is recommended that recorded seizures should be demonstrated to patients and their relatives to determine if the recorded attack is indeed the habitual seizure.

Taking the history

It has long been known that dissociative seizures often occur following sexual or other abuse during childhood. This association is particularly common in patients who develop recurrent pseudo status epilepticus. However, it is important to note that sexual abuse is also relatively common among women with epilepsy (with a prevalence of 10% according to Alper et al. 1993), and that it is difficult to estimate the exact prevalence of sexual abuse in the general population.

Table 13.5 Dissociative seizures

Typical History
- Avoiding, vague and contradictory description
- Belle indifférence
- Emotional triggers
- Seizures in the presence of witnesses
- Paramedical profession
- Knowledge of a person with epilepsy (model)
- History of abuse
- Other conversion symptoms
- Anticonvulsant drug resistance

Recent studies have highlighted the role of traumatic life-events in a broader sense for the development of dissociative seizures, and a coincidence with post-traumatic stress disorder (PTSD) has been reported to be as high as 38%. (For a review and meta-analysis of studies, see Fiszman et al. 2004.)

Many patients with dissociative seizures know a person with epilepsy; they have a "model" in their familial or professional surroundings. This is one explanation why persons who work in health-related occupations are overrepresented among people with dissociative seizures. A positive family history is therefore not necessarily an indication for a genetic seizure predisposition. In one study, 38% of patients with dissociative seizures had a family member with epilepsy (Lancman et al. 1993).

When patients have been misdiagnosed with epilepsy for a long time, there is a high risk that they have "learned" how to present a typical history of epilepsy, often supported by the suggestive way many doctors interview their patients. An example being the common question for epigastric auras: "Do you experience a rising discomfort in your stomach before a seizure?"

Pharmacoresistance to anti-epileptic drugs is not an argument against epilepsy, and we also know the pro-convulsive effects of anticonvulsants when used in inappropriate syndromes. However, this is a relatively rare phenomenon, whereas in patients with dissociative seizures the observation of paradoxical treatment reactions is quite typical. An important aspect of the history is the occurrence of other somatoform signs in the neurological examination or other unexplained medical symptoms, or a history of multiple abdominal or gynecological surgical interventions (Table 13.5).

Experienced neurologists recognize dissociative patients in the peculiar way these patients present

167

Table 13.6 Typical differences between epileptic seizures and dissociative seizures

	Epileptic seizure	Dissociative seizure
Trigger	Defined reflex mechanisms or sleep withdrawal	Emotional
Prodrome	Stereotypical, short	Variable, prolonged
Eyes	Initially eyes open	Eyes closed, Bell phenomenon, geotropic gaze
Falls	Abrupt	Protective movements, no injuries
Mydriasis	Mydriatic pupils without light reflex	Mydriasis occurs (sympathicotonus)
Automatisms	Repetitive, oroalimentary automatisms	Undulating, changing, bizarre, symbolic, crying, head shaking, suggestible, negativistic
Convulsions	Tonic-clonic and decrescendo	Crescendo or "waxing and waning"
Injuries	Stereotypical injuries, burns	Autoaggressive injuries
Tongue bite	Lateral tongue, cheek	Tip of tongue, several bites in one seizure
Vocalization	Unnatural	Emotional, cursing, offensive
Enuresis	Possible	Possible, (encopresis rare)
Breathing	Apnea, reduced oxygenization, postictal snoring	Normal order breathing pauses without cyanosis
Facial color	Cyanotic	Normal
Duration	< 2 minutes (GTCS)	> 5 minutes
Amnesia	Complete (GTCS or CPS)	Patchy and inconsistent
Postictal behavior	Slow orientation, Todd's phenomena, Babinski sign	Astonishing awakening, crying, screaming, groaning
Headaches	Postictal	Preictal

GTCS = generalized tonic clonic seizure; CPS = complex partial seizure

their history and the typical pattern of interaction with doctors during the interview. Seizure descriptions are usually vague and contradictory, and specific questions are often not properly answered. Using a linguistic approach, Schöndienst and co-workers have systematically analyzed patients with dissociative seizures compared to patients with epilepsy and found significant differences in their narrative and communicative styles (Schwabe et al. 2008). Instead of describing their subjective experiences and feelings during a seizure, patients often point out that they do not remember anything or they describe the scene and the reactions of witnesses or medical staff. When the interviewer insists, this is responded by sparse wording, long pauses, incomplete and confusing descriptions including many negations ("It is not like..." etc.). In contrast to patients with epilepsy, patients with dissociative seizures rarely mention coping strategies and how they try to avoid or suppress seizures. Schöndienst recommends starting the interview with an open question (such as "Why did you come to see me?") and to ask patients to describe their first, their most dramatic and their most recent seizure. The diagnostic accuracy using this interview technique followed by a linguistic analysis was as high as 95% when the diagnosis was later validated with video EEG (Schöndienst 2001), a result which justifies the significant time investment (which is much less than the time investment for a video EEG).

Some patients with dissociative seizures present their histories with remarkable lack of emotion, and even the most dramatic seizure events are described with very limited emotional expression or with an incongruent affect. This phenomenon was described as "*la belle indifférence*" by Charcot (2009). However, this sign is not reliable in distinguishing organic from non-organic disorders (Stone et al. 2006).

Psychogenic seizures may be triggered by a stressful event. The majority of seizures occur in the presence of other persons (audience), particularly doctors, but this is also true for neurocardiogenic syncope.

Symptomatology of dissociative seizures

Premonitory symptoms of dissociative seizures (Table 13.6) are usually not stereotyped; they are of different duration, sometimes patients "fight" against an upcoming seizure for hours, short breath and headaches are characteristic prodromes of dissociative seizures, both of which are extremely rare in epileptic auras. When headaches occur in the context of epilepsy, this happens in the postictal period.

Symptoms of dissociative seizures may be very different in individual patients, perhaps related to different "models," perhaps related to different subconscious conflicts or past traumas. Therefore, the differential diagnosis comprises all types of epileptic seizures as well as non-epileptic paroxysmal attacks. Some seizures are restricted to purely subjective sensations and must be differentiated from simple focal seizures. Other seizures are characterized by impaired consciousness and responsiveness (differential diagnosis, complex partial seizures or absence seizures). In patients with psychogenic falls, atonic, myoclonic and tonic epileptic seizures, and also cataplexy and drop attacks must be excluded.

The classical literature distinguishes three main dissociative seizure types: tantrums, trembling seizures, and fainting attacks, seizure variants which could be confirmed using a cluster analysis of seizures recorded during video-EEG telemetry (Groppel et al. 2000). The most common type of dissociative seizure is associated with motor symptoms, either with dramatic movements including kicking and beating, which may resemble hypermotor automatisms in frontal lobe seizures, or other motor dissociative seizures manifesting with a stiffening of body and limbs and generalized shaking and trembling. Such seizures can easily be mistaken for generalized tonic-clonic seizures because they often start with a pseudo-tonic stiffening and later continue with pseudo-clonic movements.

The most important diagnostic criterion for dissociative seizures is the absence of stereotyped semiology. The seizure duration is inconsistent but usually much longer than epileptic seizures, often resulting in a dissociative status. In a video-EEG analysis of 120 generalized tonic-clonic seizures, none of the spontaneously ending seizures lasted longer than 2 minutes (Theodore et al. 1994), whereas dissociative seizures have been reported to last between 20 and 805 seconds (Gates et al. 1985).

The ictal semiology can be expressive, with bizarre or sexually flavored gestures and movements. Jerks during a dissociative seizure are often asynchronous ("out of phase"), irregular with respect to amplitude and direction, and often include purposeful elements and bizarre postures. Symptom combinations are often non-physiological, such as generalized convulsions with clear consciousness (although an exception is pure generalized myoclonic seizures in epilepsy) and without mydriasis (in a patient with pseudo status epilepticus and ictal mydriasis with absent pupillary reflexes, we found a sympathomimetic in her handbag). Mydriasis may occur during a dissociative seizure but in contrast to epileptic seizures, the pupillary light reflex is always preserved.

Diminished corneal reflex and analgesia may occur during a dissociative seizure and are therefore not very useful. Nevertheless, inducing pain or holding an arm over the face and letting it fall (often patients voluntarily avoid hitting their face) may be helpful. A psychogenic coma with intact oculomotor reflexes can be identified by covering the patient's visual field with a mirror.

Seizures can often be modified and symptoms may intensify with increased attention. Negative signs such as a geotropic lateralized eye gaze may change toward the other side when the head is turned (Woodruff's sign). The opening of closed eyes is often resisted, resulting in a Bell phenomenon (with an upward and outward gaze). There is one report in the literature of psychogenic seizures arising immediately from deep sleep (Orbach et al. 2003). However, in most cases of sleep-related dissociative seizures the simultaneous EEG demonstrates an arousal preceding the seizure ("pseudosleep" according to Benbadis et al. 1996).

The amnesia for a dissociative seizure is often incomplete, and when the interviewer insists they may be able to gradually extract recollections. The recall of events during a seizure can be facilitated using hypnosis (Kuyk et al. 1999). The reaction toward intravenous sedating and anticonvulsive medication is often paradoxical with an increase of convulsions with each injection. It is remarkable that some patients tolerate extremely high dosages of benzodiazepines without seizure inhibition and without respiratory depression.

Often only the observation of small details allows the distinction between epileptic and dissociative seizures. A generalized tonic-clonic seizure starts with maximal intensity and exhausts gradually with longer intervals between clonic jerks (decrescendo). In dissociative seizures, the opposite sequence is usually observed: seizures start with subtle phenomena and become gradually more intensive (crescendo), or they show a characteristic "waxing and waning."

Table 13.7 Atypical features of epileptic and dissociative seizures

Typical epileptic phenomena during dissociative seizures	
• Incontinence	Peguero et al. 1995
• Tongue biting	Benbadis et al. 1995
• Injuries	Peguero et al. 1995
• Seizures arising from (pseudo)-sleep	Benbadis et al. 1996
• Hippocampus sclerosis	Benbadis et al. 2000b
Typical dissociative phenomena during epileptic seizures	
• Rhythmic pelvic movements	Geyer et al. 2000
• Head shaking	Saygi et al. 1992
• Crying ("dacrystic") automatisms	Luciano et al. 1993

Eyes and mouth are typically closed, hands are often fisted and further typical symptoms of dissociative seizures are head shaking, crying and opisthotonic postures as in the hysterical arch (termed "*arc de cercle*" by Charcot 2009). But even these very typical phenomena are not pathognomonic for dissociative seizures. Although rare, they have been also reported in epileptic seizures (Table 13.7).

During epileptic seizures (generalized tonic-clonic and complex partial seizures), the heart frequency regularly increases. In a study by Opherk and Hirsch (2002), an ictal increase of cardiac frequency by 30% had a positive predictive value of 97% for epileptic seizures. The heart frequency may also rise during dissociative seizure but this is usually restricted to convulsive seizures, the tachycardia is less pronounced, starts before the onset of the seizure and ends gradually, whereas in an epileptic seizure the heart frequency rises simultaneous to the seizure onset. Although subjective fear does not distinguish epileptic and dissociative seizures, patients with dissociative seizures do report more somatic features of anxiety (Goldstein and Mellers 2006).

Some signs often presumed to indicate typical epileptic seizures such as incontinence, tongue biting and injuries occur in 40% to 44% of patients with psychogenic seizures (Peguero et al. 1995). In epilepsy, the incontinence usually happens in the early postictal phase following a grand mal seizure. Incontinence during a dissociative seizure often occurs in early phases of the seizure, and encopresis during a dissociative seizure is rare. The typical tongue bite during a grand mal seizure is localized at the side of the tongue or at the inner cheek. Tongue bites during a dissociative seizure are usually localized at the tip of the tongue. Injuries during epileptic seizures are often stereotyped, for example, when patients with tonic seizures injure themselves during falls. There are epilepsy-specific injuries due to the non-physiological muscular force during a grand mal seizure such as spinal fractures, mandibular and shoulder dislocations. Burns are more common in epilepsy, and generally the injuries during dissociative seizures are relatively mild; however, exceptions can be seen in patients with personality disorders and severe autoaggressive or suicidal tendencies. Typical for dissociative seizures are injuries due to self-harm such as biting, scratching, hitting or the so-called "carpet burns" (Fig. 13.3).

The identification of emotional triggers is not always a useful diagnostic sign. Patients with chronic dissociative seizures are often unaware of emotional triggers or they are reluctant to disclose them; at the same time, many patients with epilepsy report that their seizures are triggered by stressful events or unpleasant emotions.

The differential diagnosis between dissociative seizures and hypermotor seizures generated in the

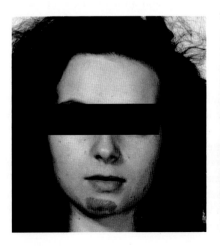
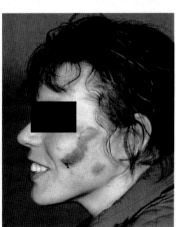

Fig. 13.3. Carpet burns.

Fig. 13.4. Diagnostic tests for retrospective diagnosis of an epileptic seizure.

Time after seizure				
0–30 Min	30 Min–24 h	24–48 h	48–72 h	72 h–1 Week
Prolactin ↑	-	-	-	-
Babinski +	-	-	-	-
Enuresis	-	-	-	-
Todd´s paresis		-	-	-
Abnormal EEG		-	-	-
Petechiae				-
Tongue bite				
-	Creatine kinase ↑			

Table 13.8 Comparison of frontal lobe seizures and dissociative seizures

	FLS	DS
High frequency	+	+
Seizure arising from sleep	+	−
Vocalization	+	+
Hypermotor automatisms rhythmic pelvic movements, rolling, kicking, cycling movements, spreading of legs	+	+
Short duration	+	−
Incomplete amnesia	+	+
Rapid reorientation	+	+

Reproduced with permission from Saygi et al. *Neurology* 1992

orbito-frontal cortex can be very difficult. The latter have been described as "pseudo-pseudo seizures" due to their often bizarre or symbolic appearance (Table 13.8). Frontal lobe seizures are typically associated with dramatic automatisms, often including rhythmic pelvic thrusting resembling sexual behaviors, and are also associated with emotional vocalizations. The seizure duration is short and consciousness is often retained, so patients are able to recall what happened during the seizures. In contrast to temporal lobe complex partial seizures, frontal lobe seizures often end abruptly and patients are almost immediately able to communicate and behave in an orderly manner. Frontal lobe seizures may include automatisms such as alternating head shaking which are otherwise typical for dissociative seizures. Three main criteria for the differential diagnosis are stereotypical automatisms, short duration and occurrence directly from sleep.

Supportive diagnostic procedures

Post-hoc diagnostic tools

A simple procedure which helps in the retrospective distinction between an epileptic generalized tonic-clonic seizure and a dissociative seizure is the measurement of the serum creatine kinase (CK). The CK level has been reported to be ten times increased after grand mal seizures in up to 90% of cases due to the massive muscle contraction during the seizure (Fig. 13.4). Following dissociative seizures, even if they last very long, the CK does not increase significantly unless falls have induced muscular injuries (Chesson et al. 1983; Wyllie et al. 1985).

It is useful to do a neurological examination as soon as possible following an epileptic seizure. After an epileptic seizure, transient focal signs such as Todd's paresis, aphasia or hemianopia point to the localization of the epileptic focus. Another transient sign after a generalized tonic-clonic seizure is a positive Babinski phenomenon and other pyramidal signs (Walczak et al. 1994). Postictal leucocytosis and fever usually occur after series or status epilepticus.

Prolactin

Serum prolactin levels increase 10 to 30 minutes following generalized tonic-clonic seizures due to a hypothalamic-pituitary seizure propagation and remain elevated for about 1 hour. Simple partial seizures do not cause a rise in prolactin levels, and prolactin measurements following complex partial seizures, particularly seizures generated in the frontal lobe, have resulted in variable and often negative results (Meierkord et al. 1992). Serum prolactin levels can be normal following repetitive seizures and in status epilepticus, perhaps because the amount of releasable prolactin is limited and exhausts rapidly with recurring seizures (Malkowicz et al. 1995). Because prolactin may be increased following syncope (see Chapter 3), the measurement is not very helpful for this differential diagnosis. Patients who take antipsychotics have an increased basis level of prolactin, which may be a reason for false-positive levels.

A postictal increase of prolactin above 700 μU/ml or a two-fold increase compared to the baseline is regarded as suspicious, and an increase above three times the baseline is considered pathological. Because prolactin levels show a significant intra- and interindividual variability, it is recommended to measure a basic reference level, which should be below 400 μU/ml. This should be done some hours following the suspicious seizure or, ideally, on a seizure-free day and, because of circadian variations, at a comparable time.

Practically, prolactin should be measured three times following a seizure: after 10 to 30 minutes, after 6 hours and after 24 hours. Using a threshold of a tenfold increase, the positive predictive value for a grand mal detection was calculated to be 89%, whereas the negative predictive value for a dissociative seizure was only 61% (Anzola 1993). This means that an increased prolactin level is a reliable marker for an epileptic seizure; however, negative values are not sufficient proof of a dissociative seizure.

Suggestion

Suggestion (e.g., an inert infusion and explaining to the patient that this is a strong seizure-provoking agent) is an effective method of inducing dissociative seizures which works in about 80% of cases (Lancman et al. 1994). Among clinicians, this method is controversial and many neurologists do not like to use it. It is not easy to explain to patients afterward that this "trick" was necessary. Therefore, this form of suggestion should only be used when other ethically unproblematic techniques have failed. Suggestion may be used in association with video-monitoring to induce a typical seizure. However, as video-monitoring has a strong seizure-provoking effect for dissociative seizures, it is essential to establish if the recorded seizure is the habitual attack. According to Parra et al. (1998), 98% of dissociative seizures occur within the first 48 hours of long-term monitoring. Unfortunately, in the experience of the author this high sensitivity does not apply to severe and chronic cases. When in-patient monitoring resources are limited (which is usually the case), it is recommended to perform video-EEGs in an out-patient setting, which is often sufficient to record dissociative seizures. Ordinary seizure-provoking methods such as sleep withdrawal, photic stimulation (especially at subthreshold frequencies) or hyperventilation also have strong suggestive effects.

EEG, imaging and neuropsychological findings

A normal interictal EEG does not exclude epilepsy, and a pathological interictal EEG does not exclude dissociation. According to Reuber et al. (2002b), pathological EEG findings are 1.8 times more common among patients with dissociative seizures compared to the normal population. In a study by Cohen and Suter (1982), 37% of patients with psychogenic seizures had a pathological EEG. Interictal epileptiform discharges are reported in 12% and 22% of patients (Cohen and Suter 1982; Reuber et al. 2002b).

There is a risk of misinterpretation of ictal EEGs. In dissociative seizures, rhythmic movement artifacts can be interpreted as epileptic discharges by inexperienced investigators. In focal epileptic seizures, without impairment of consciousness, the surface EEG often does not show epileptic discharges. Seizures which start during sleep with EEG stages III or IV without preceding arousal are unlikely to be psychogenic, although the differential diagnosis of organic seizures goes beyond epilepsy and includes the variety of paroxysmal parasomnias. A seizure with impaired consciousness and intact alpha rhythm in simultaneous EEG is very likely psychogenic.

Other neurological investigations such as functional or structural imaging may also be pathological. In one study, about a quarter of patients had a history of neurological damage, most frequently head injury (Lancman et al. 1993). Even hippocampus sclerosis has been described in four patients with definitive dissociative seizures (Benbadis et al. 2000b).

Neuropsychological tests have resulted in heterogeneous results. This may be explained by the inconsistent inclusion of patients with known learning disabilities. Also, some pathological findings may be due to variable efforts in the context of malingering or pseudo-dementia.

It is unclear why patients with pre-existing neurological problems are more prone to dissociative seizures. A psychological explanation is that patients with limited communicative skills "use" dissociative seizures as a primitive form to express protest or solve conflicts. On the other hand, the frequency of pathological findings has stimulated discussions about the organic basis of dissociation. What is the pathophysiological mechanism which underlies the production of pseudoneurological symptoms and at the same time shields this from consciousness? To identify neurological networks involved in dissociation, a number of functional imaging studies have highlighted frontal lobe regions in patients with somatoform disorders such as hemiplegia. However, this research is as yet quite preliminary and has not included patients with dissociative seizures.

Pseudo status epilepticus

In about 50% of all cases of presumed pharmacoresistent status epilepticus, the etiology is a dissociative seizure status. Pseudo status epilepticus should therefore be considered in all cases of pharmacoresistent status epilepticus – and certainly before initiating a barbiturate narcosis. One third of patients with dissociative seizures experience pseudo status epilepticus (Howell et al. 1989). One quarter of patients with pseudo status epilepticus are treated in intensive care units, and three quarters of patients with pseudo status epilepticus have recurrent status episodes (Reuber et al. 2003). The combination of pseudo status epilepticus with epilepsy is rare.

The majority of patients with pseudo status epilepticus have a severe underlying psychiatric illness; most common is a personality disorder of the borderline type (Rechlin et al. 1997). Some patients with pseudo status epilepticus suffer from a variant of the Münchhausen syndrome. This disorder belongs to a group of factitious disorders and according to the ICD-10 the diagnostic criteria include the voluntary production or simulation of symptoms, pseudologia fantastica, no apparent secondary gain and withdrawal following confrontation with the correct diagnosis.

Patients with pseudo status epilepticus are characterized by repeated admissions to intensive care units, often under dramatic conditions including transportation via helicopter. The dramatic presentation often triggers a quick initiation of invasive treatment procedures – without exploring the patient's history, without checking previous admissions and without a careful seizure analysis. These patients are often well-known in the regional epilepsy center (although they tend to move away when they become too "popular" in their local hospitals). The seizures stop usually immediately once the diagnosis becomes clear and emergency treatment is stopped. Unfortunately, patients almost always leave before they can be further explored and referred to a psychiatrist. It is not uncommon that patients suffer from iatrogenic damages following unnecessary emergency treatments. Many patients present with a permanent intravenous port system (Holtkamp et al. 2006), and a fatal case due to an unnecessary emergency treatment has been reported (Reuber et al. 2003).

Psychiatric co-morbidity

Psychiatric co-morbidity has been reported in 40% to 100% of patients, including the entire diagnostic spectrum of psychiatric disorders. In one study, 4.4 actual and 6 lifetime DSM axis I diagnoses were made (Bowman and Markand 1996). Affective disorders are most common, including both depressive and anxiety disorders. Further diagnoses comprise acute stress and post-traumatic stress disorders and personality disorders (most common is the borderline type). Particularly in female patients, an association with other somatoform complaints is suggestive of a somatization disorder with poor prognosis. Persons with intellectual disabilities are particularly prone to develop dissociative seizures. However, it should be noted that there are studies which have failed to find differences with respect to psychiatric co-morbidity comparing patients with dissociative seizures and epileptic seizures (Arnold and Privitera 1996).

Management and treatment

It is remarkable that many, and even very experienced, neurologists avoid discussing a diagnosis of dissociative seizures with their patients. Unfortunately, this avoiding tendency leads to further problems – patients are "forgotten" in the ward-round, a psychiatric consultation is requested for explaining the diagnosis or the diagnosis is not clearly spelled out, and terms like functional seizures are used which can be interpreted in many ways. The reasons for this are many. Sometimes doctors feel ashamed because they had suspected an organic diagnosis initially, and this may cause feelings of annoyance or of having

Table 13.9 How to deal with dissociative seizures

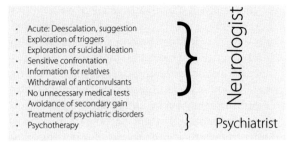

- Acute: Deescalation, suggestion
- Exploration of triggers
- Exploration of suicidal ideation
- Sensitive confrontation
- Information for relatives
- Withdrawal of anticonvulsants
- No unnecessary medical tests
- Avoidance of secondary gain
- Treatment of psychiatric disorders
- Psychotherapy

Neurologist

Psychiatrist

been cheated by the patient. These subtle and often unconscious negative emotions are noticed by patients who are usually very sensitive toward all kinds of rejection. As a consequence, the relationship between doctor and patient may become very emotional. Patients may respond in an aggressive and reproachful manner and often refuse to accept the diagnosis. To escape this unpleasant situation, doctors tend to immediate discharges or unprepared transferals. It is by no means easy to cope with patients with somatoform disorders. However, it helps to consider and discuss the differential diagnosis of dissociation in all patients with unclear seizures early on. It is also helpful to accept that dealing with pseudo-neurological disorders is primarily a neurological duty and that psychiatric specialists should only be consulted after patients have been informed and motivated for further assessment and treatment.

In the acute situation, clear communication of the diagnosis and a deescalating approach is recommended. This means that unnecessary invasive treatments are stopped (Table 13.9). At the same time, the message to the patient should be unequivocal that he and his problems are taken seriously, a positive diagnosis (of dissociative seizures) should be communicated and it should be explained that anticonvulsants are unhelpful and will be gradually withdrawn (assuming there is not a co-morbid epilepsy).

For many patients, examples of other psychologically induced somatic reactions such as palpitations, sweating and trembling in association with anxiety are helpful for better understanding the diagnosis. Quite often, plausible reasons for the seizures can be identified in a first neurological interview, and (since Charcot 2009) it has been noted that in the immediate postictal-phase patients are more likely to reveal relevant events from their biography than later. When the diagnosis is confirmed, anticonvulsants should be stepwise but completely withdrawn, and no investigations should be done which are not indicated to correct the patient's organic disease concept.

Because patients with dissociative seizures are primarily seen by neurologists and not by psychiatrists, the confrontation with the diagnosis remains a neurological task and should not be delegated to a psychotherapist or psychiatrist. Also, the primary search for an underlying psychiatric disorder or a psychological conflict or past trauma should be done by the neurologist, who should not restrict his duty to the exclusion of an organic cause. It is also important to discuss the diagnosis with relatives, who are often as reluctant to accept a non-organic explanation as the patient.

Recent studies have shown that a past history of significant trauma occurs in as many as 80% of patients with dissociative seizures (Fiszman et al. 2004). Neurologists should also screen for suicidal ideation, which is present in 39% of patients, and one study suggested as many as 19% perform suicide attempts within 18 months following the diagnosis (Ettinger et al. 1999).

Perhaps because they cannot accept a psychological diagnosis, some patients will never turn up at a recommended or even arranged psychiatric consultation, and if they turn up they often deny any psychological problems or psychiatric symptoms. When confronted with a patient with a somatoform disorder, many general psychiatrists will simply screen for obvious psychopathology, and when they fail to identify anything suggesting a major psychiatric disorder are likely to send the patient back to a neurologist with the diagnosis "no psychiatric explanation." A study has demonstrated that psychiatrists have little confidence in a video-EEG confirmed diagnosis of dissociative seizures: only 18% believed in the diagnostic reliability (Harden et al. 2003). This study stresses the importance of close interdisciplinary collaboration, and centers with specialist liaisons or neuropsychiatrists may benefit from a team approach. Patients with dissociative seizures carry a very high risk for relapse. This risk may be reduced by regular appointments with a neurologist who has no doubts with respect to the correct diagnosis.

Patients with dissociative seizures are formally not allowed to drive a vehicle, and some therapists use the driving restriction as an additional motivation for giving up seizures. A systematic study on the realistic accident risk of people with pseudo-seizures from the United States has shown that these patients do not cause more accidents than healthy drivers, and there were no severe or fatal accidents (Benbadis et al. 2000a). However, these findings may be biased by patient selection, and some patients with a tendency to self-harm may be at risk.

Because of the etiological heterogeneity of dissociative seizures, many authors have suggested an individualized approach with respect to treatment. Rigorously controlled studies are difficult to conduct, and most published studies are limited because of small sample sizes and lack of randomization or credible control treatments (Baker et al. 2007). Admittedly, it is very challenging to design a high-class treatment study because patients are quite heterogeneous with respect to their psychodynamic mechanisms and psychiatric etiologies. The success of psychotherapeutic therapies largely depends on the patient's motivation and insight and the therapist's skill. Further, it is difficult to define a relevant outcome parameter, which is not necessarily seizure frequency.

There are at least two pilot studies of structured psychotherapeutic interventions in patients with dissociative seizures. In one, 12 sessions of cognitive behavioral therapy (CBT), particularly targeting fears and avoidant behaviors, was associated with significant improvements in seizure frequency and mood variables as well as overall function. In the second, significant improvement was reported in half of the patients on a range of measures (Goldstein et al. 2004; Reuber et al. 2007).

The use of psychotropic medication is largely dependent on whether an associated psychiatric condition such as depression or PTSD can be diagnosed. There is some evidence antidepressants may be of use in patients with medically unexplained symptoms (O'Malley et al. 1999), but there are no controlled studies of their use in dissociation.

Prognosis

The prognosis of dissociative seizures is certainly worse compared to epilepsy. According to a synopsis of 16 studies, only 37% of patients reach seizure freedom following a follow-up of 39 months. In Germany, four years following diagnosis 41% of patients were still taking anticonvulsants (Reuber et al. 2003). Predictors for a poor prognosis are delayed diagnosis, lack of suffering and fixed secondary gain, severe personality disorders, hypermotor seizures and ictal aggressive behaviors. Predictors for a favorable prognosis are younger age, intact social integration, normal intelligence and acceptance of the diagnosis.

In a study, 13 out of 45 patients became and remained seizure-free after being confronted with the correct diagnosis (Kanner et al. 1999), suggesting that in many patients a psychiatric treatment or psychotherapy is not necessary. The prognostic importance of a clearly communicated diagnosis is further highlighted by a study which showed that following the video-EEG-based diagnosis there was a decrease in emergency room visits of 97%, outpatient consultations of 80% and diagnostic tests of 67% (Martin et al. 1998).

Crucial for the long-term prognosis is the early and definitive diagnosis and the undelayed, unequivocal and unemotional explanation by the responsible neurologist. If dissociative seizures are suspected, the next diagnostic step should be the referral to an experienced epileptologist. If the diagnosis remains unclear, a video-EEG monitoring should be performed as soon as possible. The approach "wait and see" and starting a trial of anticonvulsants in an unclear situation is not recommended because anticonvulsants may provoke unnecessary side-effects, the drug treatment supports the patient's organic hypothesis, once drug treatment has been established this may be interpreted as a confirmed epilepsy diagnosis by other physicians, and an underlying psychiatric condition should be treated as early as possible.

In patients with a combination of epilepsy and dissociative seizures, the course may be complicated by an alternating of different seizure types. It is not uncommon that patients with chronic epilepsy develop dissociative seizures as a form of "forced normalization" or "identity re-conceptualization" when they become seizure-free, for example, following successful epilepsy surgery. In these cases, it is important that patients and carers learn to differentiate between epileptic and psychological seizures and document this accordingly in their seizure charts.

The prognosis of patients with dissociative seizures is not simply dependent on seizure freedom. Some patients become seizure-free but instead develop other disabling somatoform disorders. On the other hand, many patients with dissociative seizures will never achieve complete seizure control but they may be able to learn to accept their seizures as a sign of psychological stress. Although they are not seizure-free, these patients still benefit from a clear diagnosis and the avoidance of unnecessary and potentially damaging treatments and investigations (see case report Ulrike M).

Case Reports

Psychogenic non epileptic seizures with onset during childhood

Case 1: Ulrike M (29 years). Following a complicated birth by forceps, the patient was diagnosed with "mild perinatal brain damage" with motor clumsiness, cognitive retardation and concentration difficulties despite normal intelligence. In addition, the patient had a severe spinal scoliosis. Following an accidental burning at the age of four, the patient was hospitalized for several months. During this in-patient treatment, she developed a transient psychogenic mutism and since then her speech has been disturbed by a heavy stutter. Seizures in the form of falls started at the age of nine and were associated with minor accidents but without serious injuries. She reported that before she fell she experienced a dream-like feeling. It was reported that during her seizures she had been unresponsive for a few seconds and that her eyes were closed. The EEG showed a right occipital dysrhythmia and the CT showed a right temporal hypodensity, which was later interpreted as a ventricle elongation. The neurologist was uncertain in his diagnosis and did not start anticonvulsants. Seizures were then observed particularly during stressful lessons at school. Symptoms included a sensation of derealization, headaches, fatigue, blurred vision, dizziness, sickness and trembling. At the age of 15, the seizures were re-evaluated. Because the EEG showed a generalized increased excitability, a trial of treatment with carbamazepine was initiated. In a hospital report the patient was quoted, "If I didn't have the problems with speech, my scoliosis and my seizures, I would have nothing left." The neurologist was still doubtful about a diagnosis of epilepsy and after the seizure frequency was unchanged, he stopped carbamazepine. He recommended a long-term EEG monitoring, which never happened.

The patient and her family moved to another town, the patient went to a new neurologist and told him that she had epilepsy and that her seizures usually start with a rising uncomfortable feeling in her stomach. She mentions that carbamazepine was stopped because she could not tolerate it. Without consulting the first neurologist, the new neurologist makes a diagnosis of "unequivocal psychomotor seizures," anticonvulsants are restarted and soon the patient takes three different drugs because of "highly drug-resistant seizures." The patient is transferred to an epilepsy center for presurgical evaluation. MRI, PET and interictal SPECT are all negative. During telemetry, three seizures were recorded and despite the fact that there were no epileptiform discharges, the diagnosis of epileptic seizures is maintained because of a background flattening prior to the seizure onset. The patient is now permanently on sick leave and deemed not fit for further training because every educational challenge was followed by a seizure exacerbation. The seizure semiology has changed again with an initial feeling of loneliness or anxiety. She describes a feeling of pins and needles and spasms in her right hand followed by a transient weakness. Seizures were often associated with crying.

Following the unexpected death of her sister, she is admitted to a hospital with a status of seizures which cannot be interrupted with benzodiazepines, and the differential diagnosis of dissociative seizures is discussed for the first time. Video-EEG is repeated and seizures are recorded which are associated with beating on the chest, screaming, kicking and shaking. The resulting diagnosis was "epilepsy plus psychogenic seizures."

In the same year, the patient required permanent retirement on health grounds and was therefore sent to an epilepsy center for medical rehabilitation. Following a re-evaluation of the history and all previous reports, the diagnosis was revised to pure dissociative seizures, which was finally – after a long-term inpatient psychotherapy – accepted by the patient. After her discharge, the patient moved to another town. Since then she has been regularly seen for five years in a seizure clinic, and in parallel she sees a psychotherapist. She has not become seizure free, and initially she repeatedly questioned the diagnosis of psychogenic seizures. Intermittently, she complaints of other symptoms such as tension headaches and abdominal pains related to stress. She does not take anticonvulsants, and she has not been admitted to an emergency room for four years. She has married and with many difficulties, drawbacks and exacerbations of her seizures, she has started a professional training which she is about to complete.

Epilepsy in a patient with borderline personality disorder

Case 2: Susanne A (38 years). The patient was adopted at the age of eight months. Seizures started at the age of 11 years and were associated with tongue biting and enuresis. The patient experienced recurrent severe injuries associated with seizures including cuts, burns and fractures. Postictally, the patient described a feeling of derealization and being split into two personalities for a couple of days. Most seizures were triggered by emotionally stressful events. For example, each burial the patient attended was followed by a seizure. After a divorce, a lesbian coming out and professional failure with heavy financial losses, she developed recurrent episodes of depression and suicidal ideation. She started psychotherapy and a diagnosis of borderline personality disorder with emotional instability was made. Seizure semiology then changed and seizures were precipitated by a swelling feeling in the throat, anxiety and trembling.

The seizures were pharmacoresistant to six anticonvulsants in monotherapy and combination. All diagnostic tests including MRI, several routine EEG and EEG following sleep withdrawal were normal. When the adopting mother was diagnosed with amyotrophic lateral sclerosis, the seizure frequency exacerbated and the patient was admitted for long-term video-EEG. After an argument with the EEG technician, she left the hospital before seizures could be recorded. Following several further unsuccessful attempts of polytherapy and repeated seizure-related severe injuries, another attempt of long-term monitoring was made, and this time several generalized tonic-clonic epileptic seizures of 3 to 4 minutes duration were recorded. The patient was put on levetiracetam and has been seizure-free from secondary generalized tonic-clonic seizures for 5 years. With respect to her emotional instability, she benefited from an additional small dose of olanzapine and is still in psychotherapy.

References

Alper K, Devisnky O, Perrine K, Vazquez B, Luciano D. Nonepileptic seizures and childhood sexual and physical abuse. *Neurology* 1993, **43**(10):1950–1953.

Anzola GP. Predictivity of plasma prolactin levels in differentiating epilepsy from pseudoseizures: a prospective study. *Epilepsia* 1993, **34**(6):1044–1048.

Arnold LM, Privitera MD. Psychopathology and trauma in epileptic and psychogenic seizure patients. *Psychosomatics* 1996, **37**(5):438–443.

Baker GA, Brooks JL, Goodfellow L, Bodde N, Aldenkamp A. Treatments for non epileptic attack disorder. *Cochrane Database Syst Rev* 2007; **24**(1):CD 006370.

Benbadis SR. How many patients with pseudoseizures receive antiepileptic drugs prior to diagnosis? *Eur Neurol* 1999, **41**(2):114–115.

Benbadis SR, Blustein JH, Sunstad L. Should patients with psychogenic nonepileptic seizures be allowed to drive? *Epilepsia* 2000a, **47**(7):895–897.

Benbadis SR, Lancman ME, King LM, Swanson SJ. Preictal pseudosleep: a new finding in psychogenic seizures. *Neurology* 1996, **47**(1):63–67.

Benbadis SR, Tatum WO, Murtagh FR, Vale FL. MRI evidence of mesial temporal sclerosis in patients with psychogenic nonepileptic seizures. *Neurology* 2000b, **55**(7):1061–1062.

Benbadis SR, Wolgamuth BR, Goren H, Brener S, Fouad-Tarazi F. Value of tongue biting in the diagnosis of seizures. *Arch Intern Med* 1995, **155**(21):2346–2349.

Blumer D, Monouris G, Hermann B. Psychiatric morbidity in seizure patients on a neurodiagnostic monitoring unit. *J. Neuropsychiatry Clin Neurosci* 1995, **7**(4):445–456.

Bowman ES, Markand ON. Psychodynamics and psychiatric diagnoses of pseudoseizure subjects. *Am J Psychiatry* 1996, **153**(1):57–63.

Charcot JM. *Lectures on the diseases of the nervous system.* Reprint. Charleston, SC: BiblioBazaar, 2009.

Chesson AL, Kasarkis EJ, Small VW. Postictal elevation of serum creatine kinase level. *Arch Neurol* 1983, **40**:315–317.

Cohen RJ, Suter C. Hysterical seizures: suggestion as a provocative EEG test. *Ann Neurol* 1982, **11**(4):391–395.

Duncan R, Oto M, Martin E, Pelosi A. Late onset psychogenic non epileptic attacks. *Neurology* 2006; **66**:1644–1647.

DSM-IV (Diagnostic and Statistical Manual of Mental Disorders). International Version, American Psychiatric Association, Washington DC, 1995.

Ettinger AB, Devinsky O, Weisbrot DM, Ramakrishna RK, Goyal A. A comprehensive profile of clinical, psychiatric, and psychosocial characteristics of patients with psychogenic nonepileptic seizures. *Epilepsia* 1999; **40**:1292–1298.

Fiszman A, Alves-Leon SV, Nunes RG, D'Andrea I, Figueira I. Traumatic events and posttraumatic stress disorder in patients with psychogenic nonepileptic seizures: a critical review. *Epilepsy Behav* 2004; **5**:818–825.

Gates JR, Ramani V, Whalen S, Loewenson R. Ictal characteristics of pseudoseizures. *Arch Neurol* 1985; **42**:1183–1187.

Geyer JD, Payne TA, Drury I. The value of pelvic thrusting in the diagnosis of seizures and pseudoseizures. *Neurology* 2000, **54**(1):227–229.

Goldstein LH, Deale A, Mitchell-O'Malley S, Toone BK, Mellers JDC. An evaluation of cognitive behavioural therapy as a treatment of dissociative seizures. *Cogn Behav Neurology* 2004; 17:41–49.

Goldstein LH, Mellers JDC. Ictal symptoms of anxiety, avoidance behaviour, and dissociation in patients with dissociative seizures *JNNP* 2006; 77:616–621.

Groppel G, Kapitany T, Baumgartner C. Cluster analysis of clinical seizure seismology of psychogenic nonepileptic seizures. *Epilepsia* 2000, 41(5):610–614.

Harden CL, Burgut FT, Kanner AM. The diagnostic significance of video-EEG monitoring findings on pseudoseizure patients differs between neurologists and psychiatrists. *Epilepsia* 2003; 44: 453–456.

Holtkamp M, Othman J, Buchheim K, Meierkord H. Diagnosis of psychogenic nonepileptic status epilepticus in the emergency setting. *Neurology* 2006; 66:1727–1729.

Howell SJ, Owen L, Chadwick DW. Pseudostatus epilepticus. *Q J Med* 1989, 71:507–519.

Kanner AM, Parra J, Frey M, Stebbins G, Pierre-Louis S, Iriarte J. Psychiatric and neurologic predictors of psychogenic pseudoseizure outcome. *Neurology* 1999, 53(5):933–938.

Kuyk J, Spinhoven P, van Dyck R. Hypnotic recall: a positive criterion in the differential diagnosis between epileptic and pseudoepileptic seizures. *Epilepsia* 1999; 40:485–491.

Lancman M, Brotherton TA, Asconape JJ, Penry JK. Psychogenic seizures in adults: a longitudinal analysis. *Seizure* 1993, 2(4):281–286.

Lancman ME, Asconape JJ, Craven WJ, Howard G, Penry JK. Predictive value of induction of psychogenic seizures by suggestion. *Ann Neurol* 1994, 35:359–361.

Lancman M, Gibson P, Ascanope J, Brotherton T. Financial cost of delayed diagnosis of pseudoseizures *Epilepsia* 1995 (Suppl. 3):179.

Luciano D, Devinsky O, Perrine K. Crying seizures. *Neurology* 1993, 43(10):2113–2117.

Malkowicz DE, Legido A, Jackel RA, Sussman NM, Eskin BA, Harner RN. Prolactin secretion following repetitive seizures. *Neurology* 1995, 45(3 Pt 1): 448–452.

Marsden CD. Hysteria – a neurologist's view. *Psychol Med* 1986, 16(2):277–288.

Martin RC, Gillam FG, Kilgore M, Faught E, Kuniekcy R. Improved health care resource utilization following video-EEG-confirmed diagnosis of nonepileptic psychogenic seizures. *Seizure* 1998, 7(5):385–390.

Meierkord H, Shorvon S, Lightman S, Trimble M. Comparison of the effects of frontal and temporal lobe partial seizures of prolactin levels. *Arch Neurol* 1992, 49(3):225–230.

O'Malley PG, Jackson JL, Santoro J, Tomkins G, Balden E, Kroenke K. Antidepressant therapy for unexplained symptoms and symptom syndromes. *J Family Practice* 1999; 48:980–990.

Opherk C, Hirsch LJ. Ictal heart rate differentiates epileptic from non-epileptic seizures. *Neurology* 2002; 58:636–638.

Orbach D, Rittaccio A, Devinsky O. Psychogenic nonepileptic seizures associated with video EEG confirmed sleep. *Epilepsia* 2003; 44:64–68.

Parra J, Kanner AM, Iriarte J, Gil-Nagel A. When should induction protocols be used in the diagnostic evaluation of patients with paroxysmal events? *Epilepsia* 1998; 39:863–867.

Peguero E, Abou-Khalil B, Fakhoury T, Mathews G. Self-injury and incontinence in psychogenic seizures. *Epilepsia* 1995, 36(6):586–591.

Rechlin T, Loew TH, Joraschky P. Pseudoseizure status. *J Psychosom Res* 1997, 42(5):495–498.

Reuber M, Burness C, Howlett S, Brazier J, Gruenewald R. Tailored psychotherapy for patients with functional neurological symptoms: results of a pilot study. *J Psychosomatic Res* 2007; 63:625–632.

Reuber M, Fernandez G, Bauer J, Helmstaedter C, Elger CE. Diagnostic delay in psychogenic nonepileptic seizures. *Neurology* 2002a, 58(3):493–495.

Reuber M, Fernandez G, Bauer J, Singh DD, Elger CE. Interictal EEG abnormalities in patients with psychogenic nonepileptic seizures. *Epilepsia* 2002b, 43(9):1013–1020.

Reuber M, Pukrop R, Bauer J, Helmstaedter C, Tessendorf N, Elger CE. Outcome in psychogenic nonepileptic seizures: 1 to 10-year follow-up in 164 patients. *Ann Neurol* 2003, 53(3):305–311.

Saygi S, Katz A, Marks DA, Spencer SS. Frontal lobe partial seizures and psychogenic seizures: comparison of clinical and ictal characteristics. *Neurology* 1992, 42(7):1274–1277.

Schöndienst M. Management of dissociative seizures in a comprehensive care setting. In: Pfaefflin M, Fraser RT, Thorbecke R, Specht U, Wolf P (eds.), *Comprehensive care for people with epilepsy*, pp. 77–85. Eastleigh, England: John Libbey, 2001.

Schwabe M, Reuber M, Schöndienst M, Gülich E. Listening to people with seizures: how can Conversation Analysis help in the differential diagnosis of seizure disorders. *Commun Med* 2008; 5(1):59–72.

Shorvon S. The outcome of tonic-clonic status epilepticus. *Curr Opin Neurol* 1994, 7(2):93–95.

Sigurdardottir KR, Olafsson E. Incidence of psychogenic seizures in adults: a population-based study in Iceland. *Epilepsia* 1998, **39**(7):749–752.

Stone J, Smyth R, Carson A, Lewis S, Prescott R, Warlow C, Sharpe M. Systematic review of misdiagnosis of conversion symptoms and "hysteria." *BMJ* 2005; **29**(331):989.

Stone J, Smyth R, Carson A, Warlow C, Sharpe M. La belle indifference in conversion symptoms and hysteria: systematic review. *Br J Psychiatry* 2006; **188**:204–209.

Theodore WH, Porter RJ, Albert P et al. The secondarily generalized tonic-clonic seizure: a videotape analysis. *Neurology* 1994, **44**(8):1403–1407.

Walczak TS, Williams DT, Berten W. Utility and reliability of placebo infusion in the evaluation of patients with seizures. *Neurology* 1994; **44**:394–399.

Wyllie E, Lueders H, Pippenger C, VanLente F. Postictal serum creatine kinase in the diagnosis of seizure disorders. *Arch Neurol* 1985, **42**(2):123–126.

Anxiety

Peter Henningsen

Definition and clinical description

Anxiety has many faces. It is an essential element of human existence and a useful signal for real danger. It is also an important symptom of many diseases. Anxiety is never an "only in the head" experience as a thought might be. Whether in health or in disease, it is frequently a paroxysmal bodily experience often associated with sweating, tremor, chest pain, gastrointestinal distress or dizziness.

Frequently, anxiety disorders are not recognized as such either by the patient or the treating physician. They are often mistaken as organic disease for long periods of time without adequate diagnosis or treatment. In contrast, it is a rare phenomenon that an organic disorder like epilepsy or brain tumor, with associated anxiety symptoms, is overlooked or the symptoms mistaken as psychogenic.

When anxiety presents with frequent paroxysmal episodes, the following classification may be useful (Table 14.1):

- Pseudoneurological anxiety manifests itself with symptoms that suggest a potential neurological disease but without ever finding evidence for such a disease following careful investigation.
- Anxiety symptoms may be a manifestation of a neurological disease. Such would be the case for anxiety as an aura in complex focal epilepsy.
- Anxiety disorders may result as a psychological reaction to a neurological disease where patients see themselves in a disabled and fear-provoking state such as Parkinson's disease.
- Anxiety symptoms may be an indirect result of medication given to treat a variety of disorders including some neurological disease

Anxiety may be an independent and truly co-morbid disorder.

The clinical phenomenology and the correlations of panic, phobic and generalized anxiety are well-characterized by the clinical diagnostic guidelines of the international classification system ICD-10, whereas the American Diagnostic and Statistical Manual (DSM-IV) differs in some minor respects.

Panic disorder

The main feature of a panic disorder is the episodic paroxysmal fear attack. These attacks are recurrent, severe and not limited to specific situations or contexts. The sudden onset of these attacks maybe associated with any or all of the following symptoms:

- Palpitations (25%)
- Chest pain (22%)
- Headache (20%)
- Dizziness (18%)
- Dyspnea (13%)
- Depersonalization (4%)

Other typical symptoms during such an attack are well-known to all of us from our own experiences with the psychophysiology of normal anxiety and fear. These symptoms include sweating, tremor, nausea, pain and gastrointestinal discomfort (33%), weakness, sensations of heat or coldness, or paraesthesia (Katon 1984). During a panic attack, fear of death or dying, fear of loss of control, or fear of going insane almost always occur as a secondary phenomenon. This subjective experience of fear is not an obligatory phenomenon for making a diagnosis of a panic attack. Single attacks normally last for several minutes, rarely longer. If a panic attack occurs in a specific situation, for example, a bus or a crowd, the patient may flee from this situation and may learn to avoid it in future, very similar to phobic aversion (see following). A panic attack

The Paroxysmal Disorders, ed. Bettina Schmitz, Barbara Tettenborn and Donald L. Schomer. Published by Cambridge University Press. © Cambridge University Press 2010.

Table 14.1 Characteristics of most important forms of anxiety disorder

	Panic disorder	Agoraphobia	Generalized anxiety disorder	Social/isolated phobia
Lead symptoms	During an attack multiple bodily symptoms; Fear of death not obligatory	Avoidance of multiple feared places and situations; Non-avoidance leads to fear up to panic	Multiple fears and worries; Muscle pains, nervousness	Avoidance of being in the focus of social attention or avoidance of specific objects. Non-avoidance leads to fear up to panic
Time course	Symptoms occur attack-like, "out of the blue." In the interval frequently fear of further attack, agoraphobic avoidance	"Successful" avoidance may lead to absence of anxiety Frequently broadening of avoidance to other situations	Continuous, "freely floating anxiety"	"Successful" avoidance may lead to absence of anxiety
Specific diagnostic difficulty	Misinterpreted as symptoms of organic disease by patients and doctors	Easily overlooked, if avoidance behavior is not specifically asked for	Overlapping with depression	Easily overlooked, if avoidance behavior is not specifically asked for. Misinterpreted as negligible problem

is frequently followed by constant fear of a further attack.

Phobia

Phobia is characterized by fear that occurs only or mainly when encountering specifically defined situations or objects that objectively are not dangerous. These situations or objects are typically avoided. Knowing that others do not consider these contexts as dangerous or fearful does not alleviate phobic fear. In terms of subjective quality, physiology and behavior, phobic fear is not different from other types of fear. Its severity ranges from mild discomfort to panic and fear of death.

Agoraphobia

Agoraphobia is the most important form of phobic fear. Beyond its literal meaning of "fear of open places," the term is used for a correlated group of frequently overlapping phobic fears which include:

- Leaving one's own house
- Entering shops
- Being in a crowd of people or in a public place
- Traveling alone in trains, buses or planes

Many patients with agoraphobia experience panic when thinking of the possibility of having a collapse or being helpless in one of these public situations. The presence of a "safe person" typically alleviates or abolishes this type of fear.

In most cases, agoraphobia is combined with a panic disorder, that is, the feared event is a panic attack. Sometimes, other fearful events like the fear of falling in someone with a gait problem trigger the development of agoraphobia, which then is called agoraphobia without panic disorder.

Social phobia

Social phobias are focused on activities performed in public, like speaking or eating out.

Specific phobias

Specific or isolated phobias cover a broad spectrum of feared objects or situations like spiders and other animals, diseases like AIDS, dentists, heights and so on. The so-called "space phobia" (Marks 1981) and the related fear of falling after prior falls (Lachman et al. 1998) in disabled and/or elderly people are specific phobias which are of particular interest for neurologists.

Hypochondriasis

In hypochondriasis, the patient predominantly suffers from the anxiously held conviction that a specific organic disease like cancer or AIDS is responsible for their unspecific bodily complaints. Patients with hypochondriasis, but not with specific phobia, are convinced of already being afflicted by the disease.

Generalized anxiety disorder

Apart from panic disorders and phobias, the third important form of anxiety disorder is generalized anxiety disorder. The cardinal symptom is an all-encompassing, enduring, free-floating anxiety with many different fears (e.g., concerning accidents, illnesses and other misadventures for oneself and one's relatives). These fears are accompanied by nervousness, bodily correlates of anxiety (see previous) and by symptoms of increased tension including muscle pain or tension headache.

For all three forms of anxiety, the pattern of psychological and bodily symptoms is not the defining feature. For panic disorder, it is the recurring, paroxysmal nature that differentiates it from generalized anxiety. It is the lack of a close relation to specifically feared situations and objects that differentiates it from the phobias. In addition, the term "panic" implies a severe reaction. However, in the other forms of anxiety disorder anxiety can be severe enough to be "panic." Such would be the experience of a person when coming near to a phobically feared object. Therefore, panic attacks can occur in phobias or in generalized anxiety disorder without calling it specifically a panic disorder (Andrews and Slade 2002).

Epidemiology of anxiety disorders

In the general population, the lifetime prevalence for panic attacks is approximately 15% (Eaton et al. 1994). The one-month prevalence for panic attacks is 3% and for panic disorder 1% to 3% (Weissman et al. 1997). Anxiety disorders are at least twice as common in women, where the onset is in early or middle adult life (Jacobi et al. 2004; Sheikh et al. 2002)

In primary care, up to 20% of a physician's patient population suffer from any anxiety disorder. Between 7% and 13% suffer from panic disorder, whereas about the same rate holds for generalized anxiety disorder (Birchall et al. 2000; Kroenke et al 2007).

In a sample of 300 consecutive neurological outpatients, the rate of anxiety disorders was as high as 31% with 7% panic disorders (Carson et al. 2000a). In patients with medically unexplained symptoms, the combined rate of anxiety and depressive disorders rose to 70%. In patients whose bodily symptoms were fully explained by organic neurological disease, the combined rate was only 32% (Carson et al. 2000b). In specific populations of neurological patients, even higher rates of anxiety disorders are found. Breslau et al.

(2001) described a lifetime prevalence of panic disorder in patients with severe non-migrainous headache as 13% and in patients with migraine of 15.9%; in controls, it was 3.6%. In patients with dizziness and vertigo, the rate of panic disorder varies between 5% and 76%. The large variance was due to both methodological and conceptual reasons (Asmundson et al. 1998). In organically unexplained dizziness, the rate of panic disorder is about double the rate seen in patients with organically explained dizziness (Sullivan et al. 1993).

Diagnosis, differential diagnosis and co-morbidity of panic-type fear

Diagnosis

Patient perspective

Unexpected panic-type fear (Fig. 14.1) is typically experienced as a threatening bodily event. The most common complaints are dizziness, chest pain or headache. About 90% of all primary-care patients with panic disorder present with these bodily complaints (Katon 1984).

Almost always, the patient attributes the simultaneous experience of intense fear (of death) as a consequence of any bodily event which, on a cognitive level, is considered possibly catastrophic (e.g., stroke, brain hemorrhage, heart attack). Even if later medical tests reveal no abnormality, it is usually difficult to convince patients that the whole threatening event was "nothing else" than fear.

Hence, patients with panic regularly "somatize" in the double sense that they primarily present bodily symptoms and that they attribute them to an organic cause. As a consequence, they primarily seek somatic medical investigations and because of the acute threatening character of their experience, they frequently present to Emergency Departments. Unfortunately, recognition and correct diagnosis of an anxiety disorder is three times less likely in patients who somatize in this way compared to the minority who accept a psychological explanation (Kirmayer et al. 1993).

The fact that only a minority of patients openly present their problem as something psychological, that is, as an anxiety attack, is not due only to the intensely bodily nature of the experience but also to the avoidance of the stigma of being seen as mentally ill. The fight for legitimacy as being "really" ill also plays an important role.

Fig. 14.1. Flow chart for the differential diagnosis of anxiety.

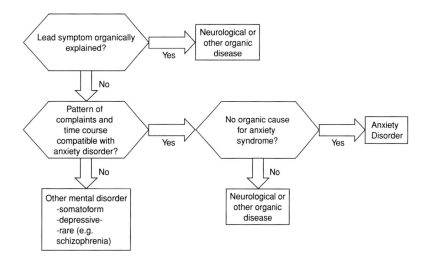

Examiner perspective

The neurologist primarily has to rule out treatable organic conditions in the many patients who present with acute symptoms like dizziness, headache or depersonalization. History and physical/neurological examinations are important tools, and laboratory and technical tests are of additional help. If there is no clear organic cause to be found, further diagnosis depends heavily on knowledge of and readiness to consider functional and potential psychosocial factors as underlying the complaint. Interestingly, this readiness is different depending on the symptoms. In vertigo, this observation is widely acknowledged. Whereas in unspecific complaints such as headache, the potential etiology of an anxiety or other mental disorder is recognized much more rarely (Preter 2001). The type of bodily complaint is not specific for a certain mental disorder. For instance, pain and fatigue, which are seen as typical bodily features of depression, also occur as the leading symptom of panic disorders (Katon 1984; Kuch et al. 1991).

It is estimated that in nine out of ten patients, anxiety disorders initially are not recognized as such (Stahl and Soefjie 1995). If an obvious organic reason is not found and a mental disorder is not recognized or thought of as a possibility, the examiner often will be uncertain as to whether a rare or difficult organic cause has been overlooked and may initiate further, more intensive diagnostic tests. This will lead the patient to feel vindicated in their fear of the presence of a serious underlying disease, making it even more difficult to change their mind in this respect.

As soon as an anxiety disorder is suspected clinically, it is important to broaden the historical data beyond the leading symptom to encompass other current and past bodily symptoms. Patients with medically unexplained symptoms complain of more bodily symptoms than patients whose complaints are organically explained (Kroenke et al. 1997). Fear (of death) must be asked for specifically as well as avoidance behavior and self-imposed limitations due to this in daily life. This is particularly important because patients with "successful" avoidance may have no or only few current anxieties or fears.

In general, patients accept an early broadening of their history taking, with an assessment of psychological symptoms and psychosocial stressors at work and in private life, more readily than if addressed later in the therapeutic relationship where it is often seen as a form of devaluating the complaints. Even when asking early for psychosocial stressors, one has to be prepared that initially the patient does not connect their acute symptoms to any psychological triggers. For them, they seem to come "out of the blue." A more detailed history of biographical factors including potential traumatizations is usually better done by a psychiatrist or psychotherapist.

Even when the examiner recognizes that the problem of the patient is an anxiety attack, the interaction with them may be difficult. The patient often resists the notion that anxiety plays a role and may decide to seek help for their suspected organic problem at other places. Consequently, patients with panic belong to the group of "high utilizers" in the health care system (Katon et al. 1992) and are similar to patients with functional somatic or somatoform disorders.

Neurological and psychiatric differential diagnosis

Two steps of neurological differential diagnosis

Neurological differential diagnosis consists of two different steps: one is symptom-based and the other is syndrome-based. At first, it is necessary to decide about the syndromatic nature, organic-neurological or psychological, of the principal symptom like dizziness, headache and tremor. At this step, if anxiety is diagnosed on the syndromatic level, it is necessary to exclude potential neurological or other organic causes for this anxiety syndrome. Only after this is done can it be seen as an anxiety disorder proper.

The first step of symptomatic differential diagnosis has been discussed previously. A specific problem frequently arises in differentiating phobic postural vertigo from panic. Some authors argue that the lack of spontaneously reported fear of death and fewer bodily symptoms would separate phobic vertigo from a panic attack (Dieterich et al. 2001; Kapfhammer et al. 1997). Others claim that both are panic because the subjective experience of fear of death is not a necessary requirement (Frommberger et al. 1994). In accordance with the research criteria of ICD-10, we suggest calling these complaints a panic attack if more than three other bodily symptoms like palpitations, sweating, tremor and so on are present apart from the vertigo, even if the patient does not report fear. If fewer than three other bodily symptoms are present, a somatoform disorder should be diagnosed. Stabb (2006) calls this syndrome "chronic subjective dizziness."

If an anxiety syndrome was entertained at this first step, it is still necessary as a second step to exclude potential organic causes for this. The likelihood for a phenomenologically complete anxiety syndrome to be due to an organic factor is much lower than the likelihood that a single leading symptom is organic in origin. From a neurological point of view, the exclusion of epilepsy with complex-partial seizures as cause for an organic ictal anxiety disorder is particularly relevant (Thompson et al. 2000). In epilepsy, the attacks may be phenomenologically similar but they are usually shorter and patients display more stereotypical behavior, including automatisms and disturbances of consciousness. In patients with established epilepsy, an interictal co-morbid anxiety disorder may also be present (Schwartz and Marsh 2000). From a general medical point of view, the exclusion of hyperthyroidism or hyperparathyroidism and of a pheochromocytoma is important.

These clinical differential diagnostic aspects are not to be confused with the scientific search for neurophysiological correlates of anxiety disorders in general. Even where these are found, their causal relevance is unclear when they are compared to psychosocial explanations for onset and maintenance of an anxiety disorder. In this respect, neither the hypothesis of vestibular dysfunctions nor the hypothesis of increased limbic excitability as underlying abnormality in panic disorders has been substantiated so far (Asmundson et al. 1998).

Psychiatric differential diagnosis

An organically unexplained principal bodily symptom like dizziness or headache does not necessarily occur within a panic or other anxiety disorder alone. Other possibilities, such as somatoform and depressive disorders, also exist.

Somatoform disorders

Following the definition in ICD-10, somatoform disorders are characterized by the repeated presentation of bodily symptoms in combination with repeated requests for medical examinations despite prior negative investigations and reassurances by doctors that the symptoms have no organic basis. Typically, the patient resists attempts to discuss the possibility of psychosocial causes, even when obvious depressive or anxiety symptoms are present. The degree of shared understanding for the nature of the symptoms is often disappointing for patients and doctors alike.

The most important form of somatoform disorders is polysymptomatic, that is, characterized by multiple organically unexplained bodily symptoms over time. Three types of complaints are most relevant:

- Pains of different locations, e.g. back, head, muscles
- Functional disorders, e.g. cardiovascular or gastrointestinal
- Fatigue

The subsuming of conversion disorders under the heading of somatoform disorders is disputed for conceptual reasons (Brown et al. 2007). Clinically, they share features with somatoform disorders, with the special feature that the functional complaints of patients with conversion disorders seem to indicate an underlying neurological disease, hence the term "pseudoneurological" for their complaints of weakness, numbness, gait disturbance and so on.

If the bodily complaints do not occur paroxysmally, that is, as attacks, and/or if they are not accompanied by the typical bodily and mental symptoms of panic or another anxiety disorder, a diagnosis of somatoform disorder is more appropriate. These constellations are particularly relevant for chest pain and palpitations and for dizziness/vertigo.

Depressive disorder

Patients with depression present primarily with bodily symptoms like fatigue, loss of appetite and headache. Questions regarding low mood or loss of joy are very good screening tools for depression. If a patient denies that these symptoms were present for more than two of the last four weeks, one can be very sure that they do not have depression. In depression, the course is more steady, without attacks, and the conviction of an underlying organic disease often is not as rigid as in an anxiety or somatoform disorder. Because there are many patients with organically unexplained bodily symptoms who are without the mental symptoms of either anxiety or depression, it is not justified to view them as examples of "masked depression" (Henningsen et al. 2003).

Although stressing the differences between anxiety, depression and somatoform disorders, one has to bear in mind that these three forms of mental disorders frequently occur together. Cases of overlap are more frequent than "pure" cases. Therefore, it is not really adequate to speak of "co-morbidity" between different "morbi" in this situation. Special attention to changes of symptoms over time will help disentangle the situation, as many patients start with one of the three disorders and later develop additional ones.

Co-morbidity of anxiety and organic neurological disease

Together with depression, anxiety disorders are a frequent co-morbid phenomenon in patients with typical neurological disease. It is often difficult to tell whether anxiety in a given patient should be seen as a psychological reaction to the experience of being ill, as a consequence of organic brain disease or as a side-effect of medication. In 40% to 65% of patients with Parkinson's disease anxiety disorders of all varieties, particularly panic disorder, occur. This rate is greater than in comparably disabling diseases. Hence, it is likely that the phenomenon is not merely a psychological reaction to the illness experience. Both disease-related neurochemical changes in the brain and side-effects of medication are discussed as relevant contributing factors (Lamberg 2001; Walsh and Bennett 2001).

"Fear of further falling" after falls due to a gait disorder which may have many different organic etiologies often goes far beyond realistic fear and leads to significant disability through avoidance, thereby fulfilling the criteria of a specific phobia. Specific phobia with fear of certain situations requiring free walking also frequently occurs in the stiff man syndrome, an autoimmune neuromuscular disorder. As the sudden painful cramps in this syndrome are accompanied mostly by intense fear but also by normal neurological findings, it is not surprising that an initial misdiagnosis of psychogenic movement disorder is very common. A pathogenetic link between this clinical picture and the proven disturbance in inhibitory neurotransmitters like GABA is possible but not proven (Henningsen and Meinck 2003).

Therapy

Management of anxiety disorders in a neurological setting

Most patients with anxiety disorders in neurology, whether associated with paroxysmal symptoms or not, have organically unexplained symptoms where the principles of clinical medicine and management apply (Henningsen et al. 2007; Stone 2005). The role of the neurologist is an active one and consists of more than recognition and referral (Lloyd 2000; Table 14.2).

Once diagnostic certainty has been achieved, it is important not to give in too easily to continuing demands by the patient for diagnostic tests just to calm them. That approach may further fixate their beliefs that there must be an organic cause underlying their symptoms. The patient should be given positive explanations of their symptoms beyond explaining the fact that nothing organically wrong has been found. A good example for this is the vicious circle

Table 14.2 Seven principles for managing patients with anxiety in neurology

1	Think of the possibility of an anxiety disorder
2	Diagnostic ascertainment as quick as possible
3	No diagnostics only for calming the patient
4	Give positive explanation of condition
5	Encourage patient to avoid avoidance
6	Talk with patient about anxiety
7	Referral to psychiatrist/psychotherapist with follow-up

between experiencing a bodily symptom like dizziness or palpitations that induces fear and that fear further induces increased uncertainty and attention to bodily processes. In turn, this creates the experience of increasing symptoms.

Giving supporting care of a coping nature to the patient is an approach which is usually more acceptable than suggesting that there is a psychological cause that has to be identified. An important part of coping with an anxiety disorder is avoiding avoidance and encouraging graded exercise and small steps instead of a "miracle cure." Initially, patients with an anxiety disorder say that their symptoms come "out of the blue." But after some time, they may realize that symptoms are more frequent in certain interpersonal situations.

In less severe cases, this type of information and counseling may be sufficient. In an acute, severe attack, it may be helpful to prescribe a benzodiazepine (e.g., lorazepam). Referrals to a psychiatrist or psychotherapist are much more successful if they are fully explained to the patient in advance and followed up afterward with a further appointment. In this way, the patient does not feel abandoned.

Psychiatric therapy and psychotherapy

Patients with anxiety disorder who present to neurological services often are reluctant to accept care by a psychiatrist or psychotherapist. Therefore, it is particularly important during the initial contacts to build up a helping alliance between patient and therapist by providing clear information and advice, as mentioned previously. Prescription of drugs may be helpful, but sole reliance on them is never adequate. Cognitive behavioral therapy in particular has been shown to be effective, especially in phobic disorders but also in panic. More recently, evidence is increasing that psychodynamic therapies are effective.

Specialized psychiatric/psychotherapeutic care has to take into account the pattern of frequent co-morbid mental disorders (in particular depression, addictive disorders, personality disorders) and the fact that despite a relatively good short-term prognosis many anxiety disorders tend toward relapses and chronification. This is exemplified by a recent study on the use of cognitive behavioral therapy in patients with phobic postural vertigo: Immediately afterward, this ten-session treatment showed significant benefit, but after one year the extent of dizziness, anxiety and depression was back to how it was before treatment (Holmberg et al. 2007).

References

Andrews G, Slade T. Agoraphobia without a history of panic disorder may be part of the panic disorder syndrome. *J Nerv Ment Dis* 2002, **190**:624–630.

Asmundson GJ, Larsen DK, Stein MB. Panic disorder and vestibular disturbance: an overview of empirical findings and clinical implications. *J Psychosom Res* 1998, **44**:107–120.

Birchall H, Brandon S, Taub N. Panic in a general practice population: prevalence, psychiatric comorbidity and associated disability. *Soc Psychiatry Psych Epidemiol* 2000, **35**:235–241.

Breslau N, Schultz LR, Stewart WF, Lipton R, Welch KM. Headache types and panic disorder: directionality and specificity. *Neurology* 2001, **56**:350–354.

Brown RJ, Cardeña E, Nijenhuis E, Sar V, Van Der Hart O. Should conversion disorder be reclassified as a dissociative disorder in DSM V? *Psychosomatics.* 2007, **48**:369–378.

Carson AJ, Ringbauer B, MacKenzie L, Warlow C, Sharpe M. Neurological disease, emotional disorder, and disability: they are related: a study of 300 consecutive new referrals to a neurology outpatient department. *J Neurol Neurosurg Psychiatry* 2000a, **68**:202–206.

Carson AJ, Ringbauer B, Stone J, McKenzie L, Warlow C, Sharpe M. Do medically unexplained symptoms matter? A prospective cohort study of 300 new referrals to neurology outpatient clinics. *J Neurol Neurosurg Psychiatry* 2000b, **68**:207–210.

Dieterich M, Krafczyk S, Querner V, Brandt T. Somatoform phobic postural vertigo and psychogenic disorders of stance and gait. *Adv Neurol* 2001, **87**:225–233.

Eaton WW, Kessler RC, Wittchen HU, Magee WJ. Panic and panic disorder in the United States. *Am J Psychiatry* 1994, **151**:413–420.

Frommberger UH, Tettenborn B, Buller R, Benkert O. Panic disorder in patients with dizziness. *Arch Intern Med* 1994, **154**:590–591.

Henningsen P, Meinck HM. Specific phobia is a frequent non-motor feature in Stiff Man Syndrome. *J Neurol Neurosurg Psychiatry* 2003, **74**:462–465.

Henningsen P, Zimmermann T, Sattel H. Medically unexplained physical symptoms, anxiety and depression: a meta-analytic review of common distress syndromes. *Psychosomatic Medicine* 2003, **65**:528–533.

Henningsen P, Zipfel S, Herzog W. Management of functional somatic syndromes. *Lancet* 2007, **369**:946–955.

Holmberg J, Karlberg M, Harlacher U, Magnusson M. One-year follow-up of cognitive behavioral therapy for phobic postural vertigo. *J Neurol* 2007, **254**:1189–1192.

Jacobi F, Wittchen HU, Holting C, Höfler M, Pfister H, Müller N, Lieb R. Prevalence, co-morbidity and correlates of mental disorders in the general population: results from the German Health Interview and Examination Survey (GHS). *Psychol Med.* 2004, **34**:597–611.

Kapfhammer HP, Mayer C, Hock U, Huppert D, Dieterich M, Brandt T. Course of illness in phobic postural vertigo. *Acta Neurol Scand* 1997, **95**:23–28.

Katon W. Panic disorder and somatization. *Am J Med* 1984, **77**:101–106.

Katon WJ, Von Korff M, Lin E. Panic disorder: relationship to high medical utilization. *Am J Med* 1992, **92**: 7S–11S.

Kirmayer LJ, Robbins JM, Dworkind M, Yaffe MJ. Somatization and the recognition of depression and anxiety in primary care. *Am J Psychiatry* 1993, **150**:734–741.

Kroenke K, Jackson JL, Chamberlin J. Depressive and anxiety disorders in patients presenting with physical complaints: clinical predictors and outcome. *Am J Med* 1997, **103**:339–347.

Kroenke K, Spitzer RL, Williams JB, Monahan PO, Löwe B Anxiety disorders in primary care: prevalence, impairment, comorbidity, and detection. *Ann Intern Med* 2007, **146**:317–325.

Kuch K, Cox BJ, Woszczyna CB, Swinson RP, Shulman I. Chronic pain in panic disorder. *J Behav Ther Exp Psychiatry* 1991, **22**:255–259.

Lachman ME, Howland J, Tennstedt S, Jette A, Assmann S, Peterson EW. Fear of falling and activity restriction: the survey of activities and fear of falling in the elderly (SAFE). *J Gerontol B Psychol Sci Soc Sci* 1998, **53**:P43–50.

Lamberg L. Psychiatric symptoms common in neurological disorders. *JAMA* 2001, **286**:15–156.

Lloyd GG. Who should treat psychiatric disorders in neurology patients? *J Neurol Neurosurg Psychiatry* 2000, **68**:134–135.

Marks I. Space "phobia": a pseudo-agoraphobic syndrome. *J Neurol Neurosurg Psychiatry* 1981, **44**:387–391.

Preter M. The interrelations of migraine, vertigo, and migrainous vertigo. *Neurology* 2001, **57**:1522.

Schwartz JM, Marsh L The psychiatric perspectives of epilepsy. *Psychosomatics* 2000, **41**:31–38.

Sheikh JI, Leskin GA, Klein DF. Gender differences in panic disorder: findings from the National Comorbidity Survey. *Am J Psychiatry* 2002, **159**:55–58.

Staab JP. Chronic dizziness: the interface between psychiatry and neuro-otology. *Curr Opin Neurol* 2006, **19**:41–48.

Stahl SM, Soefje S. Panic attacks and panic disorder: the great neurologic imposters. *Sem Neurol* 1995, **15**:126–132.

Stone J, Carson A, Sharpe M. Functional symptoms in neurology: management. *J Neurol Neurosurg Psychiatry* 2005, **76**:i13–i21.

Sullivan M, Clark MR, Katon WJ, Fischl M, Russo J, Dobie RA, Voorhees R. Psychiatric and otologic diagnoses in patients complaining of dizziness. *Arch Intern Med* 1993, **153**:1479–1484.

Thompson SA, Duncan JS, Smith SJ. Partial seizures presenting as panic attacks. *BMJ* 2000, **321**:1002–1003.

Walsh K, Bennett G. Parkinson's disease and anxiety. *Postgrad Med J* 2001, **77**:89–93.

Weissman MM, Bland RC, Canino GJ, Faravelli C, Greenwald S, Hwu HG, Joyce PR, Karam EG, Lee CK, Lellouch J, Lepine JP, Newman SC, Oakley-Browne MA, Rubio-Stipec M, Wells JE, Wickramaratne PJ, Wittchen HU, Yeh EK. The cross-national epidemiology of panic disorder. *Arch Gen Psychiatry* 1997, **54**:305–309.

Vegetative seizures

Soheyl Noachtar and Jan Rémi

Introduction

Vegetative or autonomous phenomena can occur with several different epileptic seizures. Typically with generalized tonic-clonic seizures, associated with the motor symptoms that give rise to the seizures, hypersalivation, often described as "foaming from the mouth," enuresis and occasionally encopresis occur (Noachtar and Lüders 1997). Vegetative seizures refer to phenomena where the vegetative seizure symptoms dominate (Noachtar et al. 1998). In this chapter, we will describe vegetative auras and vegetative epileptic seizures in detail. Vegetative symptoms can also occur in non-epileptic seizures, which needs to be considered in the differential diagnosis. Some disorders as pheochromocytoma, carcinoid syndrome, hyperthyroidism, syncope, panic attacks, migraine attacks as well as neurogenic hypertensive crises are examples of such conditions.

Pheochromocytoma

Pheochromocytomas are catecholamine-secreting tumors originating from chromaffin tissue. Approximately 90% develop intra-abdominally, and of these 90% develop in the adrenal medulla. The clinical symptoms are caused by permanent or attack-like stress on the body from the increased catecholamine release. Ninety-five percent of the patients suffer from hyperhidrosis or recurring tachyarrhythmias and palpitations or severe headache episodes, such that in patients with paroxysmal hypertension these symptoms should give reason to search for a pheochromocytoma. Approximately 30% of patients are normotensive, and the number of asymptomatic patients is rising as improved imaging techniques allow more incidental findings of adrenal masses.

Essential for diagnosis is the demonstration of increased autonomous production of catecholamines. This is achieved by measuring catecholamines and their degrading products like metanephrine and homovanillic mandelic acid in a 24-hour urine collection. Recently, clinical chemistry detection methods are even more refined and the products can be detected in blood plasma, but these free metanephrines can only be used to rule out plasmocytoma because of its greater sensitivity but poorer specificity (Pacak et al. 2007).

Carcinoid syndrome

The main symptoms of carcinoid syndrome are heat flushes with redness of the face and thorax that can be triggered by eating, alcohol consumption and emotional situations, and watery diarrhea and paroxysmal abdominal pain often accompanied by asthmalike dyspnea.

Flushing is very typical for the syndrome and is absent in only a few patients during an attack. Most patients with pheochromocytoma are pale during the attack because the alpha-adrenergic receptors are the first to be stimulated. Some carcinoid patients experience dyspnea as their main symptom. Carcinoid tumors are by far the most common endocrine tumors of the gastrointestinal tract. Carcinoids of the appendix and colon rarely metastasize, but when they do metastasize to the liver, they cause clinical symptoms because the mediators, mostly serotonin, histamine, tachykinins, kallikrein and prostaglandins, are released. However, up to 45 different mediators have been described that bypass their degradation in the portal liver filter system. The diagnosis can be secured by showing elevated plasma levels of serotonin and tachykinins or elevated 5-hydroxyindolacetic acid levels in the urine. Rarely, carcinoid syndromes occur

The Paroxysmal Disorders, ed. Bettina Schmitz, Barbara Tettenborn and Donald L. Schomer. Published by Cambridge University Press. © Cambridge University Press 2010.

as a paraneoplastic syndrome in neoplasms of lung, pancreas, stomach or liver tissue (Modlin et al. 2005).

Syncope, panic attacks and paroxysmal headaches are dealt with in Chapters 3, 6 and 15.

Vegetative auras and seizures

Vegetative auras should be differentiated from vegetative seizures (Noachtar 2001). Auras, including vegetative ones, by definition are purely subjective phenomena. They are seizure phenomena that are experienced only by the patient. The clinician depends on the accounts given by the patient and cannot find any objective correlates, except for psychic and emotional reactions. These reactions can encompass unrest and fear but also vegetative symptoms like an increase of heart rate or sweating. As reactions to the subjective experience of any aura, the secondary vegetative symptoms have to be carefully differentiated from vegetative auras in the stricter sense. This can be challenging if based solely on the patient history, especially in patients that have difficulty expressing themselves verbally. The vegetative aura arises, as all other auras respectively do, from epileptic activation of cortical regions. The difference in vegetative auras is that the cortical activation gives rise only to subjectively experienced vegetative symptoms.

In the stricter sense, vegetative seizures are seizures that are independent of the patient's experience but are reflected in simultaneous, objectively measurable, vegetative changes like piloerection or tachycardia (Noachtar 2001; Noachtar et al. 2000). Only the simultaneous registration of the ictal EEG can point to the cause of a vegetative symptom which might not lead to a subjective complaint. This is a rare situation that is found almost exclusively in video-EEG monitoring situations (Noachtar et al. 2003).

The term "vegetative seizure" is mostly used synonymously for an autonomic seizure. The definition varies considerably from author to author. According to the involved organ systems, vegetative seizures can loosely be grouped into:

- Cardiovascular phenomena like tachycardia, bradycardia, sinoatrial arrest, ventricular fibrillation, arterial hypertension or hypotension
- Respiratory phenomena such as hypopnea, apnea, tachypnea or pulmonary edema
- Gastrointestinal phenomena such as changes in the esophageal or gastric peristalsis, vomiting, spitting, borborygmia or encopresis

- Skin changes such as hyperhidrosis, paleness, redness or piloerection
- Pupillary phenomena such as mydriasis or miosis
- Genital or sexual phenomena such as erection or arousal
- Urinary symptoms such as urge or enuresis

Vegetative auras or seizures have to be differentiated from prodromal symptoms. This is important because prodromal symptoms can also occur in generalized epilepsies, whereas auras occur only in focal epilepsies by definition. The duration is often helpful because prodromal symptoms usually last longer than auras, typically hours. Prodromal symptoms are usually described non-specifically and remain vague. They can encompass vegetative symptoms including sweating, irregular bowel movements and heat flushes in addition to the emotional symptoms. Auras last seconds to minutes. An exception is the rare aura status. The subjective experiences that precede the tonic-clonic seizures in patients with idiopathic generalized epilepsy most likely represent an increased number of absences or myoclonic seizures that lead to the tonic-clonic seizure (So 2001). The patient's accounts of these episodes can be very elaborate and diverse, depending on the patient's psychopathology and ability to verbalize. The terms "visceral aura" or "visceral seizure" is sometimes used to describe epigastric auras. The terms abdominal aura and epigastric aura are used equivocally in English medical terminology.

The mechanisms underlying a supposedly vegetative seizure can be complex. For example, an isolated apnea can be due to seizure activity reducing respiratory drive but can also be secondary to a tonic flexion of the respiratory muscles or can be a reflex response of cardiorespiratory mechanisms to the epileptic activity. These aspects have to be taken into consideration when analyzing a vegetative epileptic seizure.

Autonomous symptoms can furthermore occur postictally. These are not a direct expression of epileptic activity in different symptomatogenic zones but rather the sequelae of the actual seizure as, for example, enuresis can be. The history is often not sufficient to differentiate the mechanisms of the actual event. In that case, speculation should be avoided and the seizure should only be labeled as a vegetative seizure if the vegetative semiology is evident and is furthermore the predominant semiology of the epileptic event. For example, during a lateralized clonic seizure the patient is hypersalivating. The hypersalivation is a vegetative symptom but the seizure will be classified as a clonic seizure because the unilateral seizure dominates the seizure semiology. In case the hypersalivation precedes clonic activity of the left face, the seizure evolution will be classified as a vegetative seizure with hypersalivation leading to a clonic seizure of the left face

It is clinically relevant whether the specific brain region is first to be involved in epileptic activity or whether the region is symptomatically affected only in the spread of epileptic activity (Noachtar et al. 1998). Rare phenomena, like lacrimation, are subject to speculation as to whether they represent direct expression of epileptic activity (O'Donovan et al. 2000).

Unspecific aura sensations that are vaguely described by patients as being "in the head" are sometimes described as cephalic auras and are counted among vegetative auras. Also, diffuse body sensations in either half of the body are in contrast to one-sided contralateral sensory disturbances, which are typically paresthesias of somatosensory origin. They are sometimes classified as vegetative auras. We regard that as being too speculative to be used in actual seizure classification because there is no evidence of a vegetative disturbance. Additionally, that situation would define vegetative symptoms too broadly.

In the following section, we will give an oversight into vegetative seizures, their importance in diagnosis and differential diagnosis, the association with the different epileptic syndromes and also their localizing value. Other paroxysmal non-epileptic vegetative events will be addressed in the section on differential diagnoses.

Epidemiology

It has been described previously that vegetative symptoms can occur in connection with epileptic auras. Gowers (1901) described vegetative auras in 18% of his patients with all auras ($n = 1145$) but included also epigastric (abdominal) auras. A comparable study several years later demonstrated a similar frequency (14.5%; Gowers 1933) but also included epigastric auras. In a study with 50 patients with temporal lobe epilepsy, 20 experienced vegetative symptoms like facial paleness or redness, urinary urge, flatulence or sweating preceding automatisms (Feindel and Penfield 1954).

More recent studies find fewer vegetative auras in cases where epigastric auras are excluded (Palmini and Gloor 1992; van Donselaar et al. 1990). In a study analyzing aura symptoms in 149 patients with a first generalized tonic-clonic seizure, only one patient was identified with a vegetative aura (cold feeling; van Donselaar et al. 1990). The other auras were mostly a feeling of dizziness or not more closely defined indisposition.

Estimates of the rate of vegetative auras differ widely, mostly because there is little agreement on the definition of vegetative seizures and because the numbers largely depend on the primary goal of the study and with the format and scrutiny of data acquisition. In a retrospective part of a study, 10 of 196 patients reported a diffuse warm sensation as an aura, whereas in the prospective part of that study none of the patients described that feeling anymore (Palmini and Gloor 1992). Differing concepts of epileptic syndromes certainly add to the difference in retro- and prospective analyses. Several epilepsy syndromes, such as the mesial temporal lobe epilepsy that is based on mesial temporal sclerosis, mesial frontal lobe epilepsy and the benign focal epilepsies of childhood, were not established disease entities until a few years ago. Hence, their clinical evaluation and retrospective data analyses is biased. Furthermore, vegetative seizure phenomena are often over powered by more dramatic seizure semiology. There are no reliable numbers on the frequency of vegetative seizures as a differentiating point between vegetative auras and vegetative seizures (Noachtar et al. 1998). Another important point is that patients can forget their auras. This is more common the more violent the seizures are, especially when tonic-clonic seizures are experienced or when there is a bilateral EEG seizure pattern (Schulz et al. 1995).

In most studies, the term vegetative aura refers to the epigastric aura and is most common in temporal lobe epilepsy (Henkel et al. 2002). This seizure disorder has clearly defined characteristics and a high localizing value, and should therefore not be classified as a vegetative aura.

Case 1: A 34-year-old patient reported that before a seizure he has a weird, hard-to-describe feeling in the stomach area, that moves to the head within seconds. Once the head is reached, he usually looses consciousness. The feeling is so characteristic that he can recognize it as the beginning of a seizure. Circumscriptions like, "It feels like being in an elevator or being on the rollercoaster," do not describe it correctly. Sometimes the rising feeling from the stomach area feels like nausea or dizziness.

Diagnosis and differential diagnosis

As mentioned previously, there are no systematic accounts of vegetative seizures in epilepsies. As for auras, there are some data because they have a high value in clinical epileptology for their localizing value. Their presence helps in differentiating non-epileptic events and supports the diagnosis of focal epilepsy.

The localizing value of the auras has been studied only sparsely (Palmini and Gloor 1992). The diagnostic yield for aura descriptions was low after a first generalized tonic-clonic seizure (van Donselaar et al. 1990). This may be due to the fact that many patients can report their auras correctly only after having experienced several of them. Most difficult to describe are the vegetative and general symptoms – diffuse auras – that have no readily corresponding physiologic sensation. The differences in valuing the importance of auras also depends on the specialization of the clinician, the verbal skills of the patients, the distribution of the epilepsy syndromes in the institution and the general frame set of the study, that is, timing, phone interviews, history-taking by non-specialists and so on.

Auras got their localizing importance from decades of clinical assessment and description of seizure semiology, especially in epilepsy surgery patients, and by comparing them to the sensations that were described during electrical cortical stimulation (Penfield and Jasper 1954). In older studies, the localization of the epileptogenic zone was often uncertain. The technical advancements in imaging techniques and video-EEG monitoring have yielded several advancements in our abilities in localization.

When analyzing stimulation results, one has to critically bear in mind that the symptoms can be an expression of the symptomatogenic zone. They can also be an expression of an electric spread to other cortex regions (Lüders and Noachtar 2001). This can only be differentiated by simultaneous electroencephalographic registration of the so-called after discharges, which in return is limited by the placement of the electrodes. For example, Penfield and Jasper did not record after discharges due to the technical restraints (Penfield and Jasper 1954).

When stimulating the insular regions, sensations that are typical for epigastric auras can arise (Penfield

and Jasper 1954). In our institution, the seizures of 491 consecutive patients were studied prospectively in a search for epigastric auras. They were then semiologically classified (Henkel et al. 2002). All patients were studied by video-EEG monitoring as well as with MRI. Of these patients, 45% had temporal lobe epilepsies, 23% had extra-temporal lobe epilepsies and in the rest the focal origin could not be localized to only a single lobe. Epigastric auras were significantly more frequent in temporal lobe epilepsies (117 of 223 patients, 52%) compared to extra-temporal lobe epilepsies (13 of 113 patients, 12%; $p < 0.0001$). They were furthermore more frequent in mesial (70 of 110 patients, 64%) than in neocortical temporal lobe patients (16 of 41 patients, 39%; $p = 0.007$). There was no side preference. The analysis of the seizure evolution allowed for better differentiate between temporal and extra-temporal epilepsies. Oral or manual automatisms (automotor seizure) followed the epigastric aura in at least one of the recorded seizures in all temporal lobe epilepsy patients (100%) but only in 2 of the 13 patients with extra-temporal lobe epilepsies (15%; $p < 0.0001$). Epigastric auras denoted a temporal lobe epilepsy with a probability of 73%. If the epigastric aura anteceded an automotor seizure, the probability rose to 98.3%. This shows that the analysis of the seizure evolution has a by far greater localizing value, as does the accounting of the single seizure form (Henkel et al. 2002).

Many epileptic seizures are accompanied by an increase in heart rate. This can be an effect of epileptic activation of the cortex, particularly the insular regions, but also as secondary reactions to emotional or motor seizure phenomena. Our institution studied so-called subclinical seizures, that up to that date showed no subjective or objective clinical symptoms but where a seizure pattern was found in the EEG. In this way, we excluded secondary reasons (emotional or motor triggers) for the tachycardia. In 22 seizures from 21 patients with focal epilepsies that were previously classified as subclinical, a heart rate increase of more than 100% was significantly more common in the temporal onset cases (8 of 13) than in extra-temporal (1 of 9) lobe EEG seizure-pattern (Weil et al. 2005). This supports findings that attribute the cortical representation of heart rate regulation near the insula. A pure ictal tachycardia is therefore of localizing value for the temporal region. Using invasive EEG recordings, an interesting phenomenon was described in temporal lobe epilepsy patients: Both left- and right-sided temporal lobe seizures showed a significant heart rate increase. Although in right-sided temporal lobe seizures, the heart rate increase started before the seizure, which was not the case in left-sided temporal lobe seizures (Saleh et al. 2000). These observations show that activating mechanisms occur in the brain that elude even invasive EEG recordings.

Bradycardia is mostly described in seizures with a temporal or frontotemporal origin (Tinuper et al. 2001). In this situation, there was a preponderance of the left hemisphere onset. Cardial bradyarrhythmias are considered as one possible cause of the sudden unexplained death in epilepsy patients (SUDEP). Several interesting vegetative seizure phenomena were described in the last few years in temporal lobe epilepsies in connection with other seizures, and will therefore not be considered as the predominant seizure semiology. These vegetative ictal phenomena have a large localizing value for seizures from the non-dominant hemisphere and include the ictal urination urge (Baumgartner et al. 2000), ictal spitting (Voss et al. 1999), ictal vomiting (Kramer et al. 1988) and postictal coughing (Wennberg 2001).

The differentiation between syncope and epileptic seizures can be difficult as syncope often shows motor symptoms such as tonic or myoclonic convulsions (see Chapter 3). Epileptic seizures too are frequently diagnosed in these situations. On the other hand, it is possible, that syncope is a consequence of a vegetative seizure, illustrated by the case of a patient with a 18q-deletion syndrome in whom epileptic activity caused a tachycardia that led to syncopal symptoms (Sturm et al. 2000).

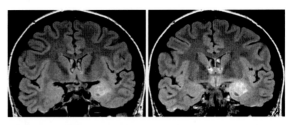

Fig. 15.1. Magnetic resonance imaging of the patient from Case 2. Two MRI-images in FLAIR sequence. Tumor in the left mesial temporal lobe.

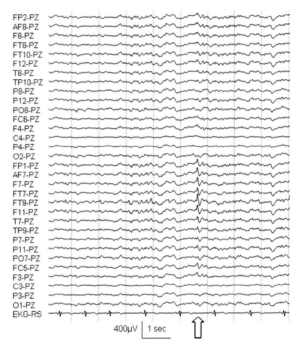

Fig. 15.2. Interictal referential EEG with mesial temporal spike. The negative electric maximum is at electrode FT9 (arrow).

Therapy

At present, the existence of vegetative seizures does not change the selection of anti-epileptic drugs (AED). However, the differentiation between focal and generalized epilepsies is crucial for choosing optimal AEDs. The presence of vegetative seizures helps in that differentiation. The clinically utility ranking of the AED is changing as some AEDs are being approved for monotherapy and newer drugs are being developed entering the market. AEDs of first choice are carbamazepine, oxcarbazepine, valproate, levetiracetam, topiramate, lamotrigine, pregabalin, gabapentin and phenytoin, in no specific order (Lhatoo and Sander 2003). The decision on a drug will depend on the situation of a given patient (elderly, female of child-bearing age, etc.), the time required to reach a maintenance dose and the side-effect profiles of the drugs.

Surgical treatment is especially successful if the epileptogenic focus can be identified and resected. This is only achieved if the epileptogenic focus is in a non-eloquent cortical area and can therefore be resected with no or only a small risk for neurological and/or neuropsychological deficits, or if the focus is in a region that is severely altered by the persisting epilepsy and therefore does not carry any significant function (Noachtar et al. 2003). Surgery on the temporal lobe is

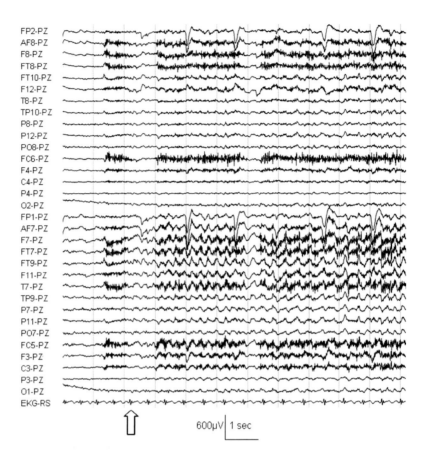

Fig. 15.3. While having the sensation of goose bumps on both arms, the EEG shows a left temporal seizure pattern, the beginning of which is marked with an arrow. Note the muscle artifacts, as the patient moved after feeling the goose bumps.

600μV | 1 sec

especially promising, with 58% becoming seizure-free. It should be considered early in patients with mesial temporal sclerosis because drug treatment is likely to fail with this pathology (Wiebe et al. 2001).

Prognosis

The prognosis of epilepsy does not depend on the seizure semiology but rather depends on the etiology and/or the epilepsy syndrome. This is also true for vegetative seizures.

In general, idiopathic generalized epilepsies have a better prognosis than symptomatic focal epilepsies. The prognosis for focal seizures with vegetative symptoms will depend on the etiology of the epilepsy and the viable therapy options. Drug treatment will not be successful in about 30% of all epilepsies. A small part of these patients can be helped with epilepsy surgery – approximately 50% to 80% seizure freedom with a 1% to 5% perisurgical morbidity (Noachtar et al. 2000).

Case 2: A 43-year-old patient reported attacks with goose bumps on both arms that lasted for several seconds. They started about two years ago. Sometimes he felt he was mentally altered during these episodes and experienced feelings which reminded him of situations of his childhood. This had reminded him of a known déjà vu sensation from his youth, and so he had not attributed any meaning to it at first. Witnesses could not report any abnormal behavior. Over the years, he had noticed that the episodes lasted longer and he was unable to speak while they were occurring. At first, he was able to compensate by leaving the situation or by using arbitrary gestures to overplay his short aphasias. Only after one of theses episodes was witnessed by his primary care physician was he subjected to further investigations. While waiting for his brain MRI, the patient suffered his first generalized tonic-clonic seizure, which was preceded by the previous symptoms. The MRI revealed a mass in the left mesial temporal lobe that was evaluated as a benign tumor of brain tissue origin (Fig. 15.1). The

interictal EEG showed left mesiotemporal epileptiform discharges (Fig. 15.2). The ictal EEG showed a left
temporal seizure pattern while he experienced goose
bumps on both arms (Fig. 15.3). He also experienced
the feeling of a known surrounding during the seizure
with goose bumps. The diagnosis was syndromic left
mesial temporal lobe epilepsy with the etiology being
a left mesial temporal tumor. His seizure pattern was
vegetative aura with goose bumps on both arms leading to a psychic aura followed by an aphasic seizure and
generalized tonic-clonic seizures. After being started
on 1.6 g of oxcarbazepine per day, he had only short
auras and rare aphasic seizures with loss of consciousness. An anterior mesial temporal lobe resection was
performed, which led to freedom from seizures. Ictal
goose bumps may have a lateralizing value, as in a case
series four of five patients with goose bumps during
their seizure had left-sided temporal lobe epilepsies
(Stefan et al. 2002).

References

Baumgartner C, Groppel G, Leutmezer F, Aull-Watschinger S, Pataraia E, Feucht M et al. Ictal urinary urge indicates seizure onset in the nondominant temporal lobe. *Neurology* 2000, **55**(3):432–434.

Feindel W, Penfield W. Localization of discharge in temporal lobe automatism. *AMA Arch Neurol Psychiatry* 1954, **72**(5):603–630.

Gowers WR. *Epilepsy and other chronic convulsive diseases: their causes, symptoms & treatment.* 2nd edn. London: J.&A. Churchill, 1901.

Gowers WR. Aura in epilepsy: a statistical review of 1,359 cases. *Arch Neurol Psychiatry* 1933, **30**:374–387.

Henkel A, Noachtar S, Pfander M, Luders HO. The localizing value of the abdominal aura and its evolution: a study in focal epilepsies. *Neurology* 2002, **58**(2):271–276.

Kramer RE, Luders H, Goldstick LP, Dinner DS, Morris HH, Lesser RP et al. Ictus emeticus: an electroclinical analysis. *Neurology* 1988, **38**(7):1048–1052.

Lhatoo SD, Sander JWAS. *The Epilepsies.* In: Kennard C (ed.). *Neurological disorders: course and treatment.* San Diego, CA: Academic Press, 2003, p. 207–234.

Lüders HO, Noachtar S. *Atlas of epileptic seizures and syndromes.* Philadelphia: Saunders, 2001.

Modlin IM, Kidd M, Latich I, Zikusoka MN, Shapiro MD. Current status of gastrointestinal carcinoids. *Gastroenterology* 2005, **128**(6):1717–1751.

Noachtar S. Seizure semiology. In: Lüders HO (ed.). *Epilepsy: comprehensive review and case discussions.* London: Martin Dunitz Publishers, 2001, p. 127–140.

Noachtar S, Lüders HO. Classification of epileptic seizures and epileptic syndromes. In: Gildenberg PL, Tasker RR. (eds.) *Textbook of stereotactic and functional neurosurgery.* New York: McGraw-Hill, 1997, pp. 1763–1774.

Noachtar S, Rosenow F, Arnold S, Baumgartner C, Ebner A, Hamer H et al. Semiologic classification of epileptic seizures. *Nervenarzt* 1998, **69**(2):117–126.

Noachtar S, Carreno M, Foldvary N, Luders HO. Seizures and pseudoseizures. *Suppl Clin Neurophysiol* 2000, **53**:259–270.

Noachtar S, Winkler PA, Lüders HO. Surgical therapy of epilepsy. In: Brandt T, Caplan C, Dichgans J, Diener J, Kennard C (eds.). *Neurological disorders: course and treatment.* 2nd edn. San Diego, CA: Academic Press, 2003, p. 235–244.

O'Donovan CA, Burgess RC, Luders HO. Autonomic auras. In: Noachtar S (ed.). *Epileptic seizures: pathophysiology and clinical semiology.* New York: Churchill Livingstone, 2000, p. 320–328.

Pacak K, Eisenhofer G, Ahlman H, Bornstein SR, Gimenez-Roqueplo AP, Grossman AB et al. Pheochromocytoma: recommendations for clinical practice from the First International Symposium. October 2005. *Nat Clin Pract Endocrinol Metab* 2007, **3**(2):92–102.

Palmini A, Gloor P. The localizing value of auras in partial epilepsies. *Neurology* 1992, **42**:801–808.

Penfield W, Jasper H. *Epilepsy and the functional anatomy of the human brain.* Boston: Brown Little & Co., 1954.

Saleh Y, Kirchner A, Pauli E, Hilz MJ, Neundorfer B, Stefan H. Temporal lobe epilepsy: effect of focus side on the autonomic regulation of heart rate. *Nervenarzt* 2000, **71**(6):477–480.

Schulz R, Luders HO, Noachtar S, May T, Sakamoto A, Holthausen H et al. Amnesia of the epileptic aura. *Neurology* 1995, **45**(2):231–235.

So NK. Epileptic auras. In: Wyllie E (ed.). *The treatment of epilepsy: principles and practice.* Philadelphia: Lippincott, Williams & Wilkins, 2001, p. 299–308.

Stefan H, Pauli E, Kerling F, Schwarz A, Koebnick C. Autonomic auras: left hemispheric predominance of epileptic generators of cold shivers and goose bumps? *Epilepsia* 2002, **43**(1):41–45.

Sturm K, Knake S, Schomburg U, Wakat JP, Hamer HM, Fritz B et al. Autonomic seizures versus syncope in 18q- deletion syndrome: a case report. *Epilepsia* 2000, **41**(8):1039–1043.

Tinuper P, Bisulli F, Cerullo A, Carcangiu R, Marini C, Pierangeli G et al. Ictal bradycardia in partial epileptic seizures: autonomic investigation in three cases and literature review. *Brain* 2001, **124**(Pt 12):2361–2371.

van Donselaar C, Geerts A, Schimsheimer R. Usefulness of an aura for classification of a first generalized seizure. *Epilepsia* 1990, **31**:529–535.

Voss NF, Davies KG, Boop FA, Montouris GD, Hermann BP. Spitting automatism in complex partial seizures: a nondominant temporal localizing sign? *Epilepsia* 1999, **40**(1):114–116.

Weil S, Arnold S, Eisensehr I, Noachtar S. Heart rate increase in otherwise subclinical seizures is different in temporal versus extratemporal seizure onset: support for temporal lobe autonomic influence. *Epileptic Disord* 2005, 7(3):199–204.

Wennberg R. Postictal coughing and noserubbing coexist in temporal lobe epilepsy. *Neurology* 2001, **56**(1):133–134.

Wiebe S, Blume WT, Girvin JP, Eliasziw M. A randomized, controlled trial of surgery for temporal-lobe epilepsy. *N Engl J Med* 2001, **345**:311–318.

Chapter 16

Episodic ataxias

Monika Jeub, Thomas Klockgether and Michael Strupp

Episodic ataxias are a clinically and genetically heterogeneous group of neurological disorders that are characterized by attacks of incoordination and imbalance. The autosomal dominantly inherited episodic ataxias type 1 (EA1) and type 2 (EA2) account for the majority of cases. In addition, there are another four types of autosomal dominantly inherited ataxias (EA3, 4, 5 and 6), which have been observed only in single families or in a single patient. The genes that have been found to be affected in EAs code for ion channels that are directly involved in control of neuronal excitability. However, a number of EAs still await genetic clarification. With a better understanding of the genetic and molecular basis of the EAs, new classifications and deeper insights into the genotype-phenotype correlation will arise.

Episodic ataxia type 1 (EA1)

Definition

EA1 is a rare, autosomal dominantly inherited disease characterized by brief attacks of ataxia and rhythmic movements. Between the spells, the patients have neuromyotonia, such as on-going, spontaneous, high-frequency muscle fiber activity due to axonal hyperactivity. EA1 is caused by mutations of the voltage-gated potassium channel KCNA1.

Epidemiology

The prevalence of EA1 is estimated to be 0.2 per 100,000. However, as the disorder may be overlooked in many families, the real prevalence may be greater.

Molecular pathogenesis

In 1994, Litt et al. demonstrated linkage of EA1 to a locus mapped to chromosome 12q near a cluster of three potassium channel genes (Litt et al. 1994). In the same year, the first mis-sense mutations associated with EA1 were discovered in KCNA1, which is one of the potassium channel genes located in chromosome 12q (Browne et al. 1994). Since then, several mis-sense mutations, one truncation mutation and one in-frame three-nucleotide deletion have been described (Browne et al. 1995; Eunson et al. 2000; Shook et al. 2007). The mutations are located throughout the gene in highly conserved regions.

The KCNA1 gene encodes for Kv1.1, the pore-forming subunit of delayed-rectifier potassium channels. Delayed-rectifier channels are tetramers of four Kv1-subunits (either homomers of Kv1.1 or heteromers consisting of Kv1.1 and other Kv1 subunits, for example, Kv1.2) combined with additional, ß-modifying subunits. Their function is to repolarize the cell membrane during an action potential and to suppress cell excitability. The Kv1.1 subunit is widely expressed in the central and peripheral nervous system. Its most pronounced expression is found in axons of cerebellar basket cells and in perinodal areas along peripheral nerves.

In gene expression systems, mutated subunits have reduced potassium currents (mostly due to a decreased expression), an increased threshold for activation, alterations in kinetic parameters, altered inactivation properties and a reduced channel open probability depending on the type of mutation (Adelman et al. 1995; Bretschneider et al. 1999; D'Adamo et al. 1998; Zerr et al. 1998). To imitate the heterozygous condition, experiments with co-expression of wild-type and mutated subunits were performed. For some mutations, it was shown that wild-type and mutated subunits assemble to form functional channels that have features between those of wild-type and mutated channels, suggesting a dominant negative effect of the

The Paroxysmal Disorders, ed. Bettina Schmitz, Barbara Tettenborn and Donald L. Schomer. Published by Cambridge University Press. © Cambridge University Press 2010.

mutation (Adelman et al. 1995; D'Adamo et al. 1998; Zerr et al. 1998).

Furthermore, the only known stop mutation, which is associated with a severe, drug-resistant phenotype, was shown to lead to defects in tetramerization and membrane targeting as well as intracellular aggregation (Manganas et al. 2001; Rea et al. 2002). These changes finally result in a reduction of the potassium current.

A homozygous knock-out mouse lacking Kv1.1 suffers from frequent epileptic seizures and problems maintaining balance and exhibits altered action potential properties in the sciatic nerve (Smart et al. 1998; Zhang et al. 1999). By using homologous recombination, Herson et al. developed an EA1 knock-in mouse model bearing the human EA1 mutation V408A. In contrast to Kv1.1-null mice, homozygous V408A mice are lethally affected. Heterozygous mice display a stress-induced loss of motor coordination that is ameliorated by acetazolamide (Herson et al. 2003). Electrophysiological studies of Kv1.1 knock-out and EA1 knock-in mice revealed an increased frequency and amplitude of spontaneous GABAergic inhibitory postsynaptic currents (sIPSC) in cerebellar Purkinje cells (Herson et al. 2003; Zhang et al. 1999). This observation led to the hypothesis that the high concentration of mutated Kv1.1 subunits on basket cell axons enhances action potential propagation, resulting in an increased GABA release at the basket cell-Purkinje cell synapse. All excitatory and inhibitory signals of the cerebellum converge at the Purkinje cells, whose GABAergic axons are the only output of the cerebellar cortex. An enhanced inhibition of the Purkinje cells via GABAergic basket cells would lead to a disinhibition and therefore activation of the downstream targets in the deep cerebellar neurons. This shift of the overall balance between excitatory and inhibitory signals of the cerebellum might underlie the behavioral deficits.

Myokymia/neuromyotonia is most probably caused by an enhanced excitability and impaired repolarization of motor axons due to a disturbed Kv1.1 channel function, leading to spontaneous, repetitive discharges scattered along the axons (Smart et al. 1998).

Clinical features

The onset of EA1 is usually in childhood, in the majority of cases between the ages of four and seven years. Attacks can start spontaneously but they are mostly provoked by sudden movements. A typical example is the start of a footrace. Fast, involuntary movements following a stumble or a long-lasting exercise like bicycling may also provoke attacks. Attacks may also follow vestibular stimuli, such as riding on a merry-go-round or after caloric irrigation of the ears. Fear, excitement, tiredness, hyperventilation, premenstrual hormone alteration and fever enhance the likelihood of attacks. Insomnia, hunger, alcohol and coffee appear to have no influence.

Attacks may be preceded by a kind of aura. Some individuals describe a click that is followed by a feeling of stiffness, slackness or weakness spreading throughout the body. Others describe a feeling of weightlessness, eye-rolling, dizziness or the impression of falling (Brunt and van Weerden 1990).

The attacks are characterized by dysarthria, ataxia of gait, stance and limbs, as well as oscillating movements, which can range from a very mild tremor to a rocking of the whole body. Sometimes movements may have dystonic and choreic features. Eating, writing and precise movements are impossible during attacks. On examination, ataxia can be recognized by a broad-based gait, impaired tandem gait, uncoordinated and dysmetric limb movements, slowing of rapidly alternating movements and slurred speech. Some patients describe impaired or double vision. However, a spontaneous or gaze-evoked nystagmus is absent. Classic vertigo, nausea or vomiting are also absent. Vegetative symptoms or headaches are rare, and consciousness is always clear. To alleviate and shorten attacks, most patients sit or lie down and avoid moving. Normally, attacks last between seconds and several minutes, very rarely over several hours. After an attack, there is a refractory period that varies in duration. The attack frequency ranges from more than 20 in one day to less than once in a month, with a rather large inter- and intra-individual variation.

Between attacks, EA1 is characterized by myokymia, which is caused by axonal hyperexcitability (see previous). Myokymia are spontaneous involuntary muscle fiber group contractions visible as vermiform movements of the overlying skin. They are mainly localized around the eyes or in the hands. Some patients exhibit a continuous adduction-opposition position of the thumbs called "priest's hand" or a hand-and-foot posture resembling a carpal-pedal spasm (Brunt and van Weerden 1990). In other patients, myokymia is not visible and is only detected by palpation or by electromyography. The degree of myokymia varies intra-individually. It is increased during attacks, after exertion or in the cold.

There are a number of phenotypic variants such as episodic ataxia without myokymia, episodic ataxia with paroxysmal dyspnea and isolated myokymia, which can be associated with skeletal deformities (Eunson et al. 2000; Kinali et al. 2004; Lee et al. 2004; Shook et al. 2007).

A number of EA1 patients have concomitant epilepsy that manifests as complex partial seizures, partial seizures with generalization and generalized seizures (Zuberi et al. 1999). Members of one family exhibited only partial epilepsy and myokymia without ataxia episodes (Eunson et al. 2000). The prevalence of epilepsy in EA1 patients is approximately ten times that in the general population. A direct relation between altered Kv1.1 function and epilepsy is suggested by the occurrence of spontaneous seizures in the Kv1.1-knockout mouse model (Smart et al. 1998). Moreover, Kv1.1 blockers have pro-convulsive actions.

Diagnosis

Even if an attack is not directly observed, EA1 can be suspected on the basis of medical history, family history and clinical examination. In some cases, an attack can be directly observed after provocation with appropriate stimuli in the hospital. One may also ask the patient to provide a home video of a typical attack. A definite diagnosis can be made by molecular genetic testing, which is commercially available.

To support a suspected diagnosis, the patient should undergo electromyography for myokymia. The resting motor unit activity consists of regularly repeated duplets and triplets, but single spikes and multiplets may also be seen. In addition to rhythmic activity, irregularly repeated single potentials and complex bursts of about 50 to 100 ms may also be found. The intensity of resting activity may reach intermediate interference pattern. The basic frequency is usually constant, between 2 and 5 Hz, with a range of 0.5 to 8 Hz. The burst duration ranges from about 5 ms for a single spike to 25 ms for multiplets. The spike frequency within a burst is usually between 100 and 200 Hz. The period during which an individual myokymic discharge continues ranges from seconds to hours and probably many weeks. Apart from the first spike of each burst, the amplitude of the myokymic potentials is rather low (up to 600 μV) in comparison with voluntarily recruited action potentials. This

is explained by partial involvement of the motor unit in successive spikes of a burst. Strong voluntary contraction of the affected muscle suppresses myokymic activity for 5 to 20 seconds. Distal nerve block leads to a complete and proximal nerve block to a partial stop of myokymic activity. The detection of resting motor unit activity in patients without visible myokymia is best achieved by using surface electrodes because of their large registration area. The best results can be obtained by examining the small hand muscles, as the resting motor unit activity is usually most pronounced there and almost always present. Myokymia can be provoked or enhanced by local ischemia caused by cuff inflation (Brunt and van Weerden 1990).

Except for an occasionally slight elevation of creatine kinase (CK), routine blood parameters, cerebrospinal fluid parameters, electrophysiological examinations other than electromyography, CT and MRI of the brain are normal. In patients with epilepsy, the EEG can show typical epilepsy patterns.

Differential diagnosis

- Other EAs (see following and Table 16.1)
- Vestibular migraine: Vestibular migraine is a subtype of basilar migraine characterized by reversible attacks of vertigo, gait and stance ataxia with or without occipital headache and brainstem symptoms. A differential diagnosis can be complicated, as migraine headaches can be missing. There is probably some overlap between vestibular migraine and EAs, and some patients diagnosed with vestibular migraine may in fact have an EA, in particular EA2.
- Vestibular paroxysms: On analogy with trigeminal neuralgia, atherosclerotic elongated arteries can lead to neurovascular compression of the eighth cranial nerve, resulting in short attacks of vertigo. Typically, they are provoked by defined head positions or a change of the head position. The onset of symptoms is usually later in life. An MRI may reveal the artery-nerve contact.
- Transient ischemic attacks of the vertebral-basilar system: These are marked by the sudden onset of brain stem neurological signs. They usually start later in life. Helpful ancillary tests are MRI, MR-angiography, ultrasound of the cerebral arteries and cardiac investigation.
- Multiple sclerosis with paroxysmal phenomena: Short-lasting attacks of ataxia or dysarthria can

Table 16.1 Episodic ataxia type 1 (EA1) and episodic ataxia type 2 (EA2)

	Episodic ataxia type 1	Episodic ataxia type 2
Mode of inheritance	autosomal dominant	autosomal dominant
Gene	KCNA1 (12p13)	CACNA1A (19p13)
Age of onset	infancy	infancy up to early adulthood
Triggers	movement, startle	emotional stress, exertion, caffeine, alcohol
Attacks	dysarthria, gait, stance and limb ataxia, tremor, rarely dystonic and choreic movements	dysarthria, gait, stance and limb ataxia, nystagmus, headache, nausea, vomiting
Duration	seconds to minutes	minutes to hours (days)
Interictal myokymia	yes	no
Progressive ataxia	no	yes
Therapy	acetazolamide, phenytoin, carbamazepine, valproic acid	4-aminopyridine, acetazolamide, sulthiame, flunarizine, valproic acid
Additional symptoms	epilepsy, paroxysmal dyspnea, skeletal deformities	epilepsy, muscle weakness, interictal dystonia, mental retardation

also appear in multiple sclerosis. They are caused by ephaptic activation of axons located in partly demyelinated lesions. Helpful ancillary tests are cMRI and cerebrospinal fluid investigation.

- Paroxysmal non-kinesigenic dyskinesia and episodic kinesigenic dyskinesia (Lee et al. 2004; Tomita et al. 1999). These autosomal dominantly inherited diseases are characterized by attacks of involuntary dystonic, choreoathetoid or ballistic movements without ataxia.
- Focal epilepsy: To distinguish EA1 from focal epilepsies, a detailed medical history, EEG (interictal and ictal) and a MRI should be performed. Patients who suffer from EA1 and epilepsy can distinguish their ataxia attacks from epileptic seizures usually without any problems.
- Diseases with continuous muscle activity/myokymia of other etiology: Myokymia and epilepsy caused by mutations of other potassium channels, myokymia caused by antibodies against voltage-gated potassium channels.

Therapy

Once the diagnosis is made, careful counseling of the patient is mandatory. It should be explained that EA1 is in principle a benign condition. By understanding the provoking stimuli, patients may learn how to prevent attacks.

If medical treatment is required, the carbonic anhydrase inhibitor acetazolamide (500–750 mg per day) is the first choice, although it is less effective than in EA2 (for a detailed description see EA2, therapy). Second-line medications include carbamazepine, phenytoin and valproic acid. Owing to myokymia, some patients have abnormal postures of their hands and feet. As these postures resolve mostly spontaneously with age, surgical correction should be avoided.

Natural history

EA1 does not result in permanent disability and therefore has a good prognosis. Attacks usually become milder with increasing age. In one patient, a progressive replacement of episodic ataxia attacks by myokymia was observed (Poujois et al. 2006). Nevertheless, many patients feel limited in their activities of daily life and suffer from the reaction of other people. Cases of traffic accidents or near-drownings during attacks have been reported.

Episodic ataxia type 2 (EA2)

Definition

EA2 is an autosomal dominantly inherited neurological disease characterized by episodes of ataxia that last for hours and sometimes days. Between attacks patients present with cerebellar symptoms, which range from a gaze-evoked nystagmus to a slowly progressive cerebellar ataxia syndrome later in life. EA2 is caused by mutations of the calcium channel gene CACNA1A.

Epidemiology

EA2 is by far the most common episodic ataxia but precise data about the prevalence are missing. As there is a large clinical overlap between the other two allelic disorders of the CACNA1A gene, the familial hemiplegic migraine type 1 (FHM1) and the spinocerebellar ataxia type 6 (SCA6), it is particularly difficult to estimate their prevalence.

Molecular pathogenesis

In 1995, the disease locus of EA2 was mapped to chromosome 19p (Kramer et al. 1995). In 1996, Ophoff et al. identified causative truncation (frameshift and splice site) mutations in the calcium channel gene CACNA1A (Ophoff et al. 1996). Currently, more than 30 mutations have been described with a distribution throughout the gene. Most of them are non-sense or frameshift mutations leading to a disruption of the reading frame or intronic mutations that predict aberrant splicing.

There are two other allelic disorders of CACNA1A: the familial hemiplegic migraine type 1, an inherited form of migraine with aura, and SCA6, a slowly progressive ataxia disorder with cerebellar degeneration. As a general rule, FHM1 mutations are missense mutations (Ophoff et al. 1996), EA2 mutations are non-sense mutations and SCA6 is caused by small expansion of a CAG repeat within the last exon of CACNA1A (Zhuchenko et al. 1997). However, the genotype-phenotype correlation is not strict, as there are also reports of mis-sense mutations and CAG repeat expansions leading to an EA2 phenotype (Denier et al. 2001; Guida et al. 2001; Jodice et al. 1997). Furthermore, there is considerable clinical overlap between EA2, FHM1 and SCA6. EA2 patients have headache, nausea and vomiting as in classic migraine (Jen et al. 2004) or they suffer in advanced age from a slowly progressive ataxia as in SCA6. Migraine attacks in FHM1 may have features of episodic ataxia. FHM1 patients may also develop a permanent cerebellar ataxia (Ducros et al. 2001). Some SCA6 patients report attacks of ataxia or migraine prior to the onset of progressive ataxia.

CACNA1A encodes for Cav2.1, the main subunit (α_{1A} subunit) of the P/Q-type voltage-gated calcium channel. The P-type current (Purkinje cell type) and the Q-type current (granule cell type) exhibit slightly different pharmacological and inactivation characteristics caused by alternative splicing of Cav2.1. One α_{1A} subunit acts as voltage sensor and channel pore, whereas additional subunits (β, $\alpha<\sigma\beta>2</\sigma\beta>\delta$, γ) have modulating effects. As most EA2 mutations are truncation mutations, it is conceivable that they result in a loss of function of the affected channels. Indeed, in heterologous expression systems truncation mutations were completely devoid of channel function and exerted dominant negative effects on co-expressed wild-type α1A subunits (Jouveceau et al. 2001; Wappl et al. 2002). In contrast to FHM1 mis-sense mutations, which have been shown to exhibit a gain of function, mis-sense mutations in EA2 not causing protein truncations led to drastically impaired or completely lost channel currents and displayed dominant-negative effects on the wild-type CACNA1A proteins (Guida et al. 2001; Jeng et al. 2006; Tottene et al. 2002; Wappl et al. 2002). In addition to altered channel function, it has been shown that the mis-folded mutant proteins impair plasma membrane trafficking of wild-type CACNA1A proteins in a negative dominant way (Jeng et al. 2008).

The CACNA1A gene is widely expressed but the greatest expression is found in the cerebellum and presynaptically at the neuromuscular junction. The P/Q-type calcium channels mediate the main presynaptic calcium influx leading to transmitter release. Their localization on dendrites and neural somata suggests an additional postsynaptic role. As P/Q-type calcium currents and channel densities are reduced in heterologous expression systems, it is conceivable that symptoms are caused by impaired neurotransmission due to an impaired release of neurotransmitters, namely GABA in Purkinje cells and acetylcholine at the neuromuscular junction. Indeed, electromyographic studies of EA2 patients demonstrated a reduced safety factor of neuromuscular transmission and an increased jitter and blocking on voluntary single-fiber electromyography (Jen et al. 2001). In vitro microelectrode studies revealed a marked reduction of endplate potential quantal content (Maselli et al. 2003), confirming a presynaptic defect in neuromuscular transmission.

The spontaneous recessive mouse models of CACNA1A tottering, leaner and rolling Nagoya display a complex phenotype of epilepsy, dystonia and ataxia and are used as animal models of EA2 (Fletcher et al. 1996; Mori et al. 2000). Electrophysiological studies of all mutants showed reduced P/Q calcium currents of Purkinje cells, which is consistent with the loss-of-function hypothesis for Cav2.1 in human EA2 mutations (Mori et al. 2000; Wakamori et al. 1998).

More recently, it was shown that the precision of Purkinje cell pace-making is lost in these mouse models, which results in a significant degradation of the synaptic information encoded in the Purkinje cell activity. The irregular pace-making was caused by a decreased activation of calcium-activated potassium channels (K_{Ca}) and could be reversed pharmacologically by the K_{Ca}-channel agonist EBIO. Chronic in vivo perfusion of EBIO significantly improved motor performance of mutated mice (Walter et al. 2006). The tottering mouse suffers – similar to patients with EA2 – from episodic attacks of dyskinesia induced by clinically relevant precipitants such as emotional stress and caffeine (Fureman et al. 2002). This animal model is most appropriate to analyze the mechanism of attack precipitation and the principles of treatment systematically. EA2 mutations not only lead to changes in ion currents and neurotransmitter release. Changes in pH and metabolism were also demonstrated, which may be related to the attack induction and neurodegeneration.

On magnetic resonance spectroscopy, untreated EA2 patients showed decreased high-energy phosphate ratios in the brain and increased pH in the cerebellum and brain, which normalized under acetazolamide. 1H magnetic resonance spectra demonstrated high lactate peaks. These metabolic alterations on cerebellar MRI spectroscopy have been interpreted as an intracellular alkalosis and may be characteristic for EA2 (Sappey-Marinier et al. 1999). Furthermore, proton MR spectroscopy showed reduced cerebellar total creatine in non-ataxic EA2 patients compared to healthy controls, possibly reflecting an early sign of calcium-channel dysfunction in EA2 (Harno et al. 2005).

Clinical features

EA2 begins in early childhood, most often before the age of 20 years but may rarely manifest in patients older than 50 years. Such late onset may be related to certain mutations, for example, multiple-base pair insertion in CACNA1A (Imbrici et al. 2005). Clinically, EA2 is characterized by recurrent attacks of ataxia which are provoked by exercise, emotional stress, alcohol and caffeine. The duration of an attack is typically longer than in EA1 and ranges from hours to days. Attacks may occur daily or over longer intervals, even years in some patients.

Episodes can vary from pure cerebellar ataxia to combinations of symptoms suggesting the additional involvement of the brain stem and even the cortex. Vertigo, nausea and vomiting are the most commonly associated symptoms, being present in more than 50% of patients. About half of patients report headaches that meet the International Headache Society (IHS) criteria for migraine. On examination during an ataxia attack, patients typically exhibit a nystagmus not seen during interictal examination or a strong enhancement of an interictal nystagmus.

Between spells, more than 90% of patients exhibit central ocular motor disturbances. The most common finding is a gaze-evoked nystagmus with features typical of a rebound nystagmus. More than 50% of patients exhibit a vertical nystagmus, most commonly a downbeat nystagmus (Sasaki et al. 2003). Downbeat nystagmus may begin as a positional downbeat nystagmus in the head-hanging position and gradually evolve into a downbeat nystagmus syndrome. Other central ocular motor disturbances are impaired smooth pursuit, saccade dysmetria, gaze-holding deficits, impaired visual suppression of the vestibular-ocular reflex or, rarely, bilateral internuclear ophthalmoplegia (Baloh et al. 1997; Rucker et al. 2005). Later in life, EA2 patients can develop subtle and slowly progressive limb ataxia and postural imbalance.

There are phenotypic variants with additional neurological symptoms. In some patients, fluctuating muscle weakness resembling myasthenia during or between ataxia attacks can be found, which may be caused by an abnormal neuromuscular transmission due to presynaptic failure (see previous; Jen et al. 2001).

In 2001, a patient with a de novo truncating mutation of the CACNA1A gene was described who presented a complex phenotype consisting of episodic and progressive ataxia as well as epilepsy (Jouvenceau et al. 2001). Until now, further EA2 families with absence epilepsy or idiopathic focal epilepsy and migraine were reported (Holtmann et al. 2002; Imbrici et al. 2004). Furthermore, EEG abnormalities in patients with acetazolamide-responsive ataxia without epilepsy have been described (Vance et al. 1984). As a rare symptom, interictal dystonia was described in two EA2 patients in the late course of the disease, possibly associated with cerebellar degeneration (Spacey et al. 2005).

Mental retardation has also been reported (Mochizuki et al. 2004). The most recent large case series from Jen et al. described the clinical spectrum in 18 families and 9 sporadic cases. All but 2 of the 64 genetically defined patients reported episodes of ataxia. Two members of one family only had progressive ataxia. All but one had onset before the age of 20 years, and all but four had interictal nystagmus. Migraine headaches occurred in more than half. Vertigo and weakness accompanied the ataxia in more than half of the genetically defined patients (Jen et al. 2004).

Diagnosis and differential diagnosis

As mentioned previously, the onset of EA2 is in childhood, almost always before the age of 20 years but may rarely manifest in patients older than 50 years. Therefore, an onset beyond 20 years is unlikely but does not rule out the diagnosis.

When examined between spells, more than 90% of patients exhibit central ocular motor disturbances (see previous). Later in the course, limb ataxia and postural imbalance may be seen. In other words, if a patient has a normal ocular motor examination the diagnosis of EA2 is unlikely.

Laboratory examinations

EEG abnormalities have been reported in patients with acetazolamide-responsive ataxia (Van Bogaert and Szliwowski 1996). A typical 3-Hz spike-wave pattern was found in a family with a combination of absence epilepsy and cerebellar ataxia (Imbrici et al. 2004). Cerebellar atrophy, especially of the anterior vermis, can be detected on MRI (Vighetto et al. 1988). As genetic testing is commercially available, patients with clinically probable EA2 should be genetically tested to confirm the diagnosis. It has to be pointed out that no mutation of the CACNA1A gene can be detected in about 30% to 50% of all patients with typical clinical features of EA2 (Jen et al. 2004). In some of these patients, other "EA genes" have been postulated, for example, on chromosome 1q42 (peak two-point lod score = 4.14; Cader et al. 2005). Further, a novel mutation of the KCNA1 gene causes "EA without myokymia," highlighting the heterogeneity of phenotypic effects (see previous; Lee et al. 2004).

Differential diagnosis

For differential diagnosis, see also EA1. As migraine headaches occur in more than half of EA2 patients,

a differentiation from vestibular migraine is often impossible (Jen et al. 2004).

Therapy

Based on the pathophysiological understanding of EA2, two pharmacologic approaches were established. They focus on modulation of the pH level and membrane ion conductance.

Acetazolamide

Today, so far acetazolamide is the drug of choice for the preventive treatment of EA2 (dosages of 250 to 1000 mg per day), although its efficacy has never been proven in a randomized controlled trial. It is a carbonic anhydrase inhibitor, which was initially shown to decrease the number of attacks in hypokalemic periodic paralysis patients. Its efficacy was discovered by serendipity in a patient with EA2 misdiagnosed as periodic paralysis and was later confirmed by others (Griggs et al. 1978). Acetazolamide effectively prevents or attenuates the attacks in about 50% to 75% of all patients. However, clinical experience shows that in the long term many patients stop the treatment with this agent because it is either not effective any more or they develop adverse effects (unpublished observation).

Acetazolamide has several effects. It inhibits the carbonic anhydrase interconversion of $CO_2 + H_2O \leftrightarrow H_2CO_3$. It produces diuresis, initial kaliuresis and metabolic acidosis. Acetazolamide also lowers serum bicarbonate levels and reduces the amount of brain lactate and pyruvate, resulting in subsequent brain acidosis (Zasorin et al. 1983). Prevention of the attacks by acetazolamide – most likely via changes in pH – may be one key to understanding the pathological mechanism of the disease, and especially how the attacks are triggered. Changes in the extra- and intracellular pH cause alterations of the transmembrane conductance, for instance, a decrease in intracellular pH reduces potassium conductance and an increase in pH raises it. Thus, one hypothesis is that attacks are secondary to abnormally large intracellular pH values, and by reducing this pH level acetazolamide may prevent attacks (Brandt and Strupp 1997). Thus, the excitability and resting activity of neurons are restored.

Observed adverse effects of acetazolamide are nephrocalcinosis, hyperhydrosis, paresthesia, muscle stiffening with easy fatigability and gastrointestinal disturbances. Side-effects are dose-related and can be partially reduced by potassium chloride supplementation. Of the other carbonic anhydrase-inhibiting drugs, sulthiame has also been used successfully. It caused fewer side-effects and was most effective in dosages between 50 and 300 mg daily (Brunt and van Weerden 1990). Nevertheless, acetazolamide is the drug of first choice and sulthiame an alternative treatment option. Scoggan et al. identified a new mis-sense mutation in exon 12 of the CACNA1A gene from a patient with EA2 whose symptoms were controlled with a combination of acetazolamide and valproic acid (Scoggan et al. 2006). It was also demonstrated that acetazolamide may improve neuro-otological abnormalities in a family with EA2, such as saccadic hypermetria and gaze-evoked nystagmus.

4-aminopyridine (4-AP)

It has recently been shown that aminopyridines (as potassium channel blockers) improve downbeat nystagmus, most likely by increasing the inhibitory influence of the Purkinje cells, a hypothesis supported by animal experiments (Etzion and Grossman 2001; Strupp et al. 2003). Because Purkinje cell function is assumed to be impaired in EA2 and downbeat nystagmus, the effects of 4-AP on the occurrence of attacks were evaluated in three patients with EA2. Attacks of ataxia were completely prevented in two patients with EA2 (who no longer responded to acetazolamide) and markedly reduced in a third by the potassium channel blocker 4-AP. All patients fulfilled the diagnostic criteria for EA2 recently published (Jen et al. 2004); the diagnosis was confirmed in two patients by detecting mutations in the CACNA1A gene. Cessation of the treatment led to a recurrence within 1 to 2 days. Subsequent therapy with 4-AP alleviated the symptoms. In the meantime, four patients with EA2 (genetically proven) and two patients with the clinical picture of EA2 were treated with 4-AP, five of them having a full response.

4-AP may prevent attacks in EA2 (and improve downbeat nystagmus) by increasing the release of GABA in the Purkinje cells. The following mechanisms appear to be involved: Animal experiments have shown that 4-AP increases the excitability of Purkinje cells; 1 to 10 micromolar concentrations of 4-AP markedly shortened the latency of calcium-spike firing after the onset of depolarizing pulses (Etzion and Grossman 2001); 4-AP prolongs the duration of action potentials and increases the release of neurotransmitters by blocking several potassium currents, for example, the A-current and the delayed-rectifier. These effects of 4-AP in EA2 were further evaluated in animal models of EA2. It is remarkable that in the tottering mouse, 4-AP was observed to completely prevent attacks of ataxia but did not affect the severity of "breakthrough" attacks that occurred in the presence of a drug. These results suggest that the aminopyridines increase the threshold for attack initiation without mitigating the character of the attack (Weisz et al. 2005). From a clinical point of view, a prospective randomized controlled study is necessary to prove the short- and long-term effects of 4-AP and to compare them with acetazolamide, which is still the standard treatment of EA2.

Mouse models of EA2 may provide the basis for the development of future therapeutics. In tottering mice, attacks were prevented by drugs that blocked noradrenergic neurotransmission but agents that facilitated noradrenergic transmission failed to induce attacks (Fureman and Hess 2005). These results suggest that whereas noradrenergic neurotransmission may be necessary for attacks, an increase in norepinephrine is not sufficient to induce attacks. As mentioned previously, EBIO reversed the irregular pacemaking of Purkinje cells of CACNA1A mutants and improved motor performance. Thus, drugs that activate K_{CA} channels might be effective in controlling ataxic attacks in EA2 patients. Interestingly, therapeutic concentrations of acetazolamide activate K_{CA} channels, which could be another mechanism of action of acetazolamide in EA2.

Natural history

In contrast to EA1, EA2 is associated with progressive ataxia. However, compared to other progressive ataxias, its progression is slow.

Other episodic ataxias

Episodic ataxia type 3 (EA3)

An autosomal dominant disorder with attacks of vestibular ataxia, vertigo, tinnitus and interictal myokymia has been described in a large Canadian kindred. Attacks last several minutes and are responsive to acetazolamide. Disease onset varies and can also occur in adolescence. The disease is clinically distinct from EA1 because of the presence of vertigo and tinnitus, and from EA2 due to the absence of interictal nystagmus and shorter episodes. Although vertigo and tinnitus are prominent in EA4 (see following), EA4 is distinguished by having abnormal eye movements, no response to acetazolamide and no interictal myokymia. Linkage analyses excluded linkage to EA1 and EA2 loci and revealed linkage to a 4-cm region on chromosome 1q42. This disease was first described as EA4 but, in the current classification according to OMIM, it is referred to as EA3 (Cader et al. 2005; Steckley et al. 2001).

Episodic ataxia type 4 (EA4)

In two North Carolina kindreds, an autosomal dominantly inherited episodic ataxia with vertigo and diplopia as well as interictal defective smooth pursuit, gaze-evoked nystagmus and inability to suppress the vestibulo-ocular reflex has been described. This disorder was formerly designated as periodic vestibulocerebellar ataxia. Disease onset is between the third and sixth decade. Attacks last hours and are not responsive to acetazolamide (Farmer and Mustian 1963; Vance et al. 1984). Linkage to EA1 and EA2 loci was ruled out (Damji et al. 1996), but so far no genome-wide scan has been reported. EA4 can be clinically distinguished from EA3 by abnormal interictal eye movements, lack of response to acetazolamide and absence of interictal myokymia.

Episodic ataxia type 5 (EA5)

In a family with an EA2 phenotype, a mis-sense mutation in the calcium channel ß$_4$ subunit (CACNB4) was found (Escayg et al. 2000). Beta subunits are accessory subunits that have modulating effects on calcium channels and are highly expressed in the cerebellum. EA5 is clinically characterized by attacks of vertigo, ataxia and seizures. The onset of symptoms is in the third and fourth decade. The attacks last hours (sometimes weeks); between the attacks, patients have downbeat nystagmus, postural imbalance and ataxia. Symptoms respond to acetazolamide.

Interestingly, an unrelated family carrying the same mutation suffers from generalized epilepsy (Escayg et al. 2000). Another mutation of the CACNB4 gene causes juvenile myoclonic epilepsy (Escayg et al. 2000).

Episodic ataxia type 6 (EA6)

A child with episodic and progressive ataxia, seizures, migraine and alternating hemiplegia was found to have a de novo heterozygous mutation in SLC1A3. SLC1A3 is a transporter molecule that regulates neurotransmitter concentrations at the excitatory glutamatergic synapses of the central nervous system. Gene-expression studies showed a decreased expression of the mutated protein and a dominant negative effect on the wild-type allele leading to a reduced glial glutamate uptake, which may result in neural hyperexcitability (Jen et al. 2005).

Episodic ataxia associated with ATPase6 gene mutation

Recently, a patient with episodic ataxia and hemiplegia was found to have a mutation in the mitochondrial ATPase6 gene (m.8993T → C), which is normally known to cause Leigh syndrome in childhood and ataxia and polyneuropathy in adulthood (Craig et al. 2007).

Sporadic late-onset paroxysmal cerebellar ataxia

Julien et al. reported on four unrelated patients with a sporadic late-onset paroxysmal cerebellar ataxia who experienced recurrent attacks of episodic cerebellar ataxia starting in the sixth decade. Attacks lasted from a few minutes to 1 to 2 hours and were not responsive to acetazolamide. As the disease progressed, a slowly progressive ataxia developed. Neuropathological examination of one patient revealed a dramatic loss of Purkinje cells in the vermis and a strong staining of granular neurons with anti-tau protein serum. Because of the clinical resemblance to EA2, a molecular analysis of the CACNA1A gene was performed and mutations of this gene were excluded (Julien et al. 2001).

Other episodic ataxias

It has to be emphasized that other diseases with the clinical presentation of episodic ataxia have not been formally assigned to EA yet. For example, episodic ataxia with paroxysmal choreoathetosis, paresthesias and spasticity has been linked to a locus on chromosome 1p. Attacks are precipitated by emotional and physical stress as well as alcohol and fatigue and last for about 20 minutes. Frequency is highly variable (Auburger et al. 1996). Patients respond to acetazolamide.

Example case

A six-year-old boy had attacks since the age of four. Attacks were characterized by unstable gait and severe motor incoordination of his arms and hands. Sometimes his head or even his body shook, and his speech was very slurred. These attacks started suddenly but sometimes they were preceded by a strange feeling. Consciousness was never disturbed. Attack intensity varied, and the duration was 3 to 5 minutes. The frequency of attacks changed from once in a month to 10 times a day. The attacks started sometimes without a clear trigger but mostly they were elicited by physical effort, especially in combination with startle or exertion. The boy described an example of an attack occurring when he rode his bicycle and competed with his friends. The attack suddenly started when he changed directions to prevent a crash.

Pregnancy, birth, motor and mental development had been normal. His mother reported that she and her father had suffered from the same type of attacks during their childhood. Over the years the attacks had become less severe and occurred only very rarely. Her father had had little twitches around his eyes, which she had never noticed on her or her son. When she was a child no diagnosis could be made, but a trial treatment with antiepileptic drugs ameliorated her symptoms.

Neurological examination of the boy was normal. Later, when holding his hands in his lap a little tingling of the ulnar hand muscles could be observed. Routine blood parameters, MRI and EEG were normal. The EMG showed spontaneous, rhythmic activity indicating neuromyotonia/myokymia in several hand muscles. Due to the description of the attacks by the mother and the boy and the detected neuromyotonic discharges, EA1 was suspected. This was confirmed by molecular genetic testing. Therapy with acetazolamide was started. Under the treatment, the attack frequency and intensity were reduced. Some attacks were so short and mild they remained unrecognized by others. As side-effects, fatigue and paresthesias were reported by the boy. The paresthesias were ameliorated by the intake of potassium chloride.

References

Adelman JP, Bond CT, Pessia M, Maylie J. Episodic ataxia results from voltage-dependent potassium channels with altered functions. *Neuron* 1995 Dec, **15**(6):1449–1454.

Auburger G, Ratzlaff T, Lunkes A, Nelles HW, Leube B, Binkofski F, Kugel H, Heindel W, Seitz R, Benecke R, Witte OW, Voit T. A gene for autosomal dominant paroxysmal choreoathetosis/spasticity (CSE) maps to the vicinity of a potassium channel gene cluster on chromosome 1p, probably within 2 cM between D1S443 and D1S197. *Genomics* 1996 Jan 1, **31**(1):90–94.

Baloh RW, Yue Q, Furman JM, Nelson SF. Familial episodic ataxia: clinical heterogeneity in four families linked to chromosome 19p. *Ann Neurol* 1997 Jan, **41**(1):8–16.

Brandt T, Strupp M. Episodic ataxia type 1 and 2 (familial periodic ataxia/vertigo). Review. *Audiol Neurootol* 1997 Nov-Dec, **2**(6):373–383.

Bretschneider F, Wrisch A, Lehmann-Horn F, Grissmer S. Expression in mammalian cells and electrophysiological characterization of two mutant Kv1.1 channels causing episodic ataxia type 1 (EA-1). *Eur J Neurosci* 1999 Jul, **11**(7):2403–2412.

Browne DL, Gancher ST, Nutt JG, Brunt ER, Smith EA, Kramer P, Litt M. Episodic ataxia/myokymia syndrome is associated with point mutations in the human potassium channel gene, KCNA1. *Nat Genet* 1994 Oct, **8**(2):136–140.

Browne DL, Brunt ER, Griggs RC, Nutt JG, Gancher ST, Smith EA, Litt M. Identification of two new KCNA1 mutations in episodic ataxia/myokymia families. *Hum Mol Genet* 1995 Sep, **4**(9):1671–1672.

Brunt ER, van Weerden TW. Familial paroxysmal kinesigenic ataxia and continuous myokymia. *Brain* 1990 Oct, **113** (Pt 5):1361–1382.

Cader MZ, Steckley JL, Dyment DA, McLachlan RS, Ebers GC. A genome-wide screen and linkage mapping for a large pedigree with episodic ataxia. *Neurology* 2005 Jul 12, **65**(1):156–158.

Craig K, Elliott HR, Keers SM, Lambert C, Pyle A, Graves TD, Woodward C, Sweeney MG, Davis MB, Hanna MG, Chinnery PF. Episodic ataxia and hemiplegia caused by the 8993T->C mitochondrial DNA mutation. *J Med Genet* 2007 Dec, **44**(12):797–799.

D'Adamo MC, Liu Z, Adelman JP, Maylie J, Pessia M. Episodic ataxia type-1 mutations in the hKv1.1 cytoplasmic pore region alter the gating properties of the channel. *EMBO J* 1998 Mar 2, **17**(5):1200–1207.

Damji KF, Allingham RR, Pollock SC, Small K, Lewis KE, Stajich JM, Yamaoka LH, Vance JM, Pericak-Vance

MA. Periodic vestibulocerebellar ataxia, an autosomal dominant ataxia with defective smooth pursuit, is genetically distinct from other autosomal dominant ataxias. Review. *Arch Neurol* 1996 Apr, **53**(4):338–344.

Denier C, Ducros A, Durr A, Eymard B, Chassande B, Tournier-Lasserve E. Missense CACNA1A mutation causing episodic ataxia type 2. *Arch Neurol* 2001 Feb, **58**(2):292–295.

Ducros A, Denier C, Joutel A, Cecillon M, Lescoat C, Vahedi K, Darcel F, Vicaut E, Bousser MG, Tournier-Lasserve E. The clinical spectrum of familial hemiplegic migraine associated with mutations in a neuronal calcium channel. *N Engl J Med* 2001 Jul 5, **345**(1):17–24.

Escayg A, De Waard M, Lee DD, Bichet D, Wolf P, Mayer T, Johnston J, Baloh R, Sander T, Meisler MH. Coding and noncoding variation of the human calcium-channel beta4-subunit gene CACNB4 in patients with idiopathic generalized epilepsy and episodic ataxia. *Am J Hum Genet* 2000 May, **66**(5):1531–1539. Epub 2000 Apr 4.

Etzion Y, Grossman Y. Highly 4-aminopyridine sensitive delayed rectifier current modulates the excitability of guinea pig cerebellar Purkinje cells. *Exp Brain Res* 2001 Aug, **139**(4):419–425.

Eunson LH, Rea R, Zuberi SM, Youroukos S, Panayiotopoulos CP, Liguori R, Avoni P, McWilliam RC, Stephenson JB, Hanna MG, Kullmann DM, Spauschus A. Clinical, genetic, and expression studies of mutations in the potassium channel gene KCNA1 reveal new phenotypic variability. *Ann Neurol* 2000 Oct, **48**(4):647–656.

Farmer TW, Mustian VM. Vestibulocerebellar ataxia. A newly defined hereditary syndrome with periodic manifestations. *Arch Neurol* 1963 May, **8**:471–480.

Fletcher CF, Lutz CM, O'Sullivan TN, Shaughnessy JD, Hawkes R, Frankel WN, Copeland NG, Jenkins NA. Absence epilepsy in tottering mutant mice is associated with calcium channel defects. *Cell* 1996 Nov 15, **87**(4):607–617.

Fureman BE, Hess EJ. Noradrenergic blockade prevents attacks in a model of episodic dysfunction caused by a channelopathy. *Neurobiol Dis* 2005 Nov, **20**(2):227–232.

Fureman BE, Jinnah HA, Hess EJ. Triggers of paroxysmal dyskinesia in the calcium channel mouse mutant tottering. *Pharmacol Biochem Behav* 2002 Oct, **73**(3):631–637.

Griggs RC, Moxley RT, Lafrance RA, McQuillen J. Hereditary paroxysmal ataxia: response to aceta-zolamide. *Neurology* 1978 Dec, **28**(12):1259–1264.

Guida S, Trettel F, Pagnutti S, Mantuano E, Tottene A , Veneziano L, Fellin T, Spadaro M, Stauderman K,

Williams M, Volsen S, Ophoff R, Frants R, Jodice C, Frontali M, Pietrobon D. Complete loss of P/Q calcium channel activity caused by a CACNA1A missense mutation carried by patients with episodic ataxia type 2. *Am J Hum Genet* 2001 Mar, **68**(3):759–764.

Harno H, Heikkinen S, Kaunisto MA, Kallela M, Häkkinen AM, Wessman M, Färkkilä M, Lundbom N. Decreased cerebellar total creatine in episodic ataxia type 2: a 1H MRS study. *Neurology* 2005 Feb 8, **64**(3):542–544.

Herson PS, Virk M, Rustay NR, Bond CT, Crabbe JC, Adelman JP, Maylie J. A mouse model of episodic ataxia type-1. *Nat Neurosci* 2003 Apr, **6**(4):378–383.

Holtmann M, Opp J, Tokarzewski M, Korn-Merker E. Human epilepsy, episodic ataxia type 2, and migraine. *Lancet* 2002 Jan 12, **359**(9301):170–171.

Imbrici P, Jaffe SL, Eunson LH, Davies NP, Herd C, Robertson R, Kullmann DM, Hanna MG. Dysfunction of the brain calcium channel CaV2.1 in absence epilepsy and episodic ataxia. *Brain* 2004 Dec, **127**(Pt 12):2682–2692.

Imbrici P, Eunson LH, Graves TD, Bhatia KP, Wadia NH, Kullmann DM, Hanna MG. Late-onset episodic ataxia type 2 due to an in-frame insertion in CACNA1A. *Neurology* 2005 Sep 27, **65**(6):944–946.

Jen J, Wan J, Graves M, Yu H, Mock AF, Coulin CJ, Kim G, Yue Q, Papazian DM, Baloh RW. Loss-of-function EA2 mutations are associated with impaired neuromuscular transmission. *Neurology* 2001 Nov 27, **57**(10):1843–1848.

Jen J, Kim GW, Baloh RW. Clinical spectrum of episodic ataxia type 2. *Neurology* 2004 Jan 13, **62**(1):17–22.

Jen JC, Wan J, Palos TP, Howard BD, Baloh RW. Mutation in the glutamate transporter EAAT1 causes episodic ataxia, hemiplegia and seizures. *Neurology* 2005 Aug 23, **65**(4):529–534.

Jeng CJ, Chen YT, Chen YW, Tang CY. Dominant-negative effects of human P/Q-type Ca2+ channel mutations associated with episodic ataxia type 2. *Am J Physiol Cell Physiol* 2006 Apr, **290**(4):C1209– C1220.

Jeng CJ, Sun MC, Chen YW, Tang CY. Dominant-negative effects of episodic ataxia type 2 mutations involve disruption of membrane trafficking of human P/Q-type Ca2+ channels. *J Cell Physiol* 2008 Feb, **214**(2):422–433.

Jodice C, Mantuano E, Veneziano L, Trettel F, Sabbadini G, Calandriello L, Francia A, Spadaro M, Pierelli F, Salvi F, Ophoff RQA, Frants RR, Frontali M. Episodic ataxia type 2 (EA2) and spinocerebellar ataxia type 6 (SCA6) due to CAG repeat expansion in the CACNA1A gene on chromosome 19p. *Hum Mol Genet* 1997 Oct, **6**(11):1973–1978.

Jouvenceau A, Eunson LH, Spauschus A, Ramesh V, Zuberi SM, Kullmann DM, Hanna MG. Human epilepsy associated with dysfunction of the brain P/Q-type calcium channel. *Lancet* 2001 Sep 8, **358**(9284):801–807.

Julien J, Denier C, Ferrer X, Ducros A, Saintarailles J, Lagueny A, Tournier-Lasserve E, Vital C. Sporadic late onset paroxysmal cerebellar ataxia in four unrelated patients: a new disease? *J Neurol* 2001 Mar, **248**(3):209–214.

Kinali M, Jungbluth H, Eunson LH, Sewry CA, Manzur AY, Mercuri E, Hanna MG, Muntoni F. Expanding the phenotype of potassium channelopathy: severe neuromyotonia and skeletal deformities without prominent Episodic Ataxia. *Neuromuscul Disord* 2004 Oct, **14**(10):689–693.

Kramer PL, Yue Q, Gancher ST, Nutt JG, Baloh R, Smith E, Browne D, Bussey K, Lovrien E, Nelson S et al. A locus for the nystagmus-associated form of episodic ataxia maps to an 11-cM region on chromosome 19p. *Am J Hum Genet* 1995 Jul, **57**(1):182–185.

Lee H, Wang H, Jen JC, Sabatti C, Baloh RW, Nelson SF. A novel mutation in KCNA1 causes episodic ataxia without myokymia. *Hum Mutat* 2004 Dec, **24**(6): 536.

Lee HY, Xu Y, Huang Y, Ahn AH, Auburger GW, Pandolfo M, Kwiecinski H, Grimes DA, Lang AE, Nielsen JE, Averyanov Y, Servidei S, Friedman A, Van Bogaert P, Abramowicz MJ, Bruno MK, Sorensen BF, Tang L, Fu YH, Ptácek LJ. The gene for paroxysmal non-kinesigenic dyskinesia encodes an enzyme in a stress response pathway. *Hum Mol Genet* 2004 Dec 15, **13**(24):3161–3170.

Litt M, Kramer P, Browne D, Gancher S, Brunt ER, Root D, Phromchotikul T, Dubay CJ, Nutt J. A gene for episodic ataxia/myokymia maps to chromosome 12p13. *Am J Hum Genet* 1994 Oct, **55**(4):702–709.

Manganas LN, Akhtar S, Antonucci DE, Campomanes CR, Dolly JO, Trimmer JS. Episodic ataxia type-1 mutations in the Kv1.1 potassium channel display distinct folding and intracellular trafficking properties. *J Biol Chem* 2001 Dec 28, **276**(52):49427–49434.

Maselli RA, Wan J, Dunne V, Graves M, Baloh RW, Wollmann RL, Jen J. Presynaptic failure of neuromuscular transmission and synaptic remodeling in EA2. *Neurology* 2003 Dec 23, **61**(12):1743–1748.

Mochizuki Y, Kawata A, Mizutani T, Takamoto K, Hayashi H, Taki K, Morimatsu Y. Hereditary paroxysmal ataxia with mental retardation: a clinicopathological study in relation to episodic ataxia type 2. *Acta Neuropathol* 2004 Oct, **108**(4):345–349.

Mori Y, Wakamori M, Oda S, Fletcher CF, Sekiguchi N, Mori E, Copeland NG, Jenkins NA, Matsushita K, Matsuyama Z, Imoto K. Reduced voltage sensitivity of activation of P/Q-type Ca2+ channels is associated with the ataxic mouse mutation rolling Nagoya (tg(rol)). *J Neurosci* 2000 Aug 1, **20**(15):5654–5662.

Ophoff RA, Terwindt GM, Vergouwe MN, van Eijk R, Oefner PJ, Hoffman SM, Lamerdin JE, Mohrenweiser HW, Bulman DE, Ferrari M, Haan J, Lindhout D, van Ommen GJ, Hofker MH, Ferrari MD, Frants RR. Familial hemiplegic migraine and episodic ataxia type-2 are caused by mutations in the Ca2+ channel gene CACNL1A4. *Cell* 1996 Nov 1, **87**(3):543–552.

Poujois A, Antoine JC, Combes A, Touraine RL. Chronic neuromyotonia as a phenotypic variation associated with a new mutation in the KCNA1 gene. *J Neurol* 2006 Jul, **253**(7):957–959.

Rea R, Spauschus A, Eunson LH, Kullmann DM. Variable K(+) channel subunit dysfunction in inherited mutations of KCNA1. *J Physiol* 2002 Jan 1, **538**(Pt 1):5–23.

Rucker JC, Jen J, Stahl JS, Natesan N, Baloh RW, Leigh RJ. Internuclear ophthalmoparesis in episodic ataxia type 2. *Ann NY Acad Sci* 2005 Apr, **1039**:571–574.

Sappey-Marinier D, Vighetto A, Peyron R, Broussolle E, Bonmartin A. Phosphorus and proton magnetic resonance spectroscopy in episodic ataxia type 2. *Ann Neurol* 1999 Aug, **46**(2):256–259.

Sasaki O, Jen JC, Baloh RW, Kim GW, Isawa M, Usami S. Neurotological findings in a family with episodic ataxia. *J Neurol* 2003 Mar, **250**(3):373–375.

Scoggan KA, Friedman JH, Bulman DE. CACNA1A mutation in a EA-2 patient responsive to acetazolamide and valproic acid. *Can J Neurol Sci* 2006 Feb, **33**(1):68–72.

Shook SJ, Mamsa H, Jen JC, Baloh RW, Zhou L. Novel mutation in KCNA1 causes episodic ataxia with paroxysmal dyspnea. *Muscle Nerve* 2007 Oct 2.

Smart SL, Lopantsev V, Zhang CL, Robbins CA, Wang H, Chiu SY, Schwartzkroin PA, Messing A, Tempel BL. Deletion of the K(V)1.1 potassium channel causes epilepsy in mice. *Neuron* 1998 Apr, **20**(4):809–819.

Spacey SD, Materek LA, Szczygielski BI, Bird TD. Two novel CACNA1A gene mutations associated with episodic ataxia type 2 and interictal dystonia. *Arch Neurol* 2005 Feb, **62**(2):314–316.

Steckley JL, Ebers GC, Cader MZ, McLachlan RS. An autosomal dominant disorder with episodic ataxia, vertigo, and tinnitus. *Neurology* 2001 Oct 23, **57**(8):1499–1502.

Strupp M, Schüler O, Krafczyk S, Jahn K, Schautzer F, Büttner U, Brandt T. Treatment of downbeat nystagmus with 3,4-diaminopyridine: a placebo-controlled study. *Neurology* 2003 Jul 22, **61**(2):165–170.

Tomita H, Nagamitsu S, Wakui K, Fukushima Y, Yamada K, Sadamatsu M, Masui A, Konishi T, Matsuishi T,

Aihara M, Shimizu K, Hashimoto K, Mineta M, Matsushima M, Tsujita T, Saito M, Tanaka H, Tsuji S, Takagi T, Nakamura Y, Nanko S, Kato N, Nakane Y, Niikawa N. Paroxysmal kinesigenic choreoathetosis locus maps to chromosome 16p11.2-q12.1. *Am J Hum Genet* 1999 Dec, **65**(6):1688–1697.

Tottene A, Fellin T, Pagnutti S, Luvisetto S, Striessnig J, Fletcher C, Pietrobon D. Familial hemiplegic migraine mutations increase Ca(2+) influx through single human CaV2.1 channels and decrease maximal CaV2.1 current density in neurons. *Proc Natl Acad Sci USA* 2002 Oct 1, **99**(20):13284–13289.

Van Bogaert P, Szliwowski HB. EEG findings in acetazolamide-responsive hereditary paroxysmal ataxia. *Neurophysiol Clin* 1996, **26**(5):335–340.

Vance JM, Pericak-Vance MA, Payne CS, Coin JT, Olanow CW. Linkage and genetic analysis in adult onset periodic vestibulo-cerebellar ataxia: report of a new family (Abstract). *Am J Hum Genet* **36**:78S, 1984.

Vighetto A, Froment JC, Trillet M, Aimard G. Magnetic resonance imaging in familial paroxysmal ataxia. *Arch Neurol* 1988 May, **45**(5):547–549.

Wakamori M, Yamazaki K, Matsunodaira H, Teramoto T, Tanaka I, Niidome T, Sawada K, Nishizawa Y, Sekiguchi N, Mori E, Mori Y, Imoto K. Single tottering mutations responsible for the neuropathic phenotype of the P-type calcium channel. *J Biol Chem* 1998 Dec 25, **273**(52):34857–34867.

Walter JT, Alviña K, Womack MD, Chevez C, Khodakhah K . Decreases in the precision of Purkinje cell pacemaking cause cerebellar dysfunction and ataxia. *Nat Neurosci* 2006 Mar, **9**(3):389–397.

Wappl E, Koschak A, Poteser M, Sinnegger MJ, Walter D, Eberhart A, Groschner K, Glossmann H, Kraus RL, Grabner M, Striessnig J. Functional consequences of P/Q-type Ca2+ channel Cav2.1 missense mutations associated with episodic ataxia type 2 and progressive ataxia. *J Biol Chem* 2002 Mar 1, **277**(9):6960–6966.

Weisz CJ, Raike RS, Soria-Jasso LE, Hess EJ . Potassium channel blockers inhibit the triggers of attacks in the calcium channel mouse mutant tottering. *J Neurosci* 2005 Apr 20, **25**(16):4141–4145.

Zasorin NL, Baloh RW, Myers LB. Acetazolamide-responsive episodic ataxia syndrome. *Neurology* 1983 Sep, **33**(9):1212–1214.

Zerr P, Adelman JP, Maylie J. Episodic ataxia mutations in Kv1.1 alter potassium channel function by dominant negative effects or haploinsufficiency. *J Neurosci* 1998 Apr 15, **18**(8):2842–2848.

Zhang CL, Messing A, Chiu SY. Specific alteration of spontaneous GABAergic inhibition in cerebellar purkinje cells in mice lacking the potassium channel Kv1. 1. *J Neurosci* 1999 Apr 15, **19**(8):2852–2864.

Zhuchenko O, Bailey J, Bonnen P, Ashizawa T, Stockton DW, Amos C, Dobyns WB, Subramony SH, Zoghbi HY, Lee CC. Autosomal dominant cerebellar ataxia (SCA6) associated with small polyglutamine expansions in the alpha 1A-voltage-dependent calcium channel. *Nat Genet* 1997 Jan, **15**(1):62–69.

Zuberi SM, Eunson LH, Spauschus A, De Silva R, Tolmie J, Wood NW, McWilliam RC, Stephenson JB, Kullmann DM, Hanna MG. A novel mutation in the human voltage-gated potassium channel gene (Kv1.1) associates with episodic ataxia type 1 and sometimes with partial epilepsy. *Brain* 1999 May, **122** (Pt 5):817–825.

Index